Essentials of Dental Radiography and Radiology

;TH EDITION

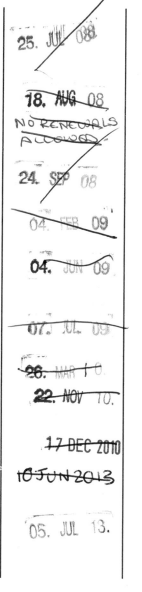

Dedication
To Catriona, Stuart, Felicity and Claudia

Commissioning Editor: Michael Parkinson
Development Editor: Clive Hewat
Project Manager: Frances Affleck
Design Direction: George Ajayi
Illustrator: Richard Tibbitts

Essentials of Dental Radiography and Radiology

FOURTH EDITION

Eric Whaites
MSc BDS(Hons) FDSRCS(Edin) FDSRCS(Eng) FRCR DDRRCR

Senior Lecturer and Honorary Consultant in Dental Radiology,
Head of the Department of Dental Radiological Imaging,
King's College London Dental Institute at Guy's, King's College and St Thomas' Hospitals, London, UK

Foreword by
R.A. Cawson MD FRCPath FDS

Emeritus Professor in Oral Medicine and Pathology in the University of London, UK

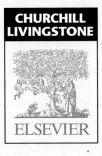

CHURCHILL LIVINGSTONE

ELSEVIER

Edinburgh   London   New York   Oxford   Philadelphia   St Louis   Sydney   Toronto 2007

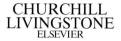

CHURCHILL
LIVINGSTONE
ELSEVIER

© Longman Group UK Limited 1992
© Pearson Professional Limited 1996
© Harcourt Publishers Limited 2002
© Elsevier Science Limited 2003
© 2007, Elsevier Limited. All rights reserved.

First edition 1992
Second edition 1996
Third edition 2002
Fourth edition 2007

ISBN 10: 0-44310168X
ISBN 13: 978-0-443-10168-7

British Library Cataloguing in Publication Data
A catalogue record for this book is available from the British Library

Library of Congress Cataloging in Publication Data
A catalog record for this book is available from the Library of Congress

Note
Knowledge and best practice in this field are constantly changing. As new research and experience broaden our knowledge, changes in practice, treatment and drug therapy may become necessary or appropriate. Readers are advised to check the most current information provided (i) on procedures featured or (ii) by the manufacturer of each product to be administered, to verify the recommended dose or formula, the method and duration of administration, and contraindications. It is the responsibility of the practitioner, relying on their own experience and knowledge of the patient, to make diagnoses, to determine dosages and the best treatment for each individual patient, and to take all appropriate safety precautions. To the fullest extent of the law, neither the Publisher nor the [Editors/Authors] [delete as appropriate] assumes any liability for any injury and/or damage to persons or property arising out or related to any use of the material contained in this book.

The Publisher

ELSEVIER your source for books,
journals and multimedia
in the health sciences
www.elsevierhealth.com

Working together to grow
libraries in developing countries

www.elsevier.com | www.bookaid.org | www.sabre.org

 ELSEVIER | BOOK AID International | Sabre Foundation

The
publisher's
policy is to use
**paper manufactured
from sustainable forests**

Printed in Spain

Contents

Foreword   vii
Preface   ix
Acknowledgements   xi

PART 1 Introduction   1

1. The radiographic image   3

PART 2 Radiation physics and equipment   13

2. The production, properties and interaction of X-rays   15

3. Dose units and dosimetry   25

4. The biological effects and risks associated with X-rays   29

5. Dental X-ray generating equipment   35

6. Image receptors   41

7. Image processing   55

PART 3 Radiation protection   67

8. Radiation protection and legislation   69

PART 4 Radiography   83

9. Dental radiography — general patient considerations including control of infection   85

10. Periapical radiography   97

11. Bitewing radiography   125

12. Occlusal radiography   135

13. Oblique lateral radiography   141

14. Skull and maxillofacial radiography   149

15. Cephalometric radiography   169

16. Tomography   179

17. Panoramic radiography (dental panoramic tomography)   187

18. The quality of radiographic images and quality assurance   207

19. Alternative and specialized imaging modalities   223

PART 5   Radiology   **243**

20. Introduction to radiological interpretation   245

21. Dental caries and the assessment of restorations   251

22. The periapical tissues   265

23. The periodontal tissues and periodontal disease   277

24. Implant assessment   289

25. Developmental abnormalities   299

26. Radiological differential diagnosis – describing a lesion   323

27. Differential diagnosis of radiolucent lesions of the jaws   329

28. Differential diagnosis of lesions of variable radiopacity in the jaws   355

29. The maxillary antra   373

30. Trauma to the teeth and facial skeleton   387

31. The temporomandibular joint   411

32. Bone diseases of radiological importance   431

33. The salivary glands   445

Bibliography and suggested reading   459

Index   463

Foreword

I am flattered to have been asked to write another Foreword to Eric Whaites' excellent text. It has been a great pleasure to see how successful this book has been. With the appearance of the first edition it was obvious that it provided an unusually clear, concise and comprehensive exposition of the subject. However, its success speaks for itself and the fact that so many reprints were demanded, has confirmed that its qualities have been appreciated. There is little therefore that one needs to add except to encourage readers to take advantage of all that this book offers.

R.A.C.
2006

Preface

Imaging in dentistry is being transformed by the development and introduction of new technology into everyday clinical practice. This new edition has given me the opportunity to embed some of these developments within the core text. Digital imaging, for example, was not mentioned in the first edition 15 years ago. It is now used extensively and is regarded as a routine imaging modality. In addition to these core text changes, I have included a brief section on Cone Beam CT, an exciting new development in dental imaging, which is already starting to replace conventional imaging in certain clinical situations.

I have updated almost every chapter and, where appropriate, have included recent classification changes as well as more examples of advanced imaging. Perhaps more importantly I have changed the emphasis in certain chapters, particularly the ones covering the maxillary antra and the temporomandibular joints, to reflect more modern approaches to investigating these areas. All the line diagrams have been professionally re-drawn and a couple of colour plates have been added. It is intended that all these changes should make this new edition feel fresh, modern and up-to-date.

The aims and objectives of this book however, remain the same, namely to provide a basic and practical account of what I consider to be the essential subject matter of both dental radiography and radiology required by undergraduate and postgraduate dental students. As in previous editions some things have inevitably had to be omitted, or sometimes, over-simplified in condensing a very large and increasingly complex subject. It therefore remains first and foremost a teaching manual, rather than a comprehensive reference book. I hope the content remains sufficiently broad and detailed to satisfy the requirement of most undergraduate and postgraduate dental examinations, but that students will build on the information acquired here by using the excellent and more comprehensive textbooks already available.

Once again, I hope that the result is a clear, logical and easily understandable text, that continues to make a positive contribution to the challenging task of teaching and learning dental radiology.

E.W.
London 2006

Acknowledgements

As with previous editions, this edition has only been possible thanks to the enormous amount of help and encouragement that I received from my family, friends and colleagues.

Firstly, I would like to thank all the members of staff in my Department for their collective help and encouragement. In particular I owe a huge debt of gratitude to my Secretary Miss Allisson Summerfield – without her help this project, along with many others, would never have been completed. Grateful thanks also to Mrs Jackie Brown, Mr Jonathan Davies, Mrs Joanne D'Emmerez de Charmoy, Mrs Nadine White, Ms Jocelyn Sewell, Miss Rita Bhowal and Mrs Olivia Richardson for their invaluable help and advice. I am indeed fortunate to continue to work with such an able and supportive team.

In addition, my thanks to the following for their help and advice with specific chapters: Mr Nicholas Drage (Chapter 7), Mr Jonathan Davies (Chapters 7 and 19), Mr Christopher Dickinson (Chapter 9), Professor Fraser Macdonald (Chapter 15), Professor Edwina Kidd and Dr Avi Banerjee (Chapter 21), Dr Mark Ide (Chapter 23), Professor Richard Palmer (Chapter 24), Professor Peter Morgan and Professor Eddie Odell (Chapters 27 and 28) and Mrs Jackie Brown (Chapters 19 and 33). My thanks also to my following colleagues for their comments and/or for providing me with new illustrations: Dr Jane Luker, Dr Julian Kabala, Mr John Rout, Mrs Laetitia Brocklebank, Professor Kostas Tsiklakis, Professor Douglas Benn, Mr Martin Payne, Professor Keith Horner and Dr Vivian Rushton.

I am also grateful to the Health Protection Agency (formerly the National Radiological Protection Board) for their permission to once again reproduce parts of the 2001 Guidance Notes (Chapter 8) and the Faculty of General Dental Practice (UK) for their permission to reproduce two summary tables from their 2004 Selection Criteria booklet.

Special thanks to Mr Andrew Dyer from the Department of Photography, Printing and Design for all his time and expertise spent on producing the new photographic material and to Miss Laura Martin for willingly sitting as the new photographic model in the new clinical illustrations. My thanks also to Mr Richard Tibbitts who spent many hours re-drawing all the line diagrams and to Mr Clive Hewat and the staff of Elsevier for their help and advice in the production process.

I must acknowledge once again Professor Rod Cawson, Professor David Smith and Mr Brian O'Riordan for all their help with previous editions and their support throughout my career.

Finally, I have to thank my family – my wife Catriona and my children Stuart, Felicity and Claudia for their love, encouragement and understanding throughout the production of this edition as, yet again, precious family time has had to be sacrificed.

PART 1

Introduction

PART CONTENTS

1. The radiographic image   3

Chapter **1**

The radiographic image

INTRODUCTION

The use of X-rays is an integral part of clinical dentistry, with some form of radiographic examination necessary on the majority of patients. As a result, radiographs are often referred to as the clinician's *main diagnostic aid*.

The range of knowledge of dental radiography and radiology thus required can be divided conveniently into four main sections:

- *Basic physics and equipment* — the production of X-rays, their properties and interactions which result in the formation of the radiographic image
- *Radiation protection* — the protection of patients and dental staff from the harmful effects of X-rays
- *Radiography* — the techniques involved in producing the various radiographic images
- *Radiology* — the interpretation of these radiographic images.

Understanding the radiographic image is central to the entire subject. This chapter provides an introduction to the nature of this image and to some of the factors that affect its quality and perception.

NATURE OF THE RADIOGRAPHIC IMAGE

Traditionally the image was produced by the X-rays passing through an object (the patient) and interacting with the photographic emulsion on a *film*, which resulted in blackening of the film. Film is gradually being replaced by a variety of *digital sensors* with the image being created in a computer. Those parts of the digital sensor that have been hit by X-rays appear black in the computer-generated image. The extent to which the emulsion or the computer-generated image is blackened depends on the number of X-rays reaching the film or sensor (either device can be referred to as an *image receptor*), which in turn depends on the density of the object.

However the final image is captured, it can be described as a two-dimensional picture made up of a variety of black, white and grey superimposed shadows and is thus sometimes referred to as a *shadowgraph* (see Fig. 1.1).

Understanding the nature of the shadowgraph and interpreting the information contained within it requires a knowledge of the following:

- The radiographic shadows
- The three-dimensional anatomical tissues
- The limitations imposed by a two-dimensional picture and superimposition.

The radiographic shadows

The amount the X-ray beam is stopped (attenuated) by an object determines the *radiodensity* of the shadows:

- The white or *radiopaque* shadows on an image represent the various dense structures within the object which have totally stopped the X-ray beam.

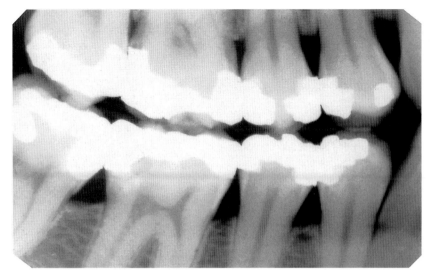

Fig. 1.1 A typical dental radiograph. The image shows the various black, grey and white radiographic shadows.

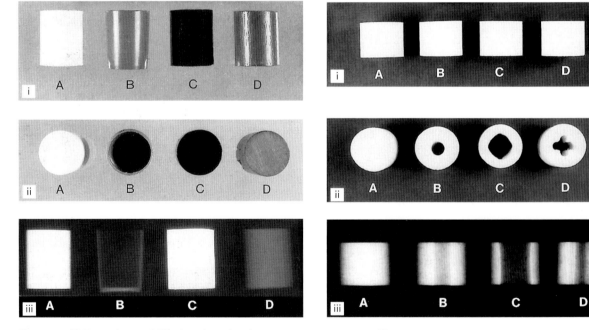

Fig. 1.2 (i) Front view and (ii) plan view of various cylinders of similar shape but made of different materials: A plaster of Paris, B hollow plastic, C metal, D wood. (iii) Radiographs of the cylinders show how objects of the same shape, but of different materials, produce different radiographic images.

Fig. 1.3 (i) Front view of four apparently similar cylinders made from plaster of Paris. (ii) Plan view shows the cylinders have varying internal designs and thicknesses. (iii) Radiographs of the apparently similar cylinders show how objects of similar shape and material, but of different densities, produce different radiographic images.

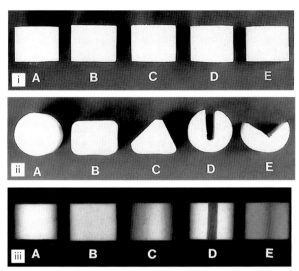

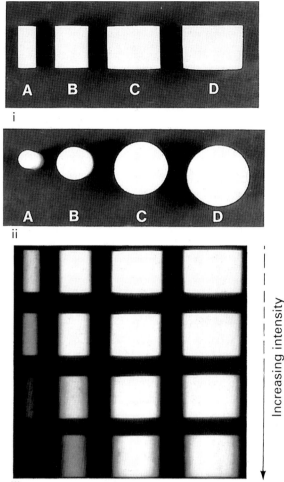

Fig. 1.4 (i) Front view of five apparently similar cylinders made from plaster of Paris. (ii) Plan view shows the objects are in fact different shapes. (iii) Radiographs show how objects of different shape, but made of the same material, produce different radiographic images.

- The black or *radiolucent* shadows represent areas where the X-ray beam has passed through the object and has not been stopped at all.
- The grey shadows represent areas where the X-ray beam has been stopped to a varying degree.

The final *shadow density* of any object is thus affected by:

- The specific type of material of which the object is made
- The thickness or density of the material
- The shape of the object
- The intensity of the X-ray beam used
- The position of the object in relation to the X-ray beam and image receptor
- The sensitivity and type of image receptor.

The effect of different materials, different thicknesses/densities, different shapes and different X-ray beam intensities on the radiographic image shadows are shown in Figures 1.2–1.5.

The three-dimensional anatomical tissues

The shape, density and thickness of the patient's tissues, principally the hard tissues, must also

Fig. 1.5 (i) Front view and (ii) plan view of four cylinders made from plaster of Paris but of different diameters. (iii) Four radiographs using different intensity X-ray beams show how increasing the intensity of the X-ray beam causes greater penetration of the object with less attenuation, hence the less radiopaque (white) shadows of the object that are produced, particularly of the smallest cylinder.

affect the radiographic image. Therefore, when viewing two-dimensional radiographic images, the three-dimensional anatomy responsible for the image must be considered (see Fig. 1.6). A sound anatomical knowledge is obviously a prerequisite for radiological interpretation (see Ch. 20).

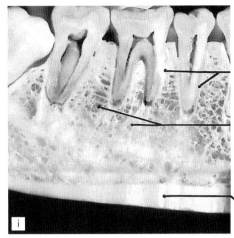

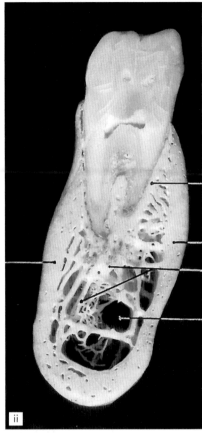

Cortical bone of the socket, producing the radiological lamina dura

Cancellous or trabecular bone, producing the radiological trabecular pattern

Dense compact bone of the lower border

Cortical bone of the socket

Buccal cortical plate

Cancellous or trabecular bone

Inferior dental canal

Lingual cortical plate

A

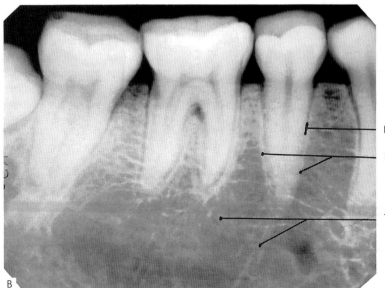

Periodontal ligament space

Lamina dura

Trabecular pattern

B

Fig. 1.6A   **(i)** Sagittal and **(ii)** coronal sections through the body of a dried mandible showing the hard tissue anatomy and internal bone pattern. **B** Two-dimensional radiographic image of the three-dimensional mandibular anatomy.

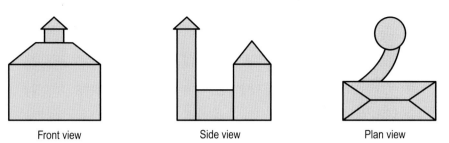

Front view   Side view   Plan view

Fig. 1.7 Diagram illustrating three views of a house. The side view shows that there is a corridor at the back of the house leading to a tall tower. The plan view provides the additional pieces of information that the roof of the tall tower is round and that the corridor is curved.

The limitations imposed by a two-dimensional image and superimposition

The main limitations of viewing the two-dimensional image of a three-dimensional object are:

- Appreciating the overall shape of the object
- Superimposition and assessing the location and shape of structures *within* an object.

Appreciating the overall shape

To visualize all aspects of any three-dimensional object, it must be viewed from several different positions. This can be illustrated by considering an object such as a *house*, and the minimum information required if an architect is to draw all aspects of the three-dimensional building in two dimensions (see Fig. 1.7). Unfortunately, it is only too easy for the clinician to forget that teeth and patients are three-dimensional. To expect one radiograph to provide *all* the required information about the shape of a tooth or patient is like asking the architect to describe the whole house from the front view alone.

Superimposition and assessing the location and shape of structures within an object

The shadows cast by different parts of an object (or patient) are superimposed upon one another on the final radiograph. The image therefore provides limited or even misleading information as to where a particular internal structure lies, or to its shape, as shown in Figure 1.8.

In addition, a dense radiopaque shadow on one side of the head may overlie an area of radiolucency on the other, so obscuring it from view, or a radiolucent shadow may make a superimposed radiopaque shadow appear less opaque.

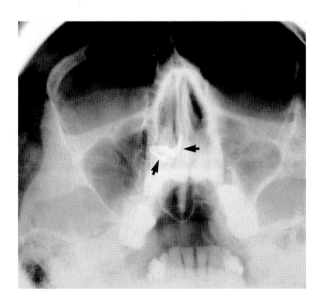

Fig. 1.8 Radiograph of the head from the front (an *occipitomental* view) taken with the head tipped back, as described later in Chapter 14. This positioning lowers the dense bones of the base of the skull and raises the facial bones so avoiding superimposition of one on the other. A radiopaque (white) object (arrowed) can be seen apparently in the base of the right nasal cavity.

One clinical solution to these problems is to take two views, at right angles to one another (see Figs 1.9 and 1.10). Unfortunately, even two views may still not be able to provide all the desired information for a diagnosis to be made (see Fig. 1.11).

These limitations of the conventional radiographic image have very important clinical implications and may be the underlying reason for a *negative radiographic report*. The fact that a particular feature or condition is not visible on one radiograph does not mean that the feature or

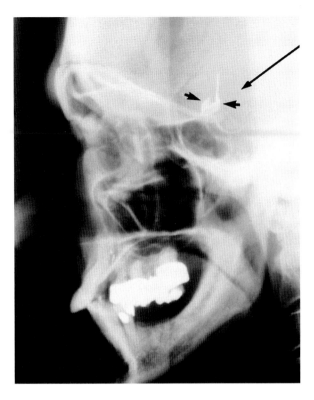

Fig. 1.9   Radiograph of the head from the side (a *true lateral skull view*) of the same patient shown in Figure 1.8. The radiopaque (white) object (arrowed) now appears intracranially just above the skull base. It is in fact a metallic aneurysm clip positioned on an artery in the Circle of Willis at the base of the brain. The long black arrow indicates the direction of the X-ray beam required to produce the radiograph in Figure 1.8, illustrating how the clip appears to be in the nose.

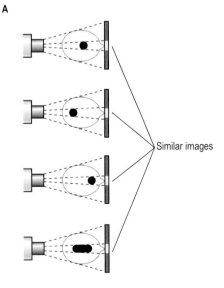

A

Similar images

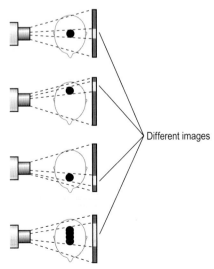

B

Different images

Fig. 1.10   Diagrams illustrating the limitations of a two-dimensional image: **A** Posteroanterior views of a head containing a variable mass. The mass appears as a similar sized opaque image on the radiograph, providing no differentiating information on its position or shape. **B** The side view provides a possible solution to the problems illustrated in **A**.

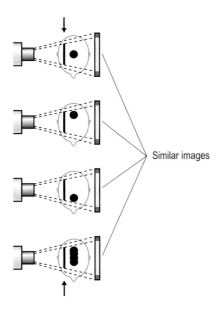

Fig. 1.11 Diagrams illustrating the problems of superimposition. Lateral views of the same masses shown in Figure 1.10 but with an additional radiodense object superimposed (arrowed). This produces a similar image in each case with no evidence of the mass. The information obtained previously is now obscured and the usefulness of using two views at right angles is negated.

condition does not exist, merely that it cannot be seen. Many of the recently developed alternative and specialized imaging modalities described in Chapter 19 have been designed to try to overcome these limitations

QUALITY OF THE RADIOGRAPHIC IMAGE

Overall image quality and the amount of detail shown on a radiographic image depend on several factors, including:

- Contrast — the visual difference between the various black, white and grey shadows
- Image geometry — the relative positions of the film, object and X-ray tubehead
- Characteristics of the X-ray beam
- Image sharpness and resolution.

These factors are in turn dependent on several variables, relating to the density of the object, the type of image receptor and the X-ray equipment. They are discussed in greater detail in Chapter 18. However, to introduce how the geometrical accuracy and detail of the final image can be influenced, two of the main factors are considered below.

Positioning of the image receptor, object and X-ray beam

The position of the X-ray beam, object and image receptor needs to satisfy certain basic geometrical requirements. These include:

- The object and the image receptor should be in contact or as close together as possible
- The object and the image receptor should be parallel to one another
- The X-ray tubehead should be positioned so that the beam meets both the object and the image receptor at right angles.

These ideal requirements are shown diagrammatically in Figure 1.12. The effects on the final image of varying the position of the object, image receptor or X-ray beam are shown in Figure 1.13.

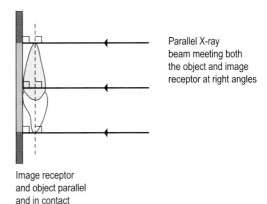

Parallel X-ray beam meeting both the object and image receptor at right angles

Image receptor and object parallel and in contact

Fig. 1.12 Diagram illustrating the ideal geometrical relationship between the image receptor, object and X-ray beam.

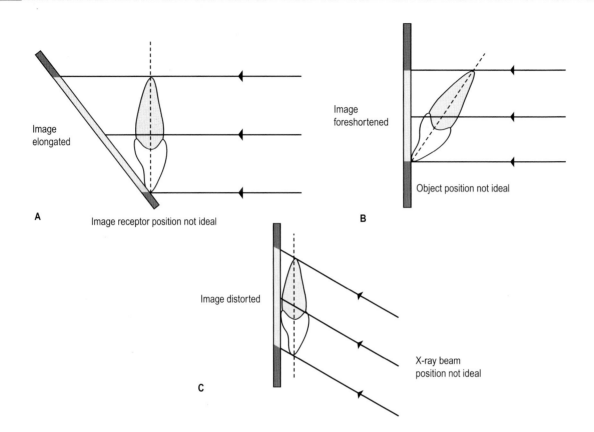

Fig. 1.13 Diagrams showing the effect on the final image of varying the position of **A** the image receptor, **B** the object and **C** the X-ray beam.

X-RAY BEAM CHARACTERISTICS

The ideal X-ray beam used for imaging should be:

- Sufficiently penetrating, to pass through the patient and react with the film emulsion or digital sensor and produce good *contrast* between the different shadows (Fig. 1.14)

- Parallel, i.e. non-diverging, to prevent magnification of the image
- Produced from a point source, to reduce blurring of the edges of the image, a phenomenon known as the *penumbra* effect.

These ideal characteristics are discussed further in Chapter 5.

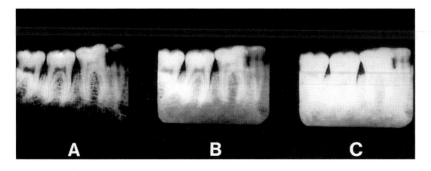

Fig. 1.14 Film-captured radiographs of the same area showing variation in contrast — the visual difference in the black, white and grey shadows due to the penetration of the X-ray beam. **A** Increased exposure (overpenetration). **B** Normal exposure. **C** Reduced exposure (underpenetration).

PERCEPTION OF THE RADIOGRAPHIC IMAGE

The verb *to perceive* means *to apprehend with the mind using one or more of the senses*. Perception is the *act* or *faculty of perceiving*. In radiology, we use our sense of sight to perceive the radiographic image, but, unfortunately, we cannot rely completely on what we see. The apparently simple black, white and grey shadowgraph is a form of optical *illusion* (from the Latin *illudere*, meaning *to mock*). The radiographic image can thus mock our senses in a number of ways. The main problems can be caused by the effects of:

- Partial images
- Contrast
- Context.

Effect of partial images

As mentioned already, the radiographic image only provides the clinician with a partial image with limited information in the form of different density shadows. To complete the picture, the clinician fills in the gaps. Unfortunately, not all clinicians necessarily do this in the same way and may therefore arrive at different conclusions. Three non-clinical examples are shown in Figure 1.15. Clinically, our differing perceptions may lead to different diagnoses.

Effect of contrast

The apparent density of a particular radiographic shadow can be affected considerably by the density of the surrounding shadows. In other words, the contrast between adjacent structures can alter the perceived density of one or both of them (see Fig. 1.16). This is of particular importance in dentistry, where metallic restorations produce densely white radiopaque shadows that can affect the apparent density of the adjacent tooth tissue. This is discussed again in Chapter 21 in relation to caries diagnosis.

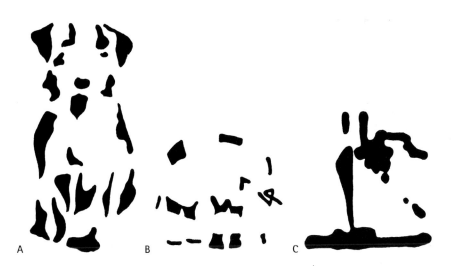

Fig. 1.15   The problem of partial images requiring the observer to fill in the missing gaps. Look at the three non-clinical pictures and what do you perceive? The objects shown are **A** a dog, **B** an elephant and **C** a steam ship. We all *see* the same partial images, but we don't necessarily *perceive* the same objects. Most people perceive the dog, some perceive the elephant while only a few perceive the ship and take some convincing that it is there. Interestingly, once observers have perceived the correct objects, it is impossible to look at the pictures again in the future without perceiving them correctly. (Figures from: Coren S, Porac C, Ward LM 1979 Sensation and perception. Harcourt Brace and Company, reproduced by permission of the publisher.)

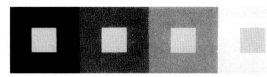

Fig. 1.16 The effect of contrast. The four small inner squares are in reality all the same grey colour, but they appear to be different because of the effect of contrast. When the surrounding square is black, the observer perceives the inner square to be very pale, while when the surrounding square is light grey, the observer perceives the inner square to be dark. (Figure from: Cornsweet TN 1970 Visual perception. Harcourt Brace and Company, reproduced by permission of the publisher.)

Effect of context

The environment or context in which we see an image can affect how we interpret that image. A non-clinical example is shown in Figure 1.17. In dentistry, the environment that can affect our perception of radiographs is that created by the patient's description of the complaint. We can imagine that we see certain radiographic changes, because the patient has conditioned our perceptual apparatus.

These various perceptual problems are included simply as a warning that radiographic interpretation is not as straightforward as it may at first appear.

COMMON TYPES OF DENTAL RADIOGRAPHS

The various radiographic images of the teeth, jaws and skull are divided into two main groups:

- *Intraoral* — the image receptor is placed *inside* the patient's mouth, including:
  - Periapical radiographs (Ch. 10)
  - Bitewing radiographs (Ch. 11)
  - Occlusal radiographs (Ch. 12)
- *Extraoral* — the image receptor is placed *outside* the patient's mouth, including:
  - Oblique lateral radiographs (Ch. 13)
  - Various skull radiographs (Chs 14 and 15)
  - Panoramic radiographs (Ch. 17).

These various radiographic techniques are described later, in the chapters indicated. The approach and format adopted throughout these radiography chapters are intended to be straightforward, practical and clinically relevant and are based upon the essential knowledge required by clinicians. This includes:

- WHY each particular projection is taken — i.e. the main clinical indications
- HOW the projections are taken — i.e. the relative positions of the patient, image receptor and X-ray tubehead
- WHAT the resultant radiographs should look like and which anatomical features they show.

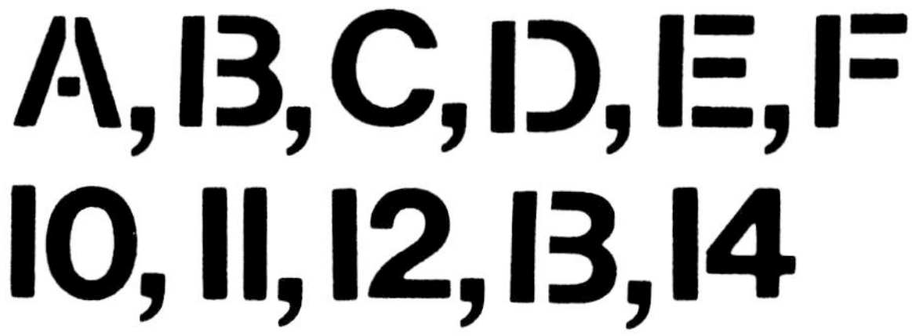

A,B,C,D,E,F
10,11,12,13,14

Fig. 1.17 The effect of context. If asked to read the two lines shown here most, if not all, observers would read the letters A,B,C,D,E,F and then the numbers 10,11,12,13,14. Closer examination shows the letter B and the number 13 to be identical. They are perceived as B and 13 because of the context (surrounding letters or numbers) in which they are seen. (Figure from: Coren S, Porac C, Ward LM 1979 Sensation and perception. Harcourt Brace and Company, reproduced by permission of the publisher.)

PART 2

Radiation physics and equipment

PART CONTENTS

2. The production, properties and interaction of X-rays   15

3. Dose units of dosimetry   25

4. The biological effects and risks associated with X-rays   29

5. Dental X-ray generating equipment   35

6. Image receptors   41

7. Image processing   55

Chapter 2

The production, properties and interactions of X-rays

INTRODUCTION

X-rays and their ability to penetrate human tissues were discovered by Röentgen in 1895. He called them X-rays because their nature was then unknown. They are in fact a form of high-energy electromagnetic radiation and are part of the electromagnetic spectrum, which also includes low-energy radiowaves, television and visible light (see Table 2.1).

X-rays are described as consisting of *wave packets* of energy. Each packet is called *a photon* and is equivalent to one *quantum* of energy. The X-ray *beam*, as used in diagnostic radiology, is made up of millions of individual photons.

To understand the production and interactions of X-rays a basic knowledge of atomic physics is essential. The next section aims to provide a simple summary of this required background information.

ATOMIC STRUCTURE

Atoms are the basic building blocks of matter. They consist of minute particles — the so-called fundamental or elementary particles — held together by electric and nuclear forces. They consist of a central dense *nucleus* made up of nuclear particles — *protons* and *neutrons* — surrounded by *electrons* in specific orbits or shells (see Fig. 2.1).

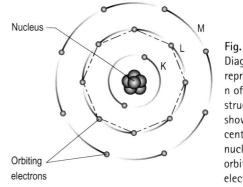

Fig. 2.1 Diagrammatic representation of atomic structure showing the central nucleus and orbiting electrons.

Table 2.1 The electromagnetic spectrum ranging from the low energy (long wavelength) radio waves to the high energy (short wavelength) X- and gamma-rays

Radiation	Wavelength	Photon energy
Radio, television and radar waves	3×10^4 m to 100 μm	4.1×10^{-11} eV to 1.2×10^{-2} eV
Infra-red	100 μm to 700 nm	1.2×10^{-2} eV to 1.8 eV
Visible light	700 nm to 400 nm	1.8 eV to 3.1 eV
Ultra-violet	400 nm to 10 nm	3.1 eV to 124 eV
X- and gamma-rays	10 nm to 0.01 pm	124 eV to 124 MeV

Useful definitions

- *Atomic number* (Z) — The number of protons in the nucleus of an atom
- *Neutron number* (N) — The number of neutrons in the nucleus of an atom
- *Atomic mass number* (A) — Sum of the number of protons and number of neutrons in an atom (A = Z + N)
- *Isotopes* — Atoms with the same atomic number (Z) but with different atomic mass numbers (A) and hence different numbers of neutrons (N)
- *Radioisotopes* — Isotopes with unstable nuclei which undergo radioactive disintegration (see Ch. 17).

Main features of the atomic particles

Nuclear particles (nucleons)

Protons
- Mass = 1.66×10^{-27} kg
- Charge = positive: 1.6×10^{-19} coulombs.

Neutrons
- Mass = 1.70×10^{-27} kg
- Charge = nil
- Neutrons act as *binding agents* within the nucleus and hold it together by counteracting the repulsive forces between the protons.

Electrons

- Mass = 1/1840 of the mass of a proton
- Charge = negative: -1.6×10^{-19} coulombs
- Electrons move in predetermined circular or elliptical shells or orbits around the nucleus
- The shells represent different *energy levels* and are labelled K,L,M,N,O outwards from the nucleus
- The shells can contain up to a maximum number of electrons per shell:
  - K ... 2
  - L ... 8
  - M ... 18
  - N ... 32
  - O ... 50

- Electrons can move from shell to shell but cannot exist between shells — an area known as the *forbidden zone*
- To remove an electron from the atom, additional energy is required to overcome the *binding energy* of attraction which keeps the electrons in their shells.

Summary of important points on atomic structure

- In the neutral atom, the number of orbiting electrons is equal to the number of protons in the nucleus. Since the number of electrons determines the chemical behaviour of an atom, the *atomic number* (Z) also determines this chemical behaviour. Each *element* has different chemical properties and thus each *element* has a different *atomic number*. These form the basis of the *periodic table*.
- Atoms in the ground state are electrically neutral because the number of positive charges (protons) is balanced by the number of negative charges (electrons).
- If an electron is removed, the atom is no longer neutral, but becomes positively charged and is referred to as a *positive ion*. The process of removing an electron from an atom is called *ionization*.
- If an electron is displaced from an inner shell to an outer shell (i.e. to a higher energy level), the atom remains neutral but is in an excited state. This process is called *excitation*.
- The unit of energy in the atomic system is the electron volt (eV), 1eV = 1.6×10^{-19} joules.

X-RAY PRODUCTION

X-rays are produced when energetic (high-speed) electrons bombard a target material and are brought suddenly to rest. This happens inside a small evacuated glass envelope called the *X-ray tube* (see Fig. 2.2).

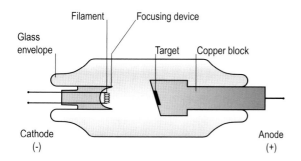

Fig. 2.2 Diagram of a simple X-ray tube showing the main components.

Main features and requirements of an X-ray tube

- The *cathode* (negative) consists of a heated *filament* of tungsten that provides the source of electrons.
- The *anode* (positive) consists of a *target* (a small piece of tungsten) set into the angled face of a large *copper block* to allow efficient removal of heat.
- A *focusing device* aims the stream of electrons at the *focal spot* on the target.
- A high-voltage (kilovoltage, kV) connected between the cathode and anode accelerates the electrons from the negative filament to the positive target. This is sometimes referred to as kVp or kilovoltage peak, as explained later in Chapter 5.
- A current (milliamperage, mA) flows from the cathode to the anode. This is a measure of the quantity of electrons being accelerated.
- A surrounding *lead casing* absorbs unwanted X-rays as a radiation protection measure since X-rays are emitted in all directions.
- Surrounding *oil* facilitates the removal of heat.

Practical considerations

The production of X-rays can be summarized as the following sequence of events:

1. The filament is electrically heated and a cloud of electrons is produced around the filament.
2. The high-voltage (potential difference) across the tube accelerates the electrons at very high speed towards the anode.

3. The focusing device aims the electron stream at the focal spot on the target.
4. The electrons bombard the target and are brought suddenly to rest.
5. The energy lost by the electrons is transferred into either *heat* (about 99%) or X-rays (about 1%).
6. The heat produced is removed and dissipated by the copper block and the surrounding oil.
7. The X-rays are emitted in all directions from the target. Those emitted through the small window in the lead casing constitute the *beam* used for diagnostic purposes.

Interactions at the atomic level

The high-speed electrons bombarding the target (Fig. 2.3) are involved in two main types of *collision* with the tungsten atoms:

- Heat-producing collisions
- X-ray-producing collisions.

Heat-producing collisions

- The incoming electron is deflected by the cloud of outer-shell tungsten electrons, with a small loss of energy, in the form of *heat* (Fig. 2.4A).
- The incoming electron collides with an outer shell tungsten electron displacing it to an even more peripheral shell (excitation) or displacing it from the atom (ionization), again with a small loss of energy in the form of *heat* (Fig. 2.4B).

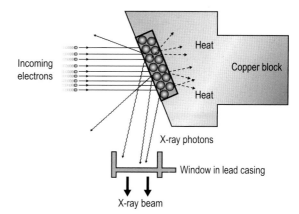

Fig. 2.3 Diagram of the anode enlarged, showing the target and summarizing the interactions at the target.

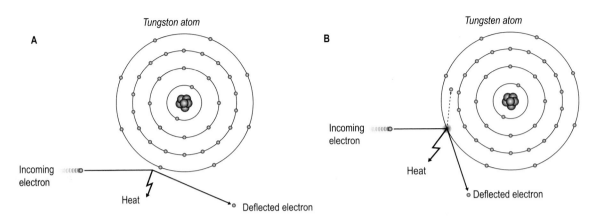

Fig. 2.4A Heat-producing collision: the incoming electron is deflected by the tungsten electron cloud. **B** Heat-producing collision: the incoming electron collides with and displaces an outer-shell tungsten electron.

Important points to note

- Heat-producing interactions are the most common because there are millions of incoming electrons and many outer-shell tungsten electrons with which to interact.
- Each individual bombarding electron can undergo many heat-producing collisions resulting in a considerable amount of heat at the target.
- Heat needs to be removed quickly and efficiently to prevent damage to the target. This is achieved by setting the tungsten target in the copper block, utilizing the high thermal capacity and good conduction properties of copper.

X-ray-producing collisions

- The incoming electron penetrates the outer electron shells and passes close to the nucleus of the tungsten atom. The incoming electron is dramatically slowed down and deflected by the nucleus with a large loss of energy which is emitted in the form of *X-rays* (Fig. 2.5A).
- The incoming electron collides with an inner-shell tungsten electron displacing it to an outer shell (excitation) or displacing it from the atom (ionization), with a large loss of energy and subsequent emission of *X-rays* (Fig. 2.5B).

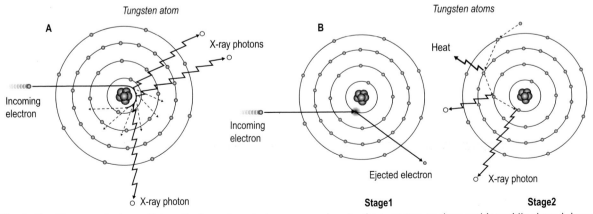

Fig. 2.5A X-ray-producing collision: the incoming electron passes close to the tungsten nucleus and is rapidly slowed down and deflected with the emission of X-ray photons. **B** X-ray-producing collision: Stage 1 — the incoming electron collides with an inner-shell tungsten electron and displaces it; Stage 2 — outer-shell electrons drop into the inner shells with subsequent emission of X-ray photons.

X-ray spectra

The two X-ray-producing collisions result in the production of two different types of *X-ray spectra*:

- Continuous spectrum
- Characteristic spectrum.

Continuous spectrum

The X-ray photons emitted by the rapid deceleration of the bombarding electrons passing close to the nucleus of the tungsten atom are sometimes referred to as *bremsstrahlung* or *braking radiation*. The amount of deceleration and degree of deflection determine the amount of energy lost by the bombarding electron and hence the energy of the resultant emitted photon. A wide range or *spectrum* of photon energies is therefore possible and is termed the *continuous spectrum* (see Fig. 2.6).

Summary of important points

- Small deflections of the bombarding electrons are the most common, producing many *low-energy* photons.
- Low-energy photons have little penetrating power and most will not exit from the X-ray tube itself. They will not contribute to the useful X-ray beam (see Fig. 2.6B). This removal of low-energy photons from the beam is known as *filtration* (see later).
- Large deflections are less likely to happen so there are relatively few *high-energy* photons.
- The maximum photon energy possible (E max) is directly related to the size of the potential difference (kV) across the X-ray tube.

Characteristic spectrum

Following the ionization or excitation of the tungsten atoms by the bombarding electrons, the orbiting tungsten electrons rearrange themselves to return the atom to the neutral or ground state. This involves electron 'jumps' from one energy level (shell) to another, and results in the emission of X-ray photons with specific energies. As stated previously, the energy levels or shells are specific for any particular atom. The X-ray photons emitted from the target are therefore described as *characteristic of tungsten atoms* and form the *characteristic* or *line spectrum* (see Fig. 2.7). The photon lines are named K and L, depending on the shell from which they have been emitted.

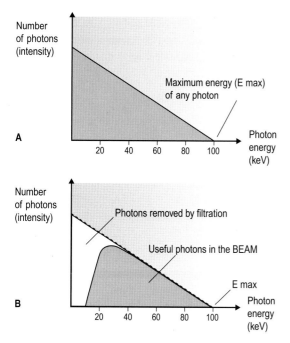

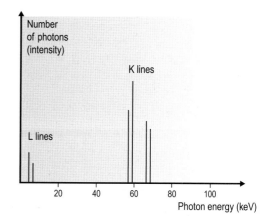

Fig. 2.6A   Graph showing the continuous X-ray spectrum at the target for an X-ray tube operating at 100 kV. **B** Graph showing the continuous spectrum in the emitted beam, as the result of *filtration*.

Fig. 2.7   Graph showing the characteristic or line spectrum at the target for an X-ray tube (with a tungsten target) operating at 100 kV.

Summary of important points

- Only the K lines are of diagnostic importance since the L lines have too little energy.
- The bombarding high-speed electron must have sufficient energy (69.5 kV) to displace a K-shell tungsten electron to produce the characteristic K line on the spectrum. (The energy of the bombarding electrons is directly related to the potential difference (kV) across the X-ray tube, see later.)
- Characteristic K-line photons are not produced by X-ray tubes with tungsten targets operating at less than 69.5 kV — referred to as the *critical voltage* (Vc).
- Dental X-ray equipment operates usually between 50 kV and 90 kV (see later).

Combined spectra

In X-ray equipment operating above 69.5 kV, the final total spectrum of the useful X-ray *beam* will be the addition of the continuous and characteristic spectra (see Fig. 2.8).

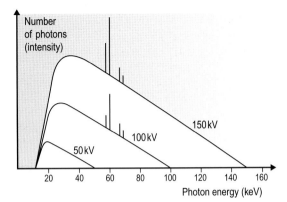

Fig. 2.8 Graphs showing the combination photon energy spectra (in the final beam) for X-ray sets operating at 50 kV, 100 kV and 150 kV.

Summary of the main properties and characteristics of X-rays

- X-rays are *wave packets* of energy of electromagnetic radiation that originate at the atomic level.
- Each *wave packet* is equivalent to a *quantum* of energy and is called a *photon*.
- An X-ray *beam* is made up of millions of photons of different energies.
- The diagnostic X-ray beam can vary in its *intensity* and in its *quality*:
  - Intensity = the number or quantity of X-ray photons in the beam
  - Quality = the energy carried by the X-ray photons which is a measure of their penetrating power.
- The factors that can affect the intensity and/or the quality of the beam include:
  - Size of the tube voltage (kV)
  - Size of the tube current (mA)
  - Distance from the target (d)
  - Time = length of exposure (t)
  - Filtration
  - Target material
  - Tube voltage waveform (see Ch. 5).
- In free space, X-rays travel in straight lines.
- Velocity in free space = 3×10^8 m s^{-1}
- In free space, X-rays obey the inverse square law:

$$\text{Intensity} = 1/d^2$$

Doubling the distance from an X-ray source reduces the intensity to $\frac{1}{4}$ (a very important principle in radiation protection, see Ch. 8).
- No medium is required for propagation.
- Shorter-wavelength X-rays possess greater energy and can therefore penetrate a greater distance.
- Longer-wavelength X-rays, sometimes referred to as *soft X-rays*, possess less energy and have little penetrating power.
- The energy carried by X-rays can be attenuated by matter, i.e. absorbed or scattered (see later).
- X-rays are capable of producing *ionization* (and subsequent biological damage in living tissue, see Ch. 4) and are thus referred to as *ionizing radiation*.
- X-rays are undetectable by human senses.
- X-rays can affect film emulsion to produce a visual image (the radiograph) and can cause certain salts to fluoresce and to emit light — the principle behind the use of intensifying screens in extraoral cassettes and digital sensors (see Ch. 6).

INTERACTION OF X-RAYS WITH MATTER

When X-rays strike matter, such as a patient's tissues, the photons have four possible fates, shown diagrammatically in Figure 2.9. The photons may be:

- Completely scattered with no loss of energy
- Absorbed with total loss of energy
- Scattered with some absorption and loss of energy
- Transmitted unchanged.

Definition of terms used in X-ray interactions

- *Scattering* — change in direction of a photon with or without a loss of energy
- *Absorption* — deposition of energy, i.e. removal of energy from the beam
- *Attenuation* — reduction in the intensity of the main X-ray beam caused by absorption and scattering

  Attenuation = Absorption + Scattering
- *Ionization* — removal of an electron from a neutral atom producing a negative ion (the electron) and a positive ion (the remaining atom).

Interaction of X-rays at the atomic level

There are four main interactions at the atomic level, depending on the energy of the incoming photon, these include:

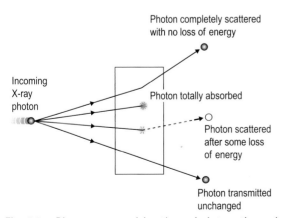

Fig. 2.9 Diagram summarizing the main interactions when X-rays interact with matter.

Photon completely scattered with no loss of energy

Incoming X-ray photon

Photon totally absorbed

Photon scattered after some loss of energy

Photon transmitted unchanged

- Unmodified or Rayleigh scattering — pure scatter
- Photoelectric effect — pure absorption
- Compton effect — scatter and absorption
- Pair production — pure absorption.

Only two interactions are important in the X-ray energy range used in dentistry:

- Photoelectric effect
- Compton effect.

Photoelectric effect

The photoelectric effect is a pure absorption interaction predominating with *low-energy* photons (see Fig. 2.10).

Summary of the stages in the photoelectric effect
1. The incoming X-ray photon interacts with a bound inner-shell electron of the tissue atom.
2. The inner-shell electron is ejected with considerable energy (now called a *photoelectron*) into the tissues and will undergo further interactions (see below).
3. The X-ray photon disappears having deposited all its energy; the process is therefore one of pure *absorption*.
4. The vacancy which now exists in the inner electron shell is filled by outer-shell electrons dropping from one shell to another.
5. This cascade of electrons to new energy levels results in the emission of excess energy in the form of light or heat.
6. Atomic stability is finally achieved by the capture of a free electron to return the atom to its neutral state.
7. The high-energy ejected *photoelectron* behaves like the original high-energy X-ray photon, undergoing many similar interactions and ejecting other electrons as it passes through the tissues. It is these ejected high-energy electrons that are responsible for the majority of the ionization interactions within tissue, and the possible resulting damage attributable to X-rays.

Important points to note
- The X-ray photon energy needs to be equal to, or just greater than, the binding energy of the inner-shell electron to be able to eject it.

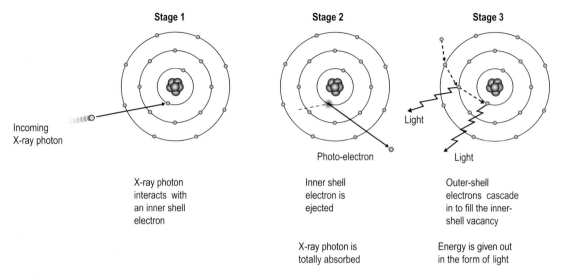

Fig. 2.10 Diagrams representing the stages in the photoelectric interaction.

- As the density (atomic number, Z) increases, the number of bound inner-shell electrons also increases. The probability of photoelectric interactions occurring is $\propto Z^3$. Lead has an atomic number of 82 and is therefore a good absorber of X-rays — hence its use in radiation protection (see Ch. 8). The approximate atomic number for soft tissue is 7 ($Z^3 = 343$) and for bone is 12 ($Z^3 = 1728$) — hence their obvious difference in radiodensity, and the *contrast* between the different tissues seen on radiographs (see Ch. 24).
- This interaction predominates with low energy X-ray photons — the probability of photo-electric interactions occurring is $\propto 1/kV^3$. This

explains why low kV X-ray equipment results in high absorption (dose) in the patient's tissues, but provides good contrast radiographs.
- The overall result of the interaction is *ionization* of the tissues.
- Intensifying screens, described in Chapter 6, function by the photoelectric effect — when exposed to X-rays, the screens emit their excess energy as *light*, which subsequently affects the film emulsion.

Compton effect
The Compton effect is an absorption *and* scattering process predominating with *higher-energy* photons (see Fig. 2.11).

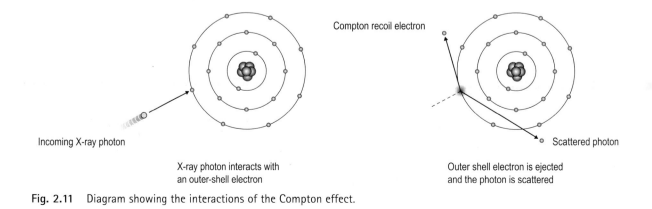

Fig. 2.11 Diagram showing the interactions of the Compton effect.

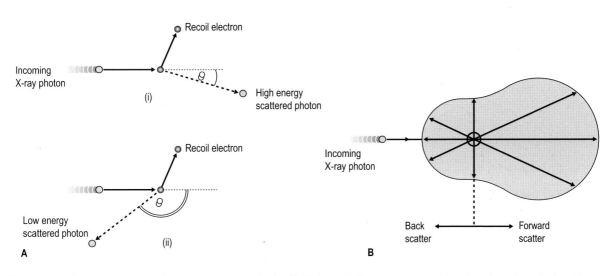

Fig. 2.12A   Diagram showing the angle of scatter θ with (i) high- and (ii) low-energy scattered photons. **B** Typical scatter distribution diagram of a 70 kV X-ray set. The length of any radius from the source of scatter indicates the relative amount of scatter in that direction. At this voltage, the majority of scatter is in a forward direction.

Summary of the stages in the Compton effect

1. The incoming X-ray photon interacts with a *free* or loosely bound outer-shell electron of the tissue atom.
2. The outer-shell electron is ejected (now called the *Compton recoil electron*) with loss of some of the energy of the incoming photon, i.e. there is some *absorption*. The ejected electron then undergoes further ionizing interactions within the tissues (as before).
3. The remainder of the incoming photon energy is deflected or *scattered* from its original path as a scattered photon.
4. The scattered photon may then:
   - Undergo further Compton interactions within the tissues
   - Undergo photoelectric interactions within the tissues
   - Escape from the tissues — it is these photons that form the *scatter radiation* of concern in the clinical environment.
5. Atomic stability is again achieved by the capture of another free electron.

Important points to note

- The energy of the incoming X-ray photon is much greater than the binding energy of the outer-shell or free electron.
- The incoming X-ray photon cannot distinguish between one free electron and another — the interaction is not dependent on the atomic number (Z). Thus, this interaction provides very little diagnostic information as there is very little discrimination between different tissues on the final radiograph.
- This interaction predominates with high X-ray photon energies. This explains why high-voltage X-ray sets result in radiographs with poor contrast.
- The energy of the scattered photon (Es) is always less than the energy of the incoming photon (E), depending on the energy given to the recoil electron (e):

$$Es = E - e$$

- Scattered photons can be deflected in any direction, but the angle of scatter (θ) depends on their energy. *High-energy* scattered photons produce *forward* scatter; *low-energy* scattered photons produce *back* scatter (see Fig. 2.12).
- Forward scatter may reach the film and degrade the image, but can be removed by using an *anti-scatter grid* (see Ch. 14).
- The overall result of the interaction is ionization of the tissues.

Chapter 3

Dose units and dosimetry

Several different terms and units have been used in dosimetry over the years. The conversion to SI units has made this subject even more confusing. However, it is essential that these terms and units are understood to appreciate what is meant by *radiation dose* and to allow meaningful comparisons between different investigations to be made. In addition to explaining the various units, this chapter also summarizes the various sources of ionizing radiation and the magnitude of *radiation doses* that are encountered.

The more important terms in dosimetry include:

- Radiation-absorbed dose (D)
- Equivalent dose (H)
- Effective dose (E)
- Collective effective dose or collective dose
- Dose rate.

RADIATION–ABSORBED DOSE (D)

This is a measure of the amount of energy absorbed from the radiation beam per unit mass of tissue.

> SI unit : Gray, (Gy) measured in joules/kg
> subunit : milligray, (mGy) ($\times 10^{-3}$)
> original unit : rad, measured in ergs/g
> conversion : 1 Gray = 100 rads

EQUIVALENT DOSE (H)

This is a measure which allows the different radiobiological effectiveness (RBE) of different types of radiation to be taken into account.

For example, alpha particles (see Ch. 19) penetrate only a few millimetres in tissue, lose all their energy and are totally absorbed, whereas X-rays penetrate much further, lose some of their energy and are only partially absorbed. The biological effect of a particular *radiation-absorbed dose* of alpha particles would be considerably more severe than a similar *radiation-absorbed dose* of X-rays.

By introducing a numerical value known as the *radiation weighting factor* W_R which represents the biological effects of different radiations, the unit of *equivalent dose (H)* provides a common unit allowing comparisons to be made between one type of radiation and another, for example:

X-rays, gamma rays and beta particles	$W_R = 1$
Fast neutrons (10 keV–100 keV) and protons	$W_R = 10$
Alpha particles	$W_R = 20$

Equivalent dose (H) = **radiation-absorbed dose (D) × radiation weighting factor (W_R)**

> SI unit : Sievert (Sv)
> subunits : millisievert (mSv) ($\times 10^{-3}$)
> microsievert (μSv) ($\times 10^{-6}$)
> original unit : rem
> conversion : 1 Sievert = 100 rems

(For X-rays, the radiation weighting factor (W_R factor) = 1, therefore the *equivalent dose (H)*, measured in *Sieverts*, is equal to the *radiation-absorbed dose (D)*, measured in *Grays*.)

EFFECTIVE DOSE (E)

This measure allows doses from different investigations of different parts of the body to be compared, by converting all doses to an *equivalent whole body dose*.

This is necessary because some parts of the body are more sensitive to radiation than others. The International Commission on Radiological Protection (ICRP) has allocated each tissue a numerical value, known as the *tissue weighting factor (W_T)*, based on its radiosensitivity, i.e. the risk of the tissue being damaged by radiation — the greater the risk, the higher the *tissue weighting factor*. The sum of the individual *tissue weighting factors* represents the *weighting factor* for the whole body. The *tissue weighting factors* recommended by the ICRP in 1990 and updated in 2005 are shown in Table 3.1.

Effective dose (E) = equivalent dose (H) × tissue weighting factor (W_T)

SI unit : Sievert (Sv)

subunit : millisievert (mSv)

When the simple term *dose* is applied loosely, it is the *effective dose (E)* that is usually being described. *Effective dose* can thus be thought of as a broad indication of the risk to health from any exposure to ionizing radiation, irrespective of the type or energy of the radiation or the part of the body being irradiated. A comparison of effective doses from different investigations is shown in Table 3.2.

COLLECTIVE EFFECTIVE DOSE OR COLLECTIVE DOSE

This measure is used when considering the total *effective dose* to a *population*, from a particular investigation or source of radiation.

Collective dose = effective dose (E) × population

SI unit : man-sievert (man-Sv)

Table 3.1 The tissue weighting factors (W_T) recommended by the ICRP in 1990 and in 2005

Tissue	1990 W_T	2005 W_T
Bone marrow	0.12	0.12
Breast	0.05	0.12
Colon	0.12	0.12
Lung	0.12	0.12
Stomach	0.12	0.12
Bladder	0.05	0.05
Oesophagus	0.05	0.05
Gonads	0.20	0.05
Liver	0.05	0.05
Thyroid	0.05	0.05
Bone surface	0.01	0.01
Brain	*	0.01
Kidneys	*	0.01
Salivary glands	----	0.01
Skin	0.01	0.01
Remainder tissues	0.05*	0.10+

*Adrenals, brain, upper large intestine, small intestine, kidney muscle, pancreas, spleen, thymus and uterus
+Adipose tissue, adrenals, connective tissue, extrathoracic airways, gall bladder, heart wall, lymphatic nodes, muscle, pancreas, prostate, SI wall, spleen, thymus and uterus/cervix

Table 3.2 Typical effective doses for a range of dental and routine medical examinations

X-ray examination	Effective dose (mSv)
CT chest	8.0
CT head	2.0
Barium swallow	1.5
Barium enema	7.0
Lumbar spine (AP)	0.7
Skull (PA)	0.03
Skull (Lat)	0.01
Chest (PA)	0.02
Chest (Lat)	0.04
Bitewing/periapical	0.001–0.008
Upper standard occlusal	0.008
Panoramic	0.004–0.03
Lateral cephalometric	0.002–0.003
CT mandible	0.36–1.2
CT maxilla	0.1–3.3

DOSE RATE

This is a measure of the dose per unit time, e.g. dose/hour, and is sometimes a more convenient, and measurable, figure than, for example, a total annual dose limit (see Ch. 8).

SI unit : microsievert/hour ($\mu Sv\ h^{-1}$)

ESTIMATED ANNUAL DOSES FROM VARIOUS SOURCES OF RADIATION

Everyone is exposed to some form of ionizing radiation from the environment in which we live. Sources include:

- Natural background radiation
  - Cosmic radiation from the earth's atmosphere
  - Gamma radiation from the rocks and soil in the earth's crust
  - Radiation from ingested radioisotopes, e.g. ^{40}K, in certain foods
  - Radon and its decay products; ^{222}Rn is a gaseous decay product of uranium that is present naturally in granite. As a gas, radon diffuses readily from rocks through soil and can be trapped in poorly ventilated houses and then breathed into the lungs. In the UK, this is of particular concern in areas of Cornwall and Scotland where houses have been built on large deposits of granite
- Artificial background radiation
  - Fallout from nuclear explosions
  - Radioactive waste discharged from nuclear establishments
- Medical and dental diagnostic radiation
- Radiation from occupational exposure.

The Radiation Protection Division of the Health Protection Agency (formerly the National Radiological Protection Board (NRPB)) has estimated the annual doses from these various sources in the UK. Table 3.3. gives a summary of the data.

An individual's average dose from background radiation is estimated at approximately **2.7 mSv per year** in the UK, while in the USA it is estimated at approximately **3.6 mSv**. These figures are useful to remember when considering the magnitude of the doses associated with various diagnostic procedures (see later).

Table 3.3   HPA(NRPB)-estimated average annual doses to the UK population from various sources of radiation

Radiation source	Average annual dose (μSv)	Approximate %
Natural background		
Cosmic rays	300	
External exposure from the earth's crust	400	
Internal radiation from certain foodstuffs	370	
Exposure to radon and its decay products	700	
Total	2.7 mSv (approx.)	87%
Artificial background		
Fallout	10	
Radioactive waste	2	>1%
Medical and dental diagnostic radiation	250	12%
Occupational exposure	9	>1%

TYPICAL DOSES ENCOUNTERED IN DIAGNOSTIC RADIOLOGY

The *European Guidelines on Radiation Protection in Dental Radiology* published in 2004 were based on an extensive review of the available evidence on all aspects of radiation protection in dentistry. They concluded that although many studies have measured doses of radiation for dental radiography, only a few had estimated effective dose. For some techniques there is no published data available and some for which very different results have been reported. The typical effective doses shown earlier in Table 3.2 are based broadly on their findings, together with a selection of typical effective doses from various medical diagnostic procedures published the in NRPB document *Guidelines on Patient Dose to Promote the Optimisation of Protection for Diagnostic Medical Exposures* in 1999.

It must be stressed that these are typical values and that a considerable range of effective doses exists in dental radiography. The main reasons for this variation are kV of equipment used, shape and size of beam, speed and type of image receptor used and the tissues included in the calculations. These factors are of great importance in radiation protection and are discussed in more detail in Chapter 8.

However, the figures do provide an indication of the comparative sizes of the various effective doses. The individual doses encountered in dental radiology may appear very small, but it must be remembered that the diagnostic burden, however small, is an additional radiation burden to that which the patient is already receiving from background radiation. This additional dose may be considerable for any individual patient. The enormous number of dental radiographs (intraoral and extraoral) taken per year (estimated at approximately 20–25 million in the UK alone) means that the *collective dose* from dental radiography is quite substantial. The risks associated with some of the diagnostic investigations are discussed in Chapter 4.

Chapter 4

The biological effects and risks associated with X-rays

CLASSIFICATION OF THE BIOLOGICAL EFFECTS

The biologically damaging effects of ionizing radiation are classified into three main categories:

- Somatic DETERMINISTIC effects
- Somatic STOCHASTIC effects.
- Genetic STOCHASTIC effects.

The somatic effects are further subdivided into:

- *Acute* or *immediate* effects — appearing shortly after exposure, e.g. as a result of large whole body doses (Table 4.1)

- *Chronic* or *long-term* effects — becoming evident after a long period of time, the so-called *latent period* (20 years or more), e.g. leukaemia.

Somatic deterministic effects

These are the damaging effects to the body of the person exposed that will **definitely** result from a specific high dose of radiation. Examples include skin reddening and cataract formation. The severity of the effect is proportional to the dose received, and in most cases a *threshold* dose exists below which there will be no effect.

Somatic stochastic effects

Stochastic effects are those that **may** develop. Their development is random and depends on the laws of chance or probability. Examples of somatic stochastic effects include leukaemia and certain tumours.

These damaging effects **may** be induced when the body is exposed to **any** dose of radiation. Experimentally it has not been possible to establish a *safe dose* — i.e. a dose below which stochastic effects do not develop. It is therefore assumed that there is *no threshold dose*, and that every exposure to ionizing radiation carries with it the **possibility** of inducing a stochastic effect.

The lower the radiation dose, the lower the probability of cell damage. However, the severity of the damage is **not related** to the size of the inducing dose. This is the underlying philosophy

Table 4.1 Summary of the main *acute effects* following large whole-body doses of radiation

Dose	Whole-body effect
0.25 Sv	Nil
0.25–1.0 Sv	Slight blood changes, e.g. decrease in white blood cell count
1–2 Sv	Vomiting in 3 hours, fatigue, loss of appetite, blood changes Recovery in a few weeks
2–6 Sv	Vomiting in 2 hours, severe blood changes, loss of hair within 2 weeks Recovery in 1 month to year for 70%
6–10 Sv	Vomiting in 1 hour, intestinal damage, severe blood changes Death in 2 weeks for 80–100%
>10 Sv	Brain damage, coma, death

behind present radiation protection recommendations (see Ch. 8).

Genetic stochastic effects

Mutations result from any sudden change to a gene or chromosome. They can be caused by external factors, such as radiation or may occur spontaneously.

Radiation to the reproductive organs **may** damage the DNA of the sperm or egg cells. This **may** result in a congenital abnormality in the offspring of the person irradiated. However, there is no certainty that these effects will happen, so all genetic effects are described as stochastic.

A cause-and-effect relationship is difficult, if not impossible, to prove. Although ionizing radiation has the potential to cause genetic damage, there are no human data that show convincing evidence of a direct link with radiation. Risk estimates have been based mainly on experiments with mice. It is estimated that a dose to the gonads of 0.5–1.0 Sv would double the spontaneous mutation rate. Once again it is assumed that there is *no threshold dose*.

Effects on the unborn child

The developing fetus is particularly sensitive to the effects of radiation, especially during the period of organogenesis (2–9 weeks after conception). The major problems are:

- Congenital abnormalities or death associated with large doses of radiation
- Mental retardation associated with low doses of radiation.

As a result, the maximum permissible dose to the abdomen of a woman who is pregnant is regulated by law. This is discussed further in Chapter 8.

Harmful effects important in dental radiology

In dentistry, the size of the doses used routinely are relatively small (see Ch. 3) and well below the threshold doses required to produce the somatic deterministic effects. However, the somatic and genetic stochastic effects can develop with **any** dose of ionizing radiation. Dental radiology does not usually involve irradiating the reproductive organs, thus in dentistry somatic stochastic effects are the damaging effects of most concern.

HOW DO X-RAYS CAUSE DAMAGE?

The action of radiation on cells and the damaging effects are illustrated in Figure 4.1. and classified as:

- *Direct action or damage* as a result of ionization of macromolecules
- *Indirect action or damage* as a result of the free radicals produced by the ionization of water.

Direct action or damage

The X-ray photons, or high-energy ejected electrons, interact directly with, and ionize, vital biologic macromolecules such as DNA, RNA, proteins and enzymes. This ionization results in the breakage of the macromolecule's chemical bonds, causing them to become abnormal structures, which may in turn lead to inappropriate chemical reactions. Rupture of one of the chemical bonds in a DNA macromolecule may sever one of the side chains of the ladder-like structure. This type of injury to DNA is called a *point mutation*. The subsequent chromosomal effects from direct damage could include:

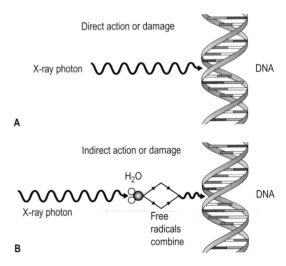

Fig. 4.1   Diagram illustrating the action and damaging effects of radiation on cells. **A** *Direct action or damage* – the X-ray photon interacts directly with the DNA. **B** *Indirect action or damage* – the X-ray photon ionizes water to produce free radicals which damage the DNA.

- Inability to pass on information
- Abnormal replication
- Cell death
- Only temporary damage — the DNA being repaired successfully before further cell division.

If the radiation directly affects somatic cells, the effects on the DNA (and hence the chromosomes) could result in a radiation-induced malignancy. If the damage is to reproductive stem cells, the result could be a radiation-induced congenital abnormality.

What actually happens in the cell depends on several factors, including:

- The type and number of nucleic acid bonds that are broken
- The intensity and type of radiation
- The time between exposures
- The ability of the cell to repair the damage
- The stage of the cell's reproductive cycle when irradiated.

Indirect action or damage

This process, which is shown in Figure 4.2, involves the breakdown of the water molecule

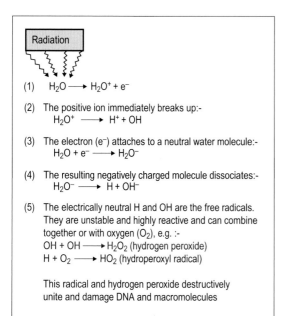

(1) $H_2O \longrightarrow H_2O^+ + e^-$

(2) The positive ion immediately breaks up:-
     $H_2O^+ \longrightarrow H^+ + OH$

(3) The electron (e^-) attaches to a neutral water molecule:-
     $H_2O + e^- \longrightarrow H_2O^-$

(4) The resulting negatively charged molecule dissociates:-
     $H_2O^- \longrightarrow H + OH^-$

(5) The electrically neutral H and OH are the free radicals. They are unstable and highly reactive and can combine together or with oxygen (O_2), e.g. :-
     $OH + OH \longrightarrow H_2O_2$ (hydrogen peroxide)
     $H + O_2 \longrightarrow HO_2$ (hydroperoxyl radical)

     This radical and hydrogen peroxide destructively unite and damage DNA and macromolecules

Fig. 4.2 A diagrammatic summary of the sequence of events following ionization of water molecules leading to *indirect damage* to the cell.

into smaller molecules, producing both ions and *free radicals* in the process. The free radicals can recombine to form hydrogen peroxide, a cellular poison, and a hydroperoxyl radical, another toxic substance. Both of these substances are highly reactive and produce biologic damage. By themselves, free radicals may transfer excess energy to other molecules, thereby breaking their chemical bonds and having an even greater effect. As about 80% of the body consists of water, the vast majority of the interactions with ionizing radiation are indirect.

ESTIMATING THE MAGNITUDE OF THE RISK OF CANCER INDUCTION

Quantifying the risk of somatic stochastic effects, such as radiation-induced cancer, is complex and controversial. Data from groups exposed to **high** doses of radiation are analysed and the results are used to provide an estimate of the risk from the **low** doses of radiation encountered in diagnostic radiology. The high-dose groups studied include:

- The survivors of the atomic explosions at Hiroshima and Nagasaki
- Patients receiving radiotherapy
- Radiation workers — people exposed to radiation in the course of their work
- The survivors of the nuclear disaster at Chernobyl.

The problem of quantifying the risk is compounded because cancer is a common disease, so in any group of individuals studied there is likely to be some incidence of cancer. In the groups listed above, that have been exposed to high doses of radiation, the incidence of cancer is likely to be increased and is referred to as the *excess cancer incidence*. From the data collected, it has been possible to construct *dose–response curves* (Fig. 4.3), showing the relationship between excess cancers and radiation dose. The graphs can be extrapolated to zero (the controversy on risk assessment revolves around exactly **how** this extrapolation should be done), and a *risk factor* for induction of cancer by low doses of radiation can be calculated.

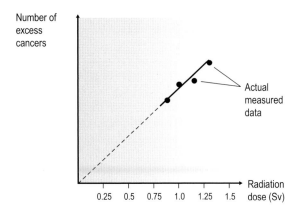

Fig. 4.3 A typical dose–response curve, showing excess cancer incidence plotted against radiation dose and a linear extrapolation of the data to zero.

A broad estimate of the magnitude of the risk of developing a fatal radiation-induced cancer, from various X-ray examinations is shown in Table 4.2. These are based broadly on the NRPB booklet *Guidelines on Patient Dose to Promote the Optimisation of Protection for Diagnostic Medical Exposures* published in the UK in 1999 and the *European Guidelines on Radiation Protection in Dental Radiology* published in 2004.

Risk is age-dependent, being highest for the young and lowest for the elderly. The risks shown in Table 4.2 are for a 30-year-old adult. The 2004 *European Guidelines* and the 2004 *Selection Criteria in Dental Radiography* booklet published by the Faculty of General Dental Practice (UK) of the Royal College of Surgeons in England, both recommend that these should be modified by the multiplication factors shown in Table 4.3 which represent averages for the two sexes. In fact at all ages, risks for females are slightly higher and risks for males slightly lower.

This epidemiological information is being updated continually and recent reports suggest that the risk from low-dose radiation may be considerably greater than thought previously. However, the present figures at least provide an idea of the comparative order of magnitude of the risk involved from different investigations. This in turn helps keep the risks associated with dental radiology in perspective.

SUMMARY

The biological effects of ionizing radiation can be extremely damaging. *Somatic deterministic effects* predominate with **high** doses of radiation, while *somatic stochastic effects* predominate with **low** doses. Dental radiology employs low doses and the risk of stochastic effects is very small. However, the number of dental radiographs is very high — estimated at between 20–25 million intraoral and extraoral radiographs per year in the UK alone. It has been estimated that the overall risk from dental radiography in the UK is in the

Table 4.2 Broad estimate of the risk of a standard adult patient developing a fatal radiation-induced malignancy from various X-ray examinations (NRPB 1999)

X-ray examination	Estimated risk of fatal cancer
Traditional bitewing/periapical (50 kV, D speed film, 10 cm fsd)	1 in 2 000 000
Modern bitewing/periapical (70 kV, F speed film, 20 cm fsd)	1 in 20 000 000
Panoramic – average (estimates range from 0.21 – 1.9)	1 in 1 000 000
Skull (PA)	1 in 670 000
Skull (Lat)	1 in 2 000 000
Chest (PA)	1 in 1 000 000
Lumbar spine (AP)	1 in 29 000
Barium swallow	1 in 13 000
Barium enema	1 in 3000
CT chest	1 in 2500
CT head	1 in 10 000

Table 4.3 The multiplication factor for risk for different age groups

Age group (years)	Multiplication factor for risk
<10	× 3
10–20	× 2
20–30	× 1.5
30–50	× 0.5
50–80	× 0.3
80+	negligible risk

order of 10 fatal malignancies per year. The various important dose-reduction and dose-limitation measures that are therefore necessary to keep all exposures *as low as reasonably practicable* (ALARP), for both patients and for dental staff, are outlined in Chapter 8.

Chapter 5

Dental X-ray generating equipment

This chapter summarizes the more important practical aspects of dental X-ray generating equipment. There are several different units available from various manufacturers. They vary in appearance, complexity and cost, but all consist of three main components:

- A tubehead
- Positioning arms
- A control panel and circuitry.

Three modern dental units, suitable for both film and digital imaging are shown in Figure 5.1. Their control panels are shown in Figure 5.6. Dental units can be either *fixed* (wall-mounted or ceiling-mounted) or *mobile* (attached to a sturdy frame on wheels).

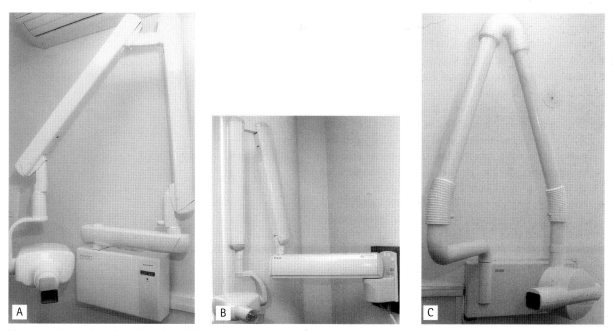

Fig. 5.1 Examples of modern dental X-ray generating equipment showing the tubeheads and positioning arms. **A** Prostyle Intra® manufactured by Planmeca. **B** Focus® manufactured by Instrumentarium Imaging. **C** Heliodent® DS manufactured by Sirona.

Ideal requirements

The equipment should be:

- Safe and accurate
- Capable of generating X-rays in the desired energy range and with adequate mechanisms for heat removal
- Small
- Easy to manoeuvre and position
- Stable, balanced and steady once the tubehead has been positioned
- Easily folded and stored
- Simple to operate and capable of both film and digital imaging
- Robust.

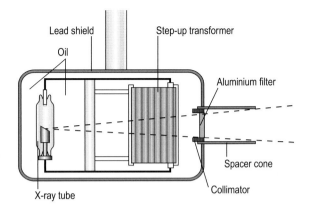

Fig. 5.2 Diagram of the tubehead of a typical dental X-ray set showing the main components.

Main components of the tubehead

A diagram of a typical tubehead is shown in Figure 5.2. The main components include:

- The *glass X-ray tube*, including the filament, copper block and the target (see Ch. 2)
- The *step-up transformer* required to step-up the mains voltage of 240 volts to the high voltage (kV) required across the X-ray tube
- The *step-down transformer* required to step-down the mains voltage of 240 volts to the low voltage current required to heat the filament
- A *surrounding lead shield* to minimize leakage
- *Surrounding oil* to facilitate heat removal
- *Aluminium filtration* to remove harmful low-energy (soft) X-rays (see Fig. 5.3)
- The *collimator* — a metal disc or cylinder with central aperture designed to shape and limit the beam size to a rectangle (the same size as intraoral film) or round with a maximum diameter of 6 cm (see Figs 5.3 and 5.4)
- The *spacer cone* or *beam-indicating device (BID)* — a device for indicating the direction of the beam and setting the ideal distance from the focal spot on the target to the skin. The required *focus to skin (fsd)* distances are:
  - 200 mm for sets operating above 60 kV
  - 100 mm for sets operating below 60 kV
  It is the length of the *focal spot to skin distance (fsd)*, that is important NOT the physical length of the spacer cone. Various designs are illustrated in Figure 5.4.

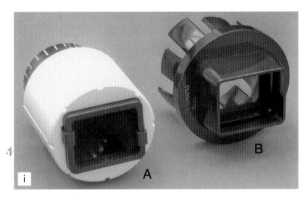

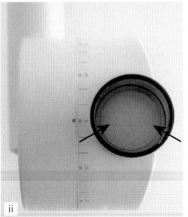

Fig. 5.3 (i) Examples of adaptors/collimators designed to change the shape of the beam from circular to rectangular. **A** Sirona Heliodent® DS collimator, **B** Dentsply's Universal collimator. (ii) Aluminium filter (arrowed) viewed from down the spacer cone on the Sirona Heliodent® DS.

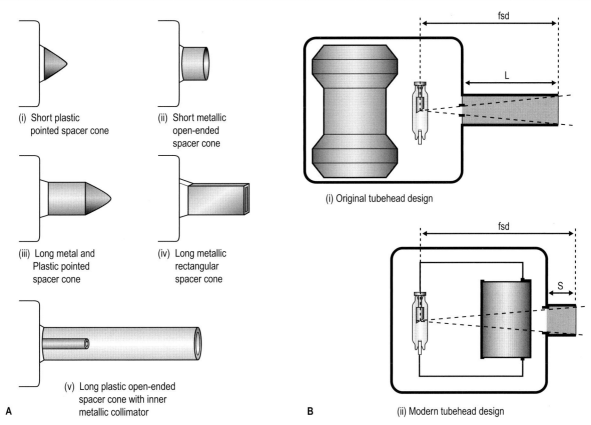

A

(i) Short plastic pointed spacer cone

(ii) Short metallic open-ended spacer cone

(iii) Long metal and Plastic pointed spacer cone

(iv) Long metallic rectangular spacer cone

(v) Long plastic open-ended spacer cone with inner metallic collimator

B

(i) Original tubehead design

(ii) Modern tubehead design

Fig. 5.4A Diagrams showing various designs and shapes of spacer cones or beam-indicating devices. **Note:** The short plastic pointed spacer cone is NOT recommended. **B** Diagrams showing (i) the original tubehead design with the X-ray tube at the **front** of the head, thus requiring a long spacer cone (L) to achieve a near-parallel X-ray beam and the correct *focus to skin distance* (fsd) and (ii) the modern tubehead design with the X-ray tube at the **back** of the head, thus requiring only a short spacer cone(S) to achieve the same *focus to skin distance* (fsd).

Focal spot size and the principle of line focus

As stated in Chapter 1, the focal spot (the source of the X-rays) should be ideally a *point source* to reduce blurring of the image — the *penumbra effect* — as shown in Figure 5.5A. However, the heat produced at the target by the bombarding electrons needs to be distributed over as large an area as possible. These two opposite requirements are satisfied by using an angled target and the principle of *line focus*, as shown in Figure 5.5B.

Main components of the control panel

Examples of three typical control panels are shown in Figure 5.6. The main components include:

- The *mains on/off* switch and *warning light*

- The *timer*, of which there are three main types:
  - electronic
  - impulse
  - clockwork (inaccurate and no longer used)
- An *exposure time selector* mechanism, usually either:
  - numerical, time selected in seconds
  - anatomical, area of mouth selected and exposure time adjusted automatically
- *Warning lights* and *audible signals* to indicate when X-rays are being generated
- Other features can include:
  - *Film speed selector*
  - *Patient size selector*
  - *Mains voltage compensator*
  - *Kilovoltage selector*
  - *Milliamperage switch*
  - *Exposure adjustment for digital imaging.*

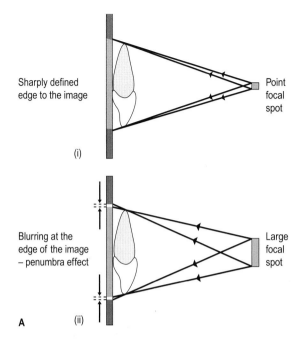

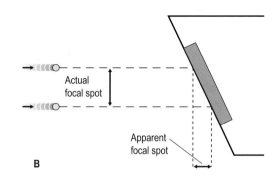

Sharply defined edge to the image

Point focal spot

(i)

Blurring at the edge of the image – penumbra effect

Large focal spot

A

(ii)

Actual focal spot

Apparent focal spot

B

Fig. 5.5A Diagrams showing the effect of X-ray beam source (focal spot) size on image blurring (i) a small or point source, (ii) a large source. **B** The principle of line focus, diagram of the target and focal spot showing how the angled target face allows a large *actual* focal spot but a small *apparent* focal spot.

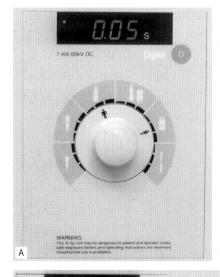

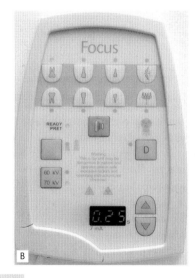

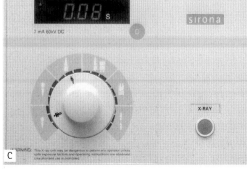

Fig. 5.6 Examples of modern dental X-ray equipment control panels. **A** Prostyle Intra® manufactured by Planmeca. **B** Focus® manufactured by Instrumentarium Imaging. **C** Heliodent® DS manufactured by Sirona. They are all anatomical timers suitable for film and digital (D) imaging.

Circuitry and tube voltage

The mains supply to the X-ray machine of 240 volts has two functions:

- To generate the high potential difference (kV) to accelerate the electrons across the X-ray tube via the step-up transformer
- To provide the low-voltage current to heat the tube filament via the step-down transformer.

However, the incoming 240 volts is an alternating current with the typical waveform shown in Figure 5.7. Half the cycle is positive and the other half is negative. For X-ray production, only the positive half of the cycle can be used to ensure that the electrons from the filament are always drawn towards the target. Thus, the stepped-up high voltage applied across the X-ray tube needs to be *rectified* to eliminate the negative half of the cycle. Four types of rectified circuits are used:

- Half-wave rectified
- Single-phase, full-wave rectified
- Three-phase, full-wave rectified
- Constant potential.

The waveforms resulting from these rectified circuits, together with graphic representation of their subsequent X-ray production, are shown in Figure 5.8. These changing waveforms mean that equipment is only working at its optimum or peak output at the top of each cycle. The kilovoltage is therefore often described as the *kV peak* or *kVp*. Thus a 50 kVp half-wave rectified X-ray set only in fact functions at 50 kV for a tiny fraction of the total time of any exposure.

Modern designs favour constant potential circuitry, often referred to as *DC units*, which keep

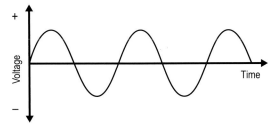

Fig. 5.7   Diagram showing the alternating current waveform.

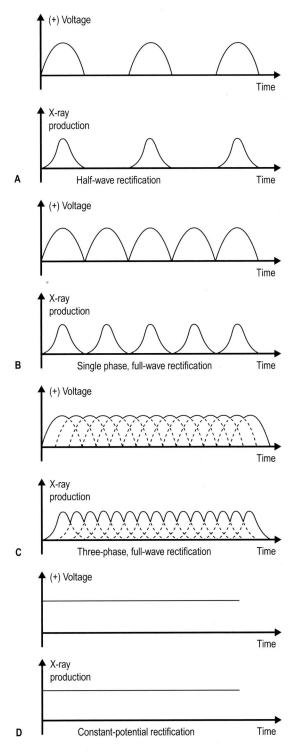

Fig. 5.8   Diagrams showing the waveforms and X-ray production graphs resulting from different forms of rectification.

the kilovoltage at kVpeak throughout any exposure, thus ensuring that:

- X-ray production per unit time is more efficient
- More high-energy, diagnostically useful photons are produced per exposure
- Fewer low energy, harmful photons are produced
- Shorter exposure times are possible.

Other X-ray generating apparatus

The other common X-ray generating equipment encountered in dentistry includes:

- Panoramic X-ray machines often combined with cephalometric skull equipment (see Ch. 17)
- Skull units, such as the Craniotome® or Orbix® (see Ch. 14)
- Various tomography units (see Chs 16 and 17).

The main features and practical components of these machines are outlined in later chapters.

Chapter 6

Image receptors

This chapter summarizes the various image receptors used in dentistry to detect X-rays. These include:

- Radiographic film
  - Direct action or packet film
  - Indirect action film used in conjunction with intensifying screens in a cassette
- Digital receptors
  - Solid-state sensors
  - Phosphor plates.

RADIOGRAPHIC FILM

Radiographic film has traditionally been employed as the image receptor in dentistry and is still widely used. There are two basic types:

- *Direct-action* or *non-screen* film (sometimes referred to as *wrapped* or *packet* film). This type of film is sensitive primarily to X-ray photons.
- *Indirect-action* or *screen* film, so-called because it is used in combination with *intensifying screens* in a *cassette*. This type of film is sensitive primarily to light photons, which are emitted by the adjacent intensifying screens. They respond to shorter exposure of X-rays, enabling a lower dose of radiation to be given to the patient.

Direct-action (non-screen) film

Uses

Direct-action film is used for intraoral radiography where the need for excellent image quality and fine anatomical detail are of importance.

Sizes

Various sizes of film are available, although only three are usually used routinely (see Fig. 6.1).

- 31 × 41 mm ⎫ for periapicals and
- 22 × 35 mm ⎭ bitewings
- 57 × 76 mm — for occlusals.

The film packet contents

The contents of a film packet are shown in Figure 6.1. It is worth noting that:

- The outer packet or wrapper is made of non-absorbent paper or plastic and is sealed to prevent the ingress of saliva.
- The side of the packet that faces towards the X-ray beam has either a pebbled or a smooth surface and is usually white.

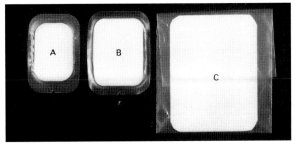

Fig. 6.1 The typical sizes of barrier-wrapped direct-action radiographic film packets available. **A** Small periapical/bitewing film. **B** Large periapical/bitewing film. **C** Occlusal film.

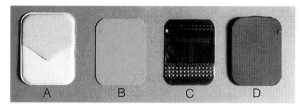

Fig. 6.2   The contents of a film packet. **A** The outer wrapper. **B** The film. **C** The sheet of lead foil. **D** The protective black paper.

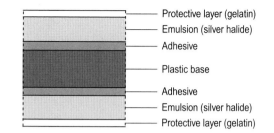

Fig. 6.3   Diagram showing the cross-sectional structure of double emulsion radiographic film.

- The reverse side is usually of two colours so there is little chance of the film being placed the wrong way round in the patient's mouth and different colours represent different film speeds.
- The black paper on either side of the film is there to protect the film from:
  - Light
  - Damage by fingers while being unwrapped
  - Saliva which may leak into the film packet.
- A thin sheet of lead foil is placed behind the film to prevent:
  - Some of the residual radiation that has passed through the film from continuing on into the patient's tissues
  - Scattered secondary radiation, from X-ray photon interactions within the tissues beyond the film, scattering back on to the film and degrading the image.
- The sheet of lead foil contains an embossed pattern so that should the film packet be placed the wrong way round, the pattern will appear on the resultant radiograph. This enables the cause of the resultant pale film to be easily identified (see Ch. 18).

The radiographic film

The cross-sectional structure and components of the radiographic film are shown in Figure 6.3. It comprises four basic components:

- A *plastic base*, made of clear, transparent cellulose acetate — acts as a support for the emulsion but does not contribute to the final image

- A thin layer of *adhesive* — fixes the emulsion to the base
- The *emulsion* on **both** sides of the base — this consists of silver halide (usually bromide) crystals embedded in a gelatin matrix. The X-ray photons *sensitize* the silver halide crystals that they strike and these sensitized silver halide crystals are later reduced to visible black metallic silver in the developer (see Ch. 7)
- A *protective layer* of clear gelatin to shield the emulsion from mechanical damage.

Film orientation

The film has an embossed *dot* on one corner that is used to help orientation. Its position is marked on the back of the packet or can be felt as a raised dot on the front. The side of the film on which the dot is raised is always placed towards the X-ray beam. When the films are mounted, this raised dot is towards the operator and the films are then arranged anatomically and viewed as if the operator were facing the patient.

Indirect–action film

Uses

Film/screen combinations are used as image detectors whenever possible because of the reduced dose of radiation to the patient (particularly when very fine image detail is not essential). The main uses include:

- Extraoral projections, including:
  - Oblique lateral radiographs (Ch. 13)
  - All skull radiographs (Ch. 14)
  - Dental panoramic radiographs (Ch. 17)
  - All routine medical radiography.

Indirect–action film construction

This type of film is similar in construction to direct-action film described above. However, the following important points should be noted:

- The silver halide emulsion is designed to be sensitive primarily to light rather than X-rays.
- Different emulsions are manufactured which are sensitive to the different colours of light emitted by different types of intensifying screens (see later). These include:
  - *Standard silver halide emulsion* sensitive to BLUE light
  - *Modified silver halide emulsion with ultraviolet sensitizers* sensitive to ULTRAVIOLET light
  - *Orthochromatic emulsion* sensitive to GREEN light
  - *Panchromatic emulsion* sensitive to RED light.

The relative spectral sensitivity of these four different film emulsions is shown in Figure 6.4.

- It is essential that the correct combination of film and intensifying screens is used.
- There is no orientation *dot* embossed in the film so some form of additional identification is required, e.g. metal letters, **L** or **R** placed on the outside of the cassette or electronic marking.

Characteristics of radiographic film

This section summarizes the more important theoretical terms and definitions used to describe how radiographic film responds to exposure to X-rays.

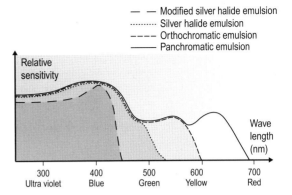

Fig. 6.4   Graph showing the relative spectral sensitivity of standard silver halide (BLUE), modified silver halide (ULTRAVIOLET), orthochromatic (GREEN) and panchromatic (RED) film emulsions.

Optical density (OD)

$$OD = \log \frac{\text{Incident light intensity}}{\text{Transmitted light intensity}}$$

Optical density is the term used for describing the degree of film blackening and can be measured directly using a densitometer. In diagnostic radiology the range of optical densities is usually 0.25–2.5. There are no units for optical density.

Characteristic curve

The characteristic curve is a graph showing the variation in optical density (degree of blackening) with different exposures. Typical characteristic curves for direct-action (non-screen) and indirect-action (screen) film are shown in Figure 6.5. This curve describes several of the film's properties.

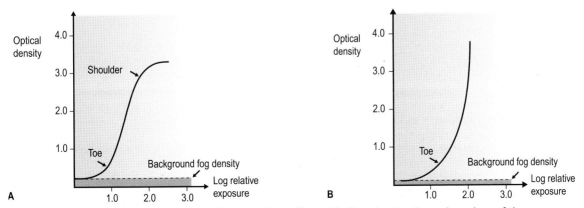

Fig. 6.5A   A typical characteristic curve of indirect-action radiographic film, showing the main regions of the curve including *background fog density, toe* and *shoulder.* B A typical characteristic curve for direct-action film.

Background fog density

This is the small degree of blackening evident even with zero exposure. This is due to:

- The colour/density of the plastic base
- The development of some unexposed silver halide crystals.

If the film has been stored correctly (see later), this background fog density should be less than 0.2 (see Fig. 6.5).

Film speed

This is the exposure required to produce an optical density of 1.0 above background fog (see Fig. 6.6). Thus, the faster the film, the less the exposure required for a given film blackening and the lower the radiation dose to the patient.

Film speed is a function of the number and size of the silver halide crystals in the emulsion. The larger the crystals, the faster the film but the poorer the image quality.

In clinical practice, the fastest films consistent with adequate diagnostic results, either D speed or more usually nowadays the faster E or F speed, should be used.

Film sensitivity

This is the reciprocal of the exposure required to produce an optical density of 1.0 above background fog. Thus, a fast film has a high sensitivity.

Film latitude

This is a measure of the range of exposures that produces distinguishable differences in optical density, i.e. the linear portion of the characteristic curve (see Fig. 6.7). The wider the film latitude the greater the range of object densities that may be seen.

Film contrast

This is the difference in optical density between two points on a film that have received different exposures (see Fig. 6.7).

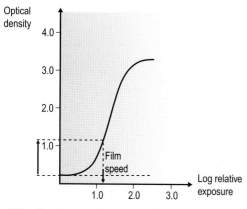

Fig. 6.6 The characteristic curve of an indirect-action (screen) film showing the *film speed* — the exposure required to produce an optical density of 1.0 above background fog.

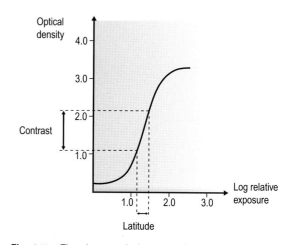

Fig. 6.7 The characteristic curve of an indirect-action film showing film *contrast* and *latitude*.

Film gamma and average gradient

Film gamma is the *maximum* gradient or slope of the linear portion of the characteristic curve. This term is often quoted but is of little value in radiology because the maximum slope (steepest) portion of the characteristic curve is usually very short.

Average gradient is a more useful measurement and is usually calculated between density 0.25 and 2.0 above background fog (see Fig. 6.8).

Thus the film *gamma* or *average gradient* measurement determines both *film latitude* and *film contrast* as follows:

- If the gamma or average gradient is **high** (i.e. a steep gradient), that film will show good contrast, but will have less latitude.
- If the film gamma or average gradient is **low** (i.e. a shallow gradient), that film will show poor contrast but will have wider latitude.

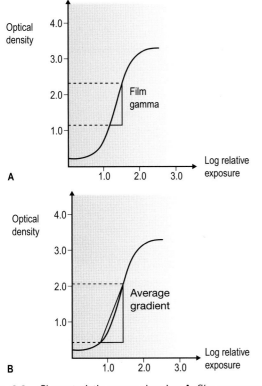

Fig. 6.8 Characteristic curves showing **A** *film gamma* and **B** *average gradient* of an indirect–action (screen) film.

Resolution

Resolution, or resolving power, is a measure of the radiograph's ability to differentiate between different structures that are close together. Factors that can affect resolution include penumbra effect (image sharpness), silver halide crystal size and contrast. It is measured in line pairs (lp) per mm. Direct-action film has a resolution of approximately 10 lp per mm and indirect-action film a resolution of about 5 lp per mm.

Intensifying screens

Intensifying screens consist of *fluorescent phosphors*, which emit light when excited by X-rays, embedded in a plastic matrix. The basic construction and components of an intensifying screen are shown in Figure 6.9.

Action

Two intensifying screens are used — one in front of the film and the other at the back. The front screen absorbs the low-energy X-ray photons and the back screen absorbs the high-energy photons. The two screens are therefore efficient at stopping the transmitted X-ray beam, which they convert into visible light by the *photoelectric effect* (described in Ch. 2). One X-ray photon will produce many light photons which will affect a relatively large area of film emulsion. Thus, the amount of radiation needed to expose the film is reduced but at the cost of fine detail; *resolution* is decreased. The ultraviolet system was developed to improve *resolution* by reducing light diffusion and having virtually no light crossover through the plastic film base (see Fig. 6.10).

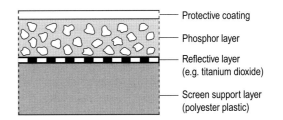

Fig. 6.9 Diagram showing the cross-sectional structure of a typical intensifying screen.

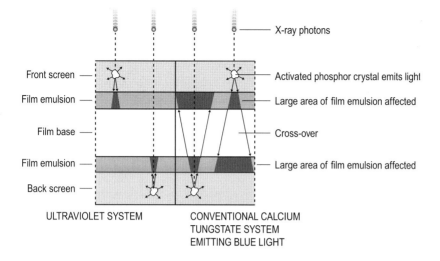

X-ray photons

Front screen — Activated phosphor crystal emits light

Film emulsion — Large area of film emulsion affected

Film base — Cross-over

Film emulsion — Large area of film emulsion affected

Back screen —

ULTRAVIOLET SYSTEM

CONVENTIONAL CALCIUM TUNGSTATE SYSTEM EMITTING BLUE LIGHT

Fig. 6.10   Diagram showing the action of conventional calcium tungstate and ultraviolet systems. Note the small cone of ultraviolet light with no cross-over through the film base, compared to the large cone of blue light and marked cross-over from the calcium tungstate phosphors. These differences result in better resolution and image sharpness with ultraviolet systems.

Useful definitions

The following terms are used to describe intensifying screens:

- *Conversion efficiency* — the efficiency with which the phosphor converts X-rays into light
- *Absorption efficiency* — the ability of the phosphor material to absorb X-rays
- *Screen efficiency* — the ability of the light emitted by the phosphor to escape from the screen and expose the film
- *Intensification factor* (IF)

$$IF = \frac{\text{Exposure required when screens are not used}}{\text{Exposure required with screens}}$$

- *Screen speed* — the time taken for the screen to emit light following exposure to X-rays. The faster the screen, the lower the radiation dose to the patient
- *Packing density* — the ability of the phosphor to pack closely together resulting in thin screens and less light divergence.

Fluorescent materials

Three main phosphor materials are, or have been, used in intensifying screens:

- Rare earth phosphors including gadolinium and lanthanum
- Yttrium (a non-rare earth phosphor but having similar properties)
- Calcium tungstate ($CaWO_4$).

Rare earth and related screens

Modern screens employ these phosphors which produce very fast screen speeds, enabling a substantial reduction in radiation dose to patients, without excessive loss of image detail. The main points can be summarized as follows:

1   The rare earth group of elements includes:
   - lanthanum (Z = 57)
   - gadolinium (Z = 64)
   - terbium (Z = 65)
   - thulium (Z = 69).
- The term *rare earth* is used because it is difficult and expensive to separate these elements from earth and from each other, not because the elements are scarce.
- These phosphors only fluoresce properly when they contain impurities of other phosphors, e.g. gadolinium plus 0.3% terbium. Typical screens include:
   - Terbium-activated gadolinium oxysulphide ($Gd_2O_1S:Tb$)
   - Thulium-activated lanthanum oxybromide (LaOBr:Tm).
- Terbium-activated screens emit GREEN light, while thulium-activated screens emit BLUE light (see Fig. 6.11).
- Yttrium (Z = 39), the rare earth related phosphor, in the form of pure yttrium tantalate ($YtaO_4$) emits ULTRAVIOLET light (see Fig. 6.11).
- Rare earth and related screens are approximately five times faster than calcium tungstate screens.

The amount of radiation required to produce an image is therefore considerably reduced, but they are relatively expensive.

- Several different screens of each phosphor, each producing a different *image system speed*, are available:

Screen type	Image system speed
Detail or Fine	100
Fast detail or Medium	200
Rapid or Fast	400
Super rapid	800

- It is important to use the appropriate films with their correctly matched screens.

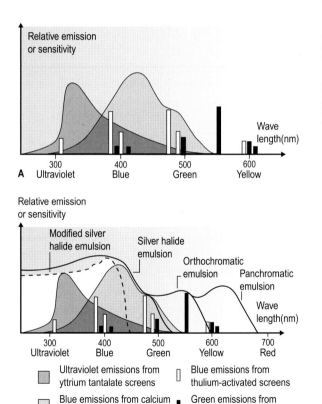

Calcium tungstate screens

The original material used but now no longer recommended. The main points can be summarized as follows:

- The speed of these screens depends upon:
  - The thickness of the phosphor layer
  - The size of the phosphor crystals
  - The presence or absence of light-absorbing dyes within the screen
  - The *conversion efficiency* of the crystals
- The faster the screen, the lower the radiation dose to the patient **but** the less the detail of the final image
- **All** calcium tungstate screens emit BLUE light and must be used with blue-light sensitive monochromatic radiographic film (see Fig. 6.11).
- Slower than rare earth screens.

Cassettes

Types

Cassettes are made in a variety of shapes and sizes for different projections. A selection is shown in Figure 6.12.

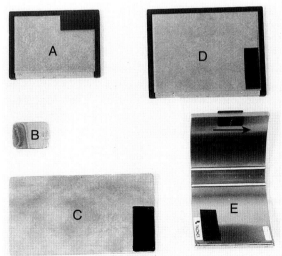

Fig. 6.11A Graph showing the relative spectral emissions of different types of intensifying screens. **B** Graph showing the spectral sensitivity of different types of film combined with the relative spectral emissions of different types of intensifying screens.

Fig. 6.12 Various cassettes for different radiographic projections. **A** Oblique lateral cassette. **B** Intraoral occlusal cassette. **C** Flat panoramic cassette. **D** Skull cassette. **E** Curved panoramic cassette.

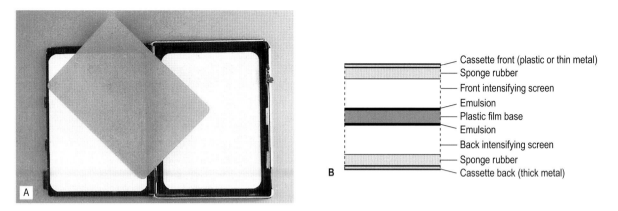

Fig. 6.13A   A standard 18 × 13 cm cassette opened up showing the white intensifying screens and the film. **B** Diagram showing the cross-sectional components in a cassette.

Construction

Despite their different shapes, the construction of the cassettes is very similar. They consist usually of a light-tight aluminium or carbon fibre container with the radiographic film sandwiched tightly between two intensifying screens (see Fig. 6.13). Any loss in film/screen contact will result in degradation of the final image.

Important practical points to note

Film storage

All radiographic film deteriorates with time and manufacturers state expiry dates on film boxes as a guide. However, this does not mean that the film automatically becomes unusable after this date. Storage conditions can have a dramatic effect on the deterioration rate. Ideally films should be stored:

- In a refrigerator in cool, dry conditions
- Away from all sources of ionizing radiation
- Away from chemical fumes including mercury and mercury-containing compounds
- With boxes placed on their edges, to prevent pressure artefacts.

Screen maintenance

Intensifying screens should last for many years if looked after correctly. Maintenance should include:

- Regular cleaning with a proprietary cleaning agent
- Careful handling to avoid scratching or damaging the surface
- Regular checks for loss of film/screen contact.

These aspects are discussed further in Chapter 18.

DIGITAL RECEPTORS

There are two types of direct digital image receptors available, namely:

- Solid-state (CCD or CMOS)
- Photostimulable phosphor storage plates.

Uses

Both types of sensors can be used for intraoral (periapical and bitewing radiograph) and extraoral radiography including panoramic and skull radiography. Only phosphor storage plates are available for occlusal and oblique lateral radiography as it is currently too expensive to manufacture sufficiently large solid-state sensors.

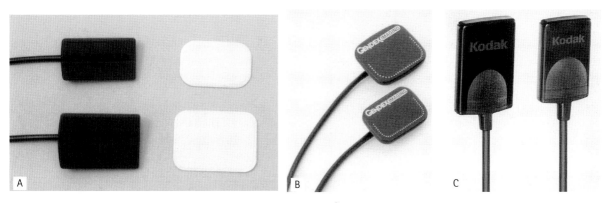

Fig. 6.14 Examples of modern solid-state sensors. **A** Planmeca dixi^2 ® and conventional film packets to show their comparative size. **B** Gendex Visualix® (kindly provided by Mr R. France). **C** Kodak RVG 6000.

Solid-state sensors

Intraoral sensors

The intraoral sensors are small, thin, flat, rigid rectangular boxes usually black in colour and similar in size to intraoral film packets as shown in Figure 6.14. They vary in thickness from about 5–7 mm. Most sensors are cabled to allow data to be transferred directly from the mouth to the computer. Several systems are now available, examples include Gendex Visualix®, Planmeca dixi^2® and Kodak RVG 6000 (see Fig. 6.14).

For ease of clinical use the sensor cables are usually 1–2 m long and plug into a remote *docking station* which can be conveniently attached to the tubehead supporting arm (see Fig. 6.15). A separate cable then connects the *docking station* to the computer.

A cable-free system is also available. The Schick CDR Wireless™ sensor transmits radiowaves from the mouth to a remote *base station* which is connected by a cable to the computer. This removes the inconvenience the cable can create clinically, but additional electronics make the sensor slightly more bulky.

The solid-state sensors are NOT autoclavable. When used clinically they all need to be covered with a protective plastic barrier envelope for infection control purposes (see Ch. 9).

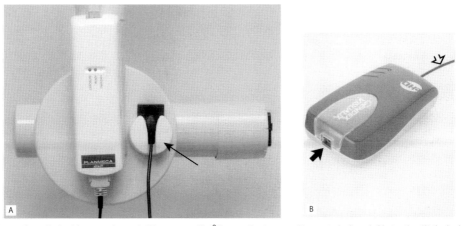

Fig. 6.15 Examples of *docking stations.* **A** Planmeca dixi^2® attached to an X-ray tubehead. Note the little holder for conveniently supporting the sensor (arrowed). **B** Gendex Visualix®. The sensor plugs into the arrowed port. The open arrowed cable connects to the computer (kindly provided by Mr R. France).

Construction and design

The sensors consist of tiny silicon chip-based pixels and their associated electronics encased in a plastic housing. Underlying technology involves either:

- CCD (charge-coupled devices)
- CMOS (complimentary metal oxide semiconductors).

CCD (charge-coupled device)

Individual pixels, consisting of a sandwich of P and N-type silicon, are arranged in rows and columns called an *array* or matrix, above which is a scintillation layer made of similar materials to the rare-earth intensifying screens. The basic design is shown in Figure 6.16. The X-ray photons that hit the scintillation layer are converted to light. The light interacts via the photoelectric effect with the silicon to create a *charge packet* for each individual pixel, which is concentrated by the electrodes.

The charge pattern formed from the individual pixels in the matrix represents the latent image. The image is read by transferring each row of pixel charges from one row to the next. At the end of its row, each charge is transferred to a read-out amplifier and transmitted down the cable as an analogue voltage signal to the computer's analogue-to-digital converter, often located in the *docking station*. Each sensor consists of between 1.5 million and 2.5 million pixels and pixel sizes vary from 20 microns to 70 microns.

CMOS (complimentary metal oxide detectors)

These sensors are similar in construction to CCDs and consist of an array of pixels but they differ from CCDs in the way that the pixel charges are read. Each CMOS pixel is isolated from its neighbour and directly connected to a transistor. The charge packet from each pixel is transferred to the transistor as a voltage enabling each individual pixel to be assessed separately.

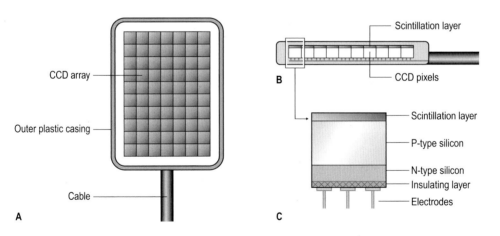

Fig. 6.16 Diagrams illustrating the basic construction of an intraoral CCD sensor. **A** The imaging surface showing the pixel array. **B** Sensor from the side showing the scintillation layer. **C** An individual pixel consisting of a sandwich of N- and P-type silicon.

Extraoral sensors

Extraoral sensors contain CCDs in long, thin linear arrays. They are a few pixels wide and many pixels long. The CCD array is incorporated into two different designs of sensor:

- Flat cassette-sized sensors designed to be retro-fitted into existing film-based panoramic equipment to replace conventional cassettes. For example, most film-based panoramic units can be converted to digital by simply installing a flat digital sensor such as the original Trophy Digipan sensor (see Fig. 6.17) or Schick CDRPan™.

- Individually designed sensors as part of completely new solely digital panoramic or skull equipment such as the Schick CDRPanX or the Planmeca dimax$^{3®}$ (see Fig. 6.18).

Although the outward appearances of these sensors is very different, both designs work in a similar fashion. The long narrow pixel array is aligned with a narrow slit-shaped X-ray beam and the equipment scans across the patient. This scanning motion takes several seconds to scan the skull and is discussed in more detail in Chapter 15.

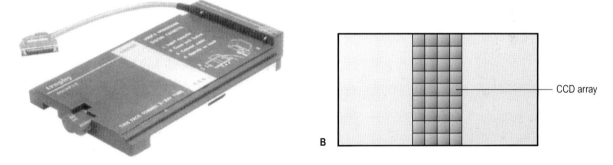

Fig. 6.17A   The original Trophy Digipan® CCD sensor for retro-fitting to panoramic equipment. **B** Diagram showing the basic with a long thin array of CCDs.

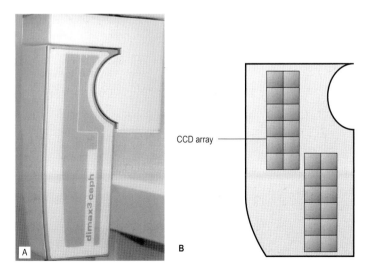

Fig. 6.18A   Specifically designed Planmeca dimax$^{3®}$ sensor for cephalometric radiography (see Ch. 15). **B** Diagram showing the basic design with two long thin arrays of CCDs.

Photostimulable phosphor storage plates

These digital sensors consist of a range of imaging plates that can be used for both intraoral and extraoral radiography. The plates are not connected to the computer by a cable. Several systems are available and include the DentOptix™ (Gendex) and the Vistascan™ (Durr) and Digora® Optime (intraoral) and PCT (extraoral) (Soredex).

A range of intraoral and extraoral plate sizes are available with these systems, identical in size to conventional periapical, occlusal, oblique lateral, panoramic and skull films (see Fig. 6.19). Once cleared (erased), the plates are reusable. Intraoral plates need to be inserted into protective barrier envelopes for control of infection purposes (see Fig. 6.20A).

Plate construction and design

The plates typically consist of a layer of barium fluorohalide phosphor on a flexible plastic backing support, as shown in Figure 6.21.

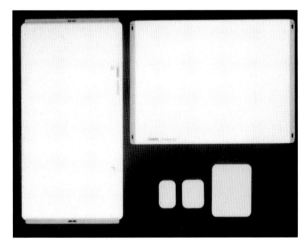

Fig. 6.19   The different sized DenOptix™ plates for panoramic, skull and intraoral radiography.

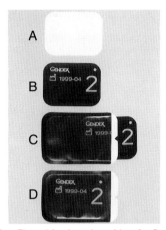

Fig. 6.20A   The white imaging side of a DenOptix™ phosphor plate. **B** The reverse side of the plate. **C** The plate being inserted into the protective barrier envelope — note the reverse side of the plate is visible through the clear side of the envelope. **D** The plate in the envelope ready for clinical use.

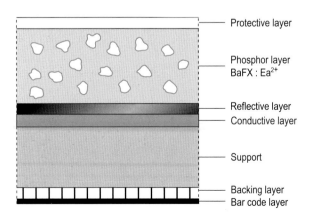

Protective layer

Phosphor layer
BaFX : Ea^{2+}

Reflective layer
Conductive layer

Support

Backing layer
Bar code layer

Fig. 6.21   Diagram showing the cross-sectional structure of a typical phosphor imaging plate.

As with using film, image production is not instantaneous with this type of image receptor. Two distinct stages are involved, namely:

- The phosphor layer absorbs and stores the X-ray energy that has not been attenuated by the patient.

- The image plate is then placed in a *reader* where it is scanned by a laser beam. The stored X-ray energy in the phosphor layer is released as light which is detected by a photo-multiplier tube and converted into a voltage which is relayed to the computer and displayed as a digital image. This is described in more detail in Chapter 7.

Chapter 7

Image processing

Processing is the general term used to describe the sequence of events required to convert the invisible *latent image*, contained in the sensitized film emulsion or in the solid-state or phosphor layer of the digital sensors, into the visible black and white radiographic film or digital image. This chapter summarizes the two methods involved, namely:

- Chemical processing
- Computer digital processing.

CHEMICAL PROCESSING

It is CRUCIAL that the stages involved in chemical processing are performed under controlled, standardized conditions with careful attention to detail. Strict quality assurance procedures must be applied (see Ch. 18). Unfortunately, all too often in dental practice poor chemical processing is the cause of radiographic films being of inadequate diagnostic quality, irrespective of how reliable and expensive the X-ray equipment or how accurate the operator's radiographic techniques.

Theory

A detailed knowledge of the chemistry involved in processing is not essential. However, a working knowledge and understanding of the theory of processing is necessary so that processing faults can be identified and corrected. A simplified approach to the stages involved in converting the green film emulsion into the black/white/grey radiograph is shown in Figure 7.1 and outlined below:

Stage 1: Development

The **sensitized** silver halide crystals in the emulsion are converted to black metallic silver to produce the *black/grey* parts of the image.

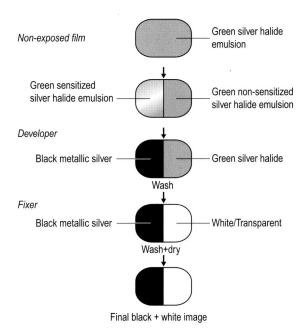

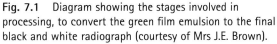

Fig. 7.1 Diagram showing the stages involved in processing, to convert the green film emulsion to the final black and white radiograph (courtesy of Mrs J.E. Brown).

Stage 2: Washing

The film is washed in water to remove residual developer solution.

Stage 3: Fixation

The **unsensitized** silver halide crystals in the emulsion are removed to reveal the *transparent* or *white* parts of the image and the emulsion is hardened.

Stage 4: Washing

The film is washed thoroughly in running water to remove residual fixer solution.

Stage 5: Drying

The resultant *black/white/grey* radiograph is dried.

Practical methods

There are three practical chemical processing methods available:

- Manual or wet processing
- Automatic processing
- Using self-developing films.

Manual processing

Manual processing is usually carried out in a *darkroom*, the general requirements of which should include:

- Absolute light-tightness
- Adequate working space
- Adequate ventilation
- Adequate washing facilities
- Adequate film storage facilities
- Safelights — positioned 1.2 m from the work surfaces with 25 W bulbs and filters suitable for the type of film being used (see Ch. 18)
- Processing equipment (see Fig. 7.2):
  - Tanks containing the various solutions
  - Thermometer
  - Immersion heater
  - An accurate timer
  - Film hangers.

Manual processing cycle

1. The exposed film packet is unwrapped and the film clipped on to a hanger.
2. The film is immersed in DEVELOPER and agitated several times in the solution to remove air bubbles and left for about five minutes at 20°C.

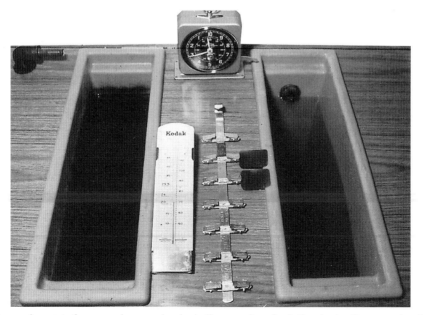

Fig. 7.2   The basic requirements for manual processing including a series of solution tanks, thermometer, timer and film.

3. The residual developer is rinsed off in water for about 10 seconds.
4. The film is immersed in FIXER for about 8–10 minutes.
5. The film is washed in running water for about 10–20 minutes to remove any residual fixer.
6. The film is allowed to dry in a dust-free atmosphere.

Processing solutions

Two different processing solutions are required, the *developer* and the *fixer*. The typical constituents of these solutions are shown in Tables 7.1 and 7.2.

Important points to note regarding development

● The alkaline developer solution should be made up to the concentration recommended in the manufacturer's instructions.

Table 7.1 The typical constituents of developer solution and their functions

Constituents	Functions
Phenidone	Helps bring out the image
Hydroquinone	Builds contrast
Sodium sulphite	Preservative – reduces oxidation
Potassium carbonate	Activator – governs the activity of the developing agents
Benzotriazole	Restrainer – prevents fog and controls the activity of the developing agents
Glutaraldehyde	Hardens the emulsion
Fungicide	Prevents bacterial growth
Buffer	Maintains pH (7+)
Water	Solvent

Table 7.2 The typical constituents of fixer solution and their functions

Constituents	Functions
Ammonium thiosulphate	Removes unsensitized silver halide crystals
Sodium sulphite	Preservative – prevents deterioration of the fixing agent
Aluminium chloride	Hardener
Acetic acid	Acidifier – maintains pH
Water	Solvent

● The developer solution is oxidized by air and its effectiveness decreased. Solutions should be used for no more than 10–14 days, irrespective of the number of films processed during that time.
● If the development process is allowed to continue for too long, more silver will be deposited than was intended and the radiograph will be too dark. Conversely, if there is too short a development time the radiograph will be too light.
● Development TIME (in fresh solutions) is dependent on the TEMPERATURE of the solution. The usual value recommended is five minutes at 20°C.
● If the temperature is too high, development is rapid, the film may be too dark and the emulsion may be damaged. If the temperature is too low, development is slowed and a pale film will result.

Important points to note regarding fixing

● Fixer solution should be made up to the concentration recommended by the manufacturer. It is an acid solution so contamination with developer should be avoided.
● Ideally films should be fixed for double the *clearing time*. The clearing time is how long it takes to remove the unsensitized silver halide crystals. Total fixing time is usually 8–10 minutes.
● Films may be removed from the fixer after 2–4 minutes for *wet* viewing but should be returned to the fixer solution to complete fixing.
● Inadequately fixed films may appear greenish yellow or milky owing to residual emulsion. In time these films may discolour further, becoming brown.

Automatic processing

This term is used when processing is carried out automatically by a machine. There are several automatic processors available which are designed to carry the film through the complete cycle usually by a system of rollers. Most have a daylight loading facility, eliminating the need for a dark-room (see Fig. 7.3), but in the interests of infection control, salivary-contaminated film packets should be wiped with a disinfecting solution such as 1% hypochlorite, before being placed into the loading facility.

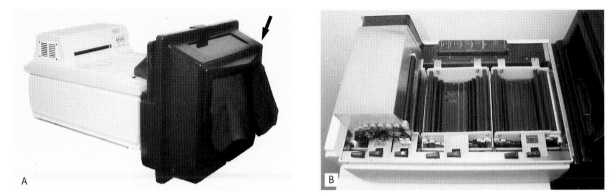

Fig. 7.3A The AP200 automatic processor fitted with its daylight loading apparatus (arrowed). **B** The internal tanks and roller system of the AP200 processor.

Automatic processing cycle

The cycle is the same as for manual processing except that the rollers squeeze off any excess developing solution before passing the film on to the fixer, eliminating the need for the water wash between these two solutions.

Advantages

The main advantages include:

- Time saving — dry films are produced in about five minutes
- The need for a darkroom is often eliminated
- Controlled, standardized processing conditions are easy to maintain
- Chemicals can be replenished automatically by some machines.

Disadvantages

The main disadvantages include:

- Strict maintenance and regular cleaning are essential; dirty rollers produce marked films
- Some models need to be plumbed in
- Equipment is relatively expensive
- Smaller machines cannot process large extraoral films.

Self–developing films

Self-developing films are an alternative to manual processing. The X-ray film is presented in a special sachet containing developer and fixer (see Fig. 7.4). Following exposure, the developer tab is pulled, releasing developer solution which is milked down towards the film and massaged around it. After about 15 seconds, the fixer tab is pulled to release the fixer solution which is similarly milked down to the film. After fixing, the used chemicals are discarded and the film is rinsed thoroughly under running water for about 10 minutes.

Advantages

The main advantages include:

- No darkroom or processing facilities are needed.
- Time saving — the final radiograph is ready in about a minute.

Disadvantages

The main disadvantages include:

- Poor overall image quality
- The image deteriorates rapidly with time
- There is no lead foil inside the film packet
- The film packet is very flexible and easily bent
- These films are difficult to use in positioning holders
- Relatively expensive.

A rigid, radiopaque plastic backing support tray for the film is manufactured, which helps to reduce the problems of flexibility and lack of lead foil.

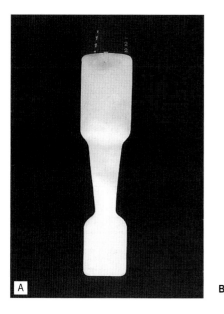

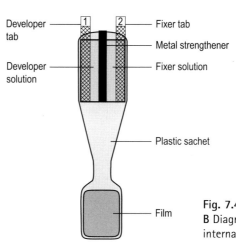

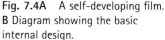

Developer tab

Developer solution

Fixer tab

Metal strengthener

Fixer solution

Plastic sachet

Film

A

B

Fig. 7.4A   A self-developing film. **B** Diagram showing the basic internal design.

COMPUTER DIGITAL PROCESSING

Digital image

The digital image is captured in pixels (tiny squares), by two different types of sensor — solid-state or photostimulable phosphor plates described in Chapter 6. However captured, the digital image is similar to a film-captured image, in that both are 2-dimensional representations of a 3-dimensional object. In digital imaging, each 2-D pixel represents a 3-D cuboid or *voxel* of the patient. This is shown diagrammatically in Figure 7.5. The depth of the cuboid is dependent on the thickness of the part of the body being X-rayed. Each pixel measures the total X-ray absorption throughout the whole of each voxel. This 2-D limitation has been overcome with the development of *cone beam computed tomography* (CBCT), also called *digital volume tomography* (see Ch. 19).

Computer input

Solid-state sensors

As explained in Chapter 6, solid-state sensors input the information from each pixel directly (usually down the cable) to the computer's analogue-to-digital converter as an analogue voltage signal.

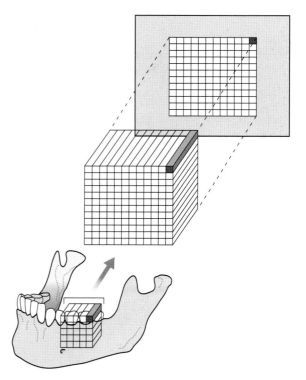

Fig. 7.5   Diagram illustrating how the 3-dimensional jaw is represented as a digital image made up of a grid or matrix of 2-dimensional pixels.

Phosphor plates

Phosphor plates are **not** directly connected to the computer and therefore an intermediary stage is required when the plate is *read*. The time taken to read the plate depends on the particular system being used, and the size of the plate, but typically varies between 5–100 seconds. Several dental systems are available including Soredex's Digora® Optime (intraoral) and PCT (extraoral), Durr's Vistascan and the Gendex® DenOptix™ (see Fig. 7.6). Although different in design they all work on the same principle, namely:

- During the radiographic procedure the phosphor layer on the plate absorbs and stores the X-ray energy that has not been attenuated by the patient.
- The plate is then placed in the reader.
- The plate is scanned by a laser beam and the stored X-ray energy is released as light.
- The light is detected by a photomultiplier tube and converted into an electrical signal (voltage) and input to the connected computer's analogue-to-digital converter
- The plate is cleared (erased) ready for reuse.

Computer processing theory

Computers deals with numbers, hence the need for the *analogue* voltage from each pixel to be changed by the analogue-to-digital converter into a discrete *numerical* digital signal. Each pixel has an x and y coordinate and is allocated a number. Typically using the grey-scale there are 256 numbers to select. These range from 0, when the voltage received is at its maximum (no X-ray attenuation in the patient), to 255 when there is no voltage (total X-ray attenuation in the patient). The computer finally allocates an appropriate colour from the grey scale (256 shades of grey from black through to white) to each pixel (0 = black, 255 = white) to create the visual image on the monitor. This concept is illustrated simply in Figure 7.7 using just eight numbers and eight shades of grey.

The number and size of the pixels, together with the number of shades of grey available, determine the amount of information in an image, the size of the image file and the resolution of the final image (see Fig. 7.8). Pixel sizes vary from 20 microns to 70 microns producing resolution between 7–25 line pairs/mm.

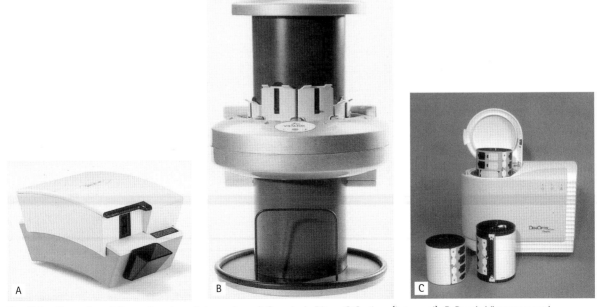

Fig. 7.6 Examples of three phosphor plate readers. **A** Soredex's Digora® Optime (intraoral), **B** Durr's Vistascan and **C** Gendex® DenOptix™.

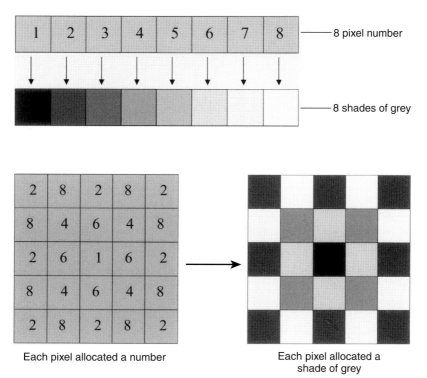

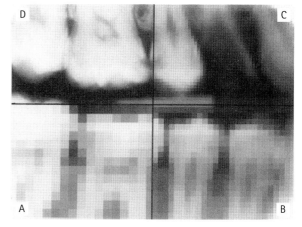

Fig. 7.7 Illustration of simple digital image creation using eight pixel numbers corresponding to eight shades of grey. Each pixel is allocated a number (dependent of the size of the input voltage) and then allocated a shade of grey to create the visual image (kindly provided by Mr N. Drage).

Image manipulation

Digital images can be changed by giving the pixels different numbers so altering the shades of grey. Different colours can be used. The coordinates of pixels may be changed or swapped, allowing different parts of the image to be moved around. These variables are the basis for image manipulation and enhancement. Software packages allow several enhancement techniques, some of which are shown in Figure 7.9. These can include:

- Alteration in contrast
- Alteration in brightness
- Inversion (reversed)
- Embossing or pseudo 3-D
- Magnification
- Automated measurement
- Pseudocolourization.

The two most frequently used enhancement functions are altering *brightness* and *contrast*.

Fig. 7.8 A bitewing radiograph showing the effect on image quality and resolution of different sized pixels gradually reducing from **A** to **D**.

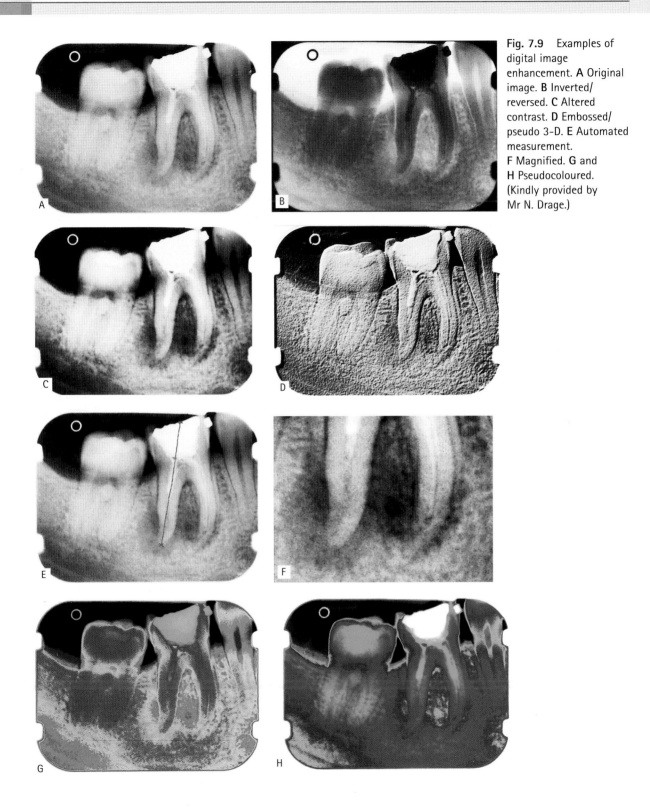

Fig. 7.9 Examples of digital image enhancement. **A** Original image. **B** Inverted/reversed. **C** Altered contrast. **D** Embossed/pseudo 3-D. **E** Automated measurement. **F** Magnified. **G** and **H** Pseudocoloured. (Kindly provided by Mr N. Drage.)

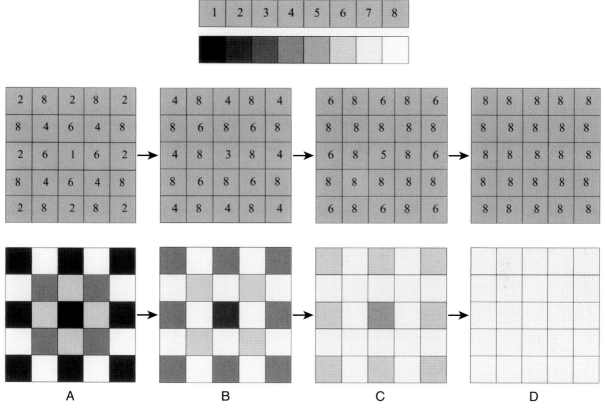

Fig. 7.10   Illustration showing the effect of increasing **brightness**. **A** The original numbers allocated to the pixels and the original black/white and grey image. **B** Pixel values increased by 2 and the resultant grey/white image. **C** Pixel values increased by 4 and the resultant brighter image. **D** Pixel values increased by 7 (i.e. to extreme end of the brightness scale) and the resultant totally white image. (Created from images kindly provided by Mr N. Drage.)

Brightness

Brightness can be regarded as equivalent to the *degree of blackening* of a film-captured image. Increasing brightness decreases the degree of blackening and makes the image lighter. This is done by increasing the numerical value of each pixel in the image and allocating it a lighter shade of grey. Taken to the extreme, every pixel would be allocated the highest number and the image will be totally white. The concept of altering brightness is illustrated in Figure 7.10, using the same simple model of eight numbers and eight shades of grey. Conversely, decreasing brightness increases the degree of blackening and makes the image darker.

Contrast

Contrast is the visual difference between black and white. Increasing contrast increases this difference. This is done by decreasing the pixel numbers in the darker half of the grey-scale and increasing the pixel numbers in the lighter half. Taken to the extreme, every pixel would be allocated either the lowest number available or the highest and the image would be black and white only containing no shades of grey. The concept of altering contrast is illustrated in Figure 7.11 using the same simple model of eight shades of grey. Conversely, decreasing contrast results in a grey image with little visual difference between the pixels.

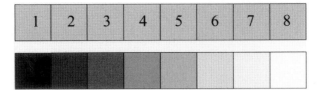

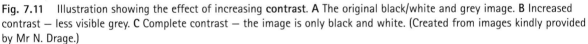

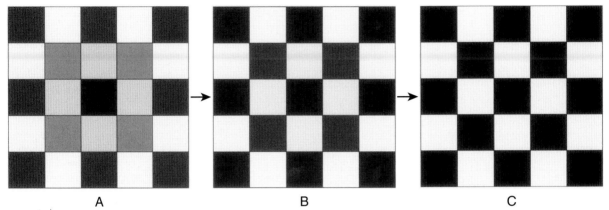

Fig. 7.11 Illustration showing the effect of increasing **contrast**. **A** The original black/white and grey image. **B** Increased contrast — less visible grey. **C** Complete contrast — the image is only black and white. (Created from images kindly provided by Mr N. Drage.)

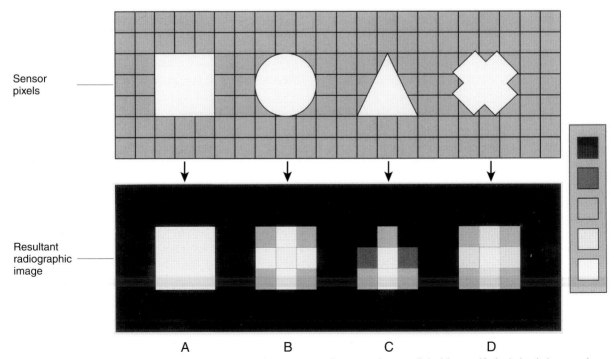

Fig. 7.12 Illustration showing how objects may not be represented accurately on a digital image if pixel size is large, using five shades of grey. **A** The square covers *exactly* and fills the sensor pixels and is therefore represented exactly radiographically. The outlines of **B** the circle, **C** the triangle and **D** the cross do not exactly cover and fill whole sensor pixels. The number and hence shade of grey allocated to an individual radiographic pixel represents the average of the total X-ray absorption within the whole pixel. Hence, the outlines and shapes of the objects are not represented accurately. (Created from images kindly provided by Mr N. Drage.)

Note: Despite being able to alter the final image, the computer cannot provide any additional information to that contained in the original image. It should be remembered that although manipulation and enhancement may make images look aesthetically more pleasing, they also may cause clinical information to be lost and diagnosis compromised.

Hard copy printed images

Hard printed copies of digital images can be obtained on glossy photographic paper by using thermal, laser or ink-jet printers. However, image quality is considerably compromised because of the printers inability to reproduce 256 shade of grey. It is possible to produce excellent quality hard copy images using expensive heat sublimation printers. These print the digital image back onto film and can reproduce all the shades of grey. The quality is comparable to film-captured images.

Advantages

- No need for chemical processing, thus avoiding all conventional processing faults (see Ch. 18) and the hazards associated with handling chemical solutions.
- Easy storage and archiving of patient information and incorporation into patient records.
- Easy transfer of images electronically.
- Image enhancement and manipulation.
- Phosphor plates have a wide latitude producing an acceptable image whether under-exposed or over-exposed.

Disadvantages

- Large pixels result in poor resolution and structures may not be represented accurately as shown in Figures 7.12 and 7.13.
- Conventional PC screens/monitors reduce or limit image quality. Diagnostic image quality screens/monitors are required for optimal viewing.
- Long-term storage of images, although this should be solved by saving them on CD or DVD.
- Digital image security and the need to back up data.

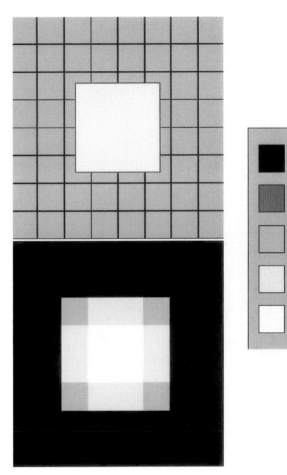

Fig. 7.13 Another illustration showing how an object may not be represented accurately on a digital image if pixel size is large, using five shades of grey. The square from Figure 7.12 is positioned so that it does **not** cover *exactly* and fill the sensor pixels. As a result it is now not accurately represented (kindly provided by Mr N. Drage.)

- Over-exposure and overloading of CCD sensors creating the phenomenon of blooming (see Fig. 7.14).
- Loss of image quality and resolution on hard copy print-outs when using thermal, laser or ink-jet printers.
- Image enhancement and manipulation:
  - operators need to understand how the image is created and being altered to avoid being misled
  - time-consuming
  - magnification is achieved by enlarging the pixels, but resolution is lost.

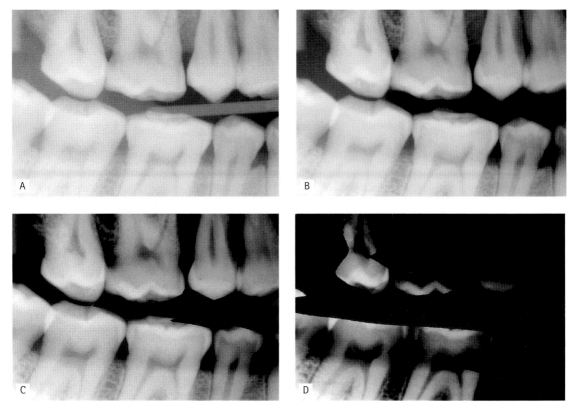

Fig. 7.14 The effect of *blooming*. Four bitewing images taken using a CCD solid-state sensor. **A** Under exposed. **B** Ideally exposed. **C** Over exposed. **D** Considerably overexposed. Some of the CCDs become over-loaded and parts of the image become black. (Kindly provided by Mr J. Davies.)

- While manufacturers provide safeguards to prevent any tampering with original images within their own software, it is relatively easy to access these images using inexpensive third party software and then to change them, as shown in Figure 7.15.

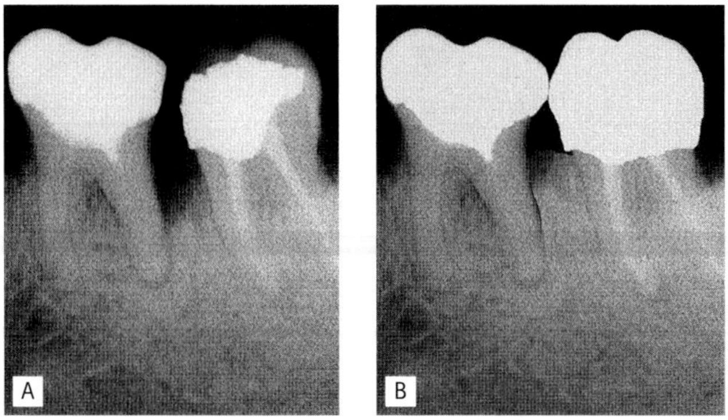

Fig. 7.15 An example of image alteration using third-party software. **A** Original image — note the bony defect between the ⌐6 and ⌐7, the lack of contact point and the restoration in ⌐7. **B** After digital manipulation and no clinical treatment. (Kindly provided by Mr N. Drage.)

PART 3

Radiation protection

PART CONTENTS

8. Radiation protection and legislation   69

Chapter 8

Radiation protection and legislation

Ionizing radiation is the subject of considerable safety legislation designed to minimize the risks to radiation workers and to patients. The International Commission on Radiological Protection (ICRP) regularly publishes data and general recommendations based on the following general principles:

- No practice shall be adopted unless its introduction produces a positive net benefit (*Justification*)
- All exposures shall be kept **as low as reasonably practicable** (ALARP), taking economic and social factors into account (*Optimization*)
- The dose equivalent to individuals shall not exceed the limits recommended by the ICRP (*Limitation*).

Their recommendations are usually incorporated eventually into national legislation and guidelines, although the precise details may vary from one country to another. By way of illustration, this chapter summarizes the current recommendations, guidelines and legislative requirements in force in the UK, together with the practical radiation protection measures that apply to patients and dental staff.

CURRENT UK LEGISLATION AND GUIDELINES

Legislation

There are two sets of regulations in the UK governing the use of ionizing radiation. They both form part of The Health and Safety at Work Act 1974 and comply with the provisions of the European Council Directives 96/29/Euratom and 97/43/Euratom:

- *The Ionising Radiations Regulations 1999 (SI 1999 No. 3232)* (IRR 99) which replace the Ionising Radiations Regulations 1985 (SI 1985 No. 1333).
- *The Ionising Radiation (Medical Exposure) Regulations 2000 (SI 2000 No. 1059)* (IR(ME) R 2000) which replace the Ionising Radiation (Protection of Persons Undergoing Medical Examination or Treatment) Regulations 1988 (SI 1988 No. 778).

Guidelines

There are three sets of guidelines, namely:

- *Guidelines on Radiological Standards in Primary Dental Care* published in 1994 by the National Radiological Protection Board (NRPB) and the Royal College of Radiologists. These guidelines and their recommendations cover all aspects of dental radiology and set out the principles of good practice.
- *Selection Criteria for Dental Radiography* 2nd edn. published in 2004 by the Faculty of General Dental Practice (UK) of the Royal College of Surgeons of England. This booklet reviews the evidence for, and provides guidance on, which radiographs are appropriate for different clinical conditions and how frequently they should be taken. The overview of their

recommendations is reproduced later in this chapter.

- *Guidance Notes for Dental Practitioners on the Safe Use of X-ray Equipment* published by the Department of Health in 2001 which brings together the requirements of IRR99 and IR(ME)R 2000 as they relate to dentists and includes the principles of good practice established in the 1994 Guidelines. The main points and various extracts from these 2001 *Guidance Notes* are reproduced below with kind permission from the Radiation Protection Division of the Health Protection Agency (formerly the National Radiological Protection Board (NRPB)).

NOTE: These points are **not** intended to cover all aspects of the guidance notes and legislation. The various publications mentioned above, particularly the 2001 *Guidance Notes* and the 2004 *Selection Criteria*, should be regarded as essential reading for all members of the dental profession, whether in general practice, dental hospitals or community clinics.

SUMMARY OF THE LEGISLATION AND EXTRACTS FROM THE 2001 GUIDANCE NOTES FOR DENTAL PRACTITIONERS ON THE SAFE USE OF X-RAY EQUIPMENT

Ionising Radiations Regulations 1999 (IRR99)

General points

- These regulations are concerned principally with the safety of workers and the general public but also address the equipment aspects of patient protection.
- They came into force on 1st January 2000.
- They replace the Ionising Radiations Regulations 1985.

Essential legal requirements

- *Authorization.* Use of dental X-ray equipment for research purposes should be in accordance with a generic authorization granted by the Health and Safety Executive (HSE).
- *Notification.* The HSE must be notified of the routine use of dental X-ray equipment and of any material changes to a notification including a change in ownership of the practice or a move to new premises.
- *Prior risk assessment.* This must be undertaken before work commences and be subject to regular review. All employers are recommended to record the findings of their risk assessment, but it is a requirement for employers with five or more employees. A five-step approach is recommended by the HSE:
  1. Identify the hazards (i.e. routine and accidental exposure to X-rays).
  2. Decide who might be harmed and how they might be affected.
  3. Evaluate the risks and decide whether existing precautions are adequate or whether more precautions need to be taken. Implement additional precautions, if needed.
  4. Record the findings of the risk assessment.
  5. Review the risk assessment and revise it, if necessary.
- *Restriction of exposure.* There is an over-riding requirement to restrict radiation doses to staff and other persons to as low as reasonably practicable (ALARP) (see later).
- *Maintenance and examination of engineering controls.* Applies particularly to safety and warning features of dental X-ray equipment.
- *Contingency plans.* These should arise out of the risk assessment and be provided within the *Local Rules* (see later).
- *Radiation Protection Adviser (RPA).* A suitably trained RPA must be appointed in writing and consulted to give advice on IRR99. The RPA should be an expert in radiation protection and will be able to advise on compliance with the Regulations and all aspects of radiation protection, including advice on:
  - controlled and designated areas for all radiation equipment
  - installation of new or modified X-ray equipment
  - periodic examination and testing of engineering controls, safety features and warning signals
  - systems of work
  - risk assessment
  - contingency plans
  - staff training

- assessment and recording of doses received by patients
- quality assurance (QA) programmes.
- *Information, instruction and training.* Must be provided, as appropriate, for all persons associated with dental radiology.
- *Designated areas.* During an exposure, a *controlled area* will normally be designated around the X-ray set as an aid to the effective control of exposures. The controlled area may be defined as within the primary X-ray beam until it has been sufficiently attenuated by distance or shielding and within 1.5 m of the X-ray tube and the patient, as shown in Figure 8.1. Normally, only the patient is allowed in this area. This can be facilitated by the use of appropriate signs, as shown in Figure 8.2.
- *Radiation Protection Supervisor (RPS).* An RPS—usually a dentist or senior member of staff in the practice—should be appointed to ensure compliance with IRR99 and the *Local Rules*. The RPS must be *adequately trained*, should be closely involved with the radiography and have the authority to adequately implement their responsibilities.
- *Local Rules.* All practices should have a written set of Local Rules relating to radiation protection measures within that practice and applying to all employees. Information should include:

- the name of the RPS
- identification and description of the *controlled area*
- summary of working instructions including the names of staff qualified to use the X-ray equipment and details of their training as well as instructions on the use of equipment
- contingency arrangements in the event of equipment malfunction and/or accidental exposure to radiation
- name of the person with legal responsibility of compliance with the regulations
- details and results of dose-investigation levels (**Note:** A dose constraint of no higher than 1mSv per year is recommended as generally appropriate for practice staff from dental radiography—see later section on dose limits)
- name and contact details of the RPA
- arrangements for personal dosimetry
- arrangements for pregnant staff
- reminder to employees of their legal responsibilities under IRR99.
- *Classified persons.* Division of staff into *classified* and *non-classified* workers and the dose limits that apply to each group are discussed later. In dental practice, most staff are non-classified unless their radiography workload is very high.
- *Duties of manufacturers.* The installer is responsible for the *critical examination and report*

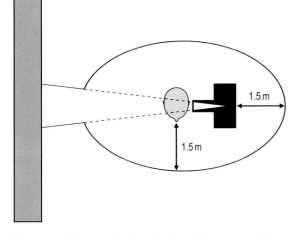

Fig. 8.1 Diagram showing the size of the *controlled area*, 1.5 m in any direction from the patient and tubehead and anywhere in the line of the main beam until it is attenuated by a solid wall.

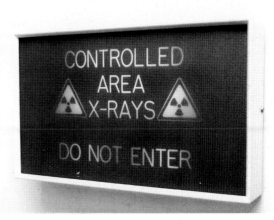

Fig. 8.2 An example of a *controlled area* warning sign. The words DO NOT ENTER are illuminated when the exposure button is pressed.

of all new or significantly modified X-ray equipment, which should include:

- a clear and unambiguous description of the equipment and its location
- an evaluation of the acceptability of the location in relation to the operator's position and the room's warning signs and signals, if applicable
- an evaluation of the acceptability of the equipment's warning signals
- an evaluation of the acceptability of the exposure control
- confirmation that the equipment's safety features are in place and operating correctly (e.g. beam dimensions and alignment, beam filtration and timer operation)
- an overall conclusion as to whether or not the equipment's safety features are operating correctly, the installation is providing sufficient protection for persons from exposure to X-rays and whether the user has been provided with 'adequate information about proper use, testing and maintenance of equipment'.

- *X-ray equipment.* All equipment must be critically examined and acceptance tested before being put into clinical use and then routinely tested as part of a QA programme (see Ch. 18). The *acceptance test*, in addition to the features covered in the *critical examination* outlined above, should include:
  - measurements to determine whether the equipment is operating within agreed performance parameters (e.g. operating potential (kV), X-ray output (mA) and timer accuracy (s))
  - an assessment of the typical patient dose for comparison with national Diagnostic Reference Levels (DRLs)
  - a review and record of film, film/screen combinations and processing details and an evaluation of the adequacy of processing.

A permanent record should be made of the results and conclusions of all tests and this should be retained as part of the QA programme and all deficiencies should be rectified.

All equipment (X-ray generating and image receptors) should comply with the general requirements in the regulations namely:

Intraoral radiography
- Tube voltage should not be lower than 50 kV. New equipment should operate within the range 60–70 kV.
- All equipment should operate within 10% of the stated or selected kV setting.
- Beam diameter should not exceed 60 mm at the patient end of the spacer cone or beam-indicating device.
- Rectangular collimation (see Ch. 5) should be provided on new equipment and fitted to existing equipment at the earliest opportunity and the beam size should not exceed 40 by 50 mm.
- Total beam filtration (inherent and added) should be 1.5 mm of aluminium for sets operating below 70 kV and 2.5 mm of aluminium for sets operating above 70 kV and should be marked on the tube housing.
- The focal spot position should be marked on the outer casing of the tubehead.
- Focal spot to skin distance (fsd) should be at least 100 mm for sets operating below 60 kV and 200 mm for sets operating above 60 kV (see Ch. 5).
- Film speed controls and finely adjustable exposure time settings should be provided.
- The fastest film available (E or F speed) that will produce satisfactory diagnostic images should be used.

Panoramic radiography (see Ch. 17)
- Equipment should have a range of tube potential settings, preferably from 60 to 90 kV.
- The beam height at the receiving slit of cassette holder should not be greater than the film in use (normally 125 mm or 150 mm). The width of the beam should not be greater than 5 mm.
- Equipment should be provided with adequate patient-positioning aids incorporating light beam markers.
- New equipment should provide facilities for field-limitation techniques.

Cephalometric radiography (see Ch. 15)
- Equipment must be able to ensure the precise alignment of X-ray beam, cassette and patient.

- The beam should be collimated to include only the diagnostically relevant area (see Ch. 15).
- To facilitate the imaging of the soft tissues, an aluminium wedge filter should be provided at the X-ray tubehead, in preference to one at the cassette.

All equipment:
- Should have a light on the control panel to show that the mains supply is switched on.
- Should be fitted with a light that gives a clear and visible indication to the operator that an exposure is taking place and audible warnings should also provide the operator with the same information
- Exposure switches (timers) should only function while continuous pressure is maintained on the switch and terminate if pressure is released
- Exposure switches should be positioned so that the operator can remain outside the controlled area and at least 2 m from the X-ray tube and patient
- Exposure times should be terminated automatically.

- *Duties of employees*. Notwithstanding the many and varied responsibilities placed on the person legally responsible, the so-called *legal person*, IRR99 places over-riding responsibilities on employees which include:
  - to not knowingly expose themselves or any other person to X-rays to an extent greater than is reasonably necessary for the purposes of their work
  - to exercise reasonable care when working on any aspect of dental radiology
  - to immediately report to the *legal person* whenever they have reasonable cause to believe that an incident or accident has occurred with the X-ray equipment and that they or some other person have received an overexposure.

Ionising Radiation (Medical Exposure) Regulations 2000 (IR(ME)R 2000)

General points

- These regulations are concerned with the safety of patients.

- They came into force on 13th May 2000.
- They replace the Ionising Radiation (Protection of Persons Undergoing Medical Examination or Treatment) Regulations 1988.
- New positions of responsibility are defined, namely:
  - the employer
  - the referrer
  - the practitioner
  - the operator.

Essential legal requirements

- *Duties of employers*. The employer (*legal person*) is the person or body corporate with natural or legal responsibility for a radiological installation. He/she is responsible for providing the overall safety of the practice and for ensuring that staff and procedures conform with the regulations. In addition, the legal person must provide a framework of *written procedures* for medical exposures which should include information on:
  - procedures for correctly identifying patients before radiography
  - identification of referrers, practitioners and operators
  - authorization and justification of all clinical exposures to ensure that the justification process has taken place
  - justification of medicolegal exposures
  - identification of pregnant patients
  - compliance with and details of QA programmes
  - assessment of patient dose
  - use of diagnostic reference levels (DRLs) – defined as 'dose levels in medical radiodiagnostic practices for typical examinations for groups of standard-sized patients or standard phantoms for broadly defined types of equipment'. As such, they should not normally be exceeded without good reason. In 1999, the NRPB recommended DRLs of 4 mGy for an adult mandibular molar periapical radiograph and 65 mGy mm for an adult panoramic radiograph
  - carrying out and recording a clinical evaluation of the outcome of each exposure
  - ensuring that the probability and magnitude of accidental or unintended doses to patients are reduced as far as reasonably practicable

- provision for carrying out clinical audits
- guidelines for referral criteria for radiographic examinations
- written protocols (guideline exposure settings) for every type of standard projection for each item of equipment
- procedures to follow if a patient is suspected of having received an excessive exposure as a result of any occurrence other than an equipment malfunction.

It is recommended that these employers *written procedures* and the *Local Rules* (see earlier) are kept together as a *radiation protection file* and that all staff are made aware of the contents.

- *Duties of the Practitioner, Operator and Referrer.*

   The referrer: a registered doctor or dentist or other health professional entitled to refer a patient to a *practitioner* for a medical exposure. The *referrer* is responsible for supplying the *practitioner* with sufficient information to justify an appropriate exposure.

   The practitioner: a registered doctor or dentist or other health professional entitled to take responsibility for a medical exposure. The *practitioner* must be adequately trained to take decisions and the responsibility for the justification of every exposure.

   The operator: the person conducting any practical aspect of a medical exposure. Practical aspects include:
   * patient identification
   * positioning the film, patient or X-ray tubehead
   * setting the exposure parameters
   * pressing the exposure switch to initiate the exposure
   * processing films
   * clinical evaluation of radiographs
   * exposing test objects as part of the QA programme.

   The *operator* must be adequately trained for his/her role in the exposure (see later).

- *Justification of individual medical exposures.* Before an exposure can take place, it must be justified (i.e. assessed to ensure that it will lead to a change in the patient's management and prognosis) by an *IRMER practitioner* and authorized as the means of demonstrating that

it has been justified. Every exposure should be justified on the grounds of:
- the availability and/or findings of previous radiographs
- the specific objectives of the exposure in relation to the history and examination of the patient
- the total potential diagnostic benefit to the patient
- the radiation risk associated with the radiographic examination
- the efficacy, benefits and risks of alternative techniques having the same objective but involving no or less exposure to ionizing radiation.

Note: The 2004 *Selection Criteria in Dental Radiography* (see later) states that there can be no possible justification for routine radiography of 'new' patients prior to clinical examination. A history and clinical examination are the only acceptable means of determining that the most appropriate, or necessary, radiographic views are requested.

- *Optimization.* All doses must be kept as low as reasonably practicable (ALARP) consistent with the intended purpose. This includes the need to apply QA procedures to the optimization of patient dose (see Ch. 18).
- *Clinical audit.* Provisions must be made for clinical audit. Suitable topics could include the various aspects of the QA programme (see Ch. 18), the appropriateness of radiographic requests and the clinical evaluation of radiographs.
- *Expert advice.* The regulations lay down the need for, and involvement of a Medical Physics Expert (MPE) who would give advice on such matters as the measurement and optimization of patient dose. However, the need for medical physics support in dental practice is fairly limited and in most cases the RPA should be able to act as the MPE.
- *Equipment.* The keeping and maintenance of an up-to-date inventory of each item of equipment is required and should include:
- name of manufacturer
- model number

- serial number or other unique identifier
- year of manufacture
- year of installation.

● *Adequate training and continuing education.* *Operators* and *practitioners* must have received adequate training and must undertake continuing education and training after qualification. The nature of this training is then specified in the *Guidance Notes*:

- *Adequate training for UK graduated practitioners:*
  An undergraduate degree conforming to the requirements for the undergraduate curriculum in dental radiology and imaging as specified by the General Dental Council and including the current core curriculum in dental radiography and radiology published by the British Society of Dental and Maxillofacial Radiology in 2002.

- *Adequate training for operators involved in selecting exposure settings and/or positioning the patient, film or X-ray tubehead:*
  * *Dentists — practitioner* training (as above)
  * *Dental nurses* — should possess a Certificate in Dental Radiography. (An appropriate curriculum, certificate, and examination was made available in 2005 by the National Examining Board for Dental Nurses (NEBDN) in conjunction with the College of Radiographers, the British Society of Dental and Maxillofacial Radiology (BSDMFR) and British Dental Association.)
  * *Dental hygienists and therapists* — should have received an equivalent level of training to that for dental nurses.

- *Adequate training for other operators*:
  Dental nurses and other such operators should preferably possess the Certificate in Dental Nursing or they must have received adequate and documented training specific to the tasks that they undertake. Dental nurses (or other staff), who simply 'press the exposure button' after the patient has been prepared by another adequately trained *operator*, may only do so in the continued presence and under the direct supervision of the *operator*.
  Continuing education and training for practitioners:

Continuing education and training in all aspects of dental radiology should be part of *practitioners* and *operators* life-long learning. To this end, it is recommended that *practitioners* attend a formal course (equivalent to 5 hours of verifiable continuing education) every 5 years covering all aspects of radiation protection including:
* principles of radiation physics
* risks of ionizing radiation
* radiation doses in dental radiography
* factors affecting doses in dental radiography
* principles of radiation protection
* statutory requirements
* selection criteria
* quality assurance.

- *Continuing education for operators involved in radiographing patients:*
  These *operators* are also recommended to attend a continuing education course every 5 years that covers:
  * principles of radiation physics
  * risks of ionizing radiation
  * radiation doses in dental radiography
  * factors affecting doses in dental radiography
  * principles of radiation protection
  * statutory requirements
  * quality assurance.

● *Lead protection.* The confusion and controversy which surrounded the use of lead protection was the main instigating factor for the 1994 NRPB/RCR guidelines. They concluded that patient protection was best achieved by implementation of practical dose reduction measures in relation to clinical judgement, equipment and radiographic technique and not by lead protection. This view has been endorsed in the 2001 *Guidance Notes* which state:
- There is no justification for the routine use of lead aprons for patients in dental radiography.
- Thyroid collars, as shown in Figure 8.3, should be used in those few cases where the thyroid may be in the primary beam. (In the author's opinion, this can include maxillary occlusal radiography, and thyroid protection is therefore shown in Ch. 12.)
- Lead aprons do not protect against radiation scattered internally within the body.

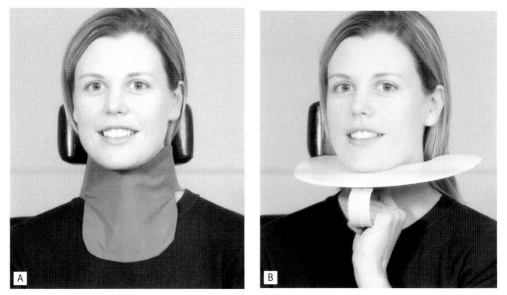

Fig. 8.3 Examples of thyroid lead protection. **A** Lead collar (0.5 mm Pb equivalent). **B** Hand-held neck shield (0.5 mm Pb equivalent).

– Protective aprons, having a lead equivalence of not less than 0.25 mm, should be provided for any adult who provides assistance by supporting a patient during radiography.
– When a lead apron is provided, it must be correctly stored (e.g. over a suitable hanger) and not folded. Its condition must be routinely checked including a visual inspection at annual intervals.

Specific requirements for women of childbearing age.

The developing fetus is most susceptible to the dangers of ionizing radiation during the period of organogenesis (2–9 weeks) — often before the woman knows that she is pregnant. IR(ME)R 2000 prohibits the carrying out of a medical exposure of a female of childbearing age without an enquiry as to whether she is pregnant **if** the primary beam is likely to irradiate the pelvic area. This is highly unlikely in dental radiography. Even so, it is recommended, essentially for psychological reasons, that the operator should enquire of all women of childbearing age whether they are pregnant or likely to be pregnant. If the answer is yes, then, in addition to the routine protective measures appropriate for all patients, the following specific points should be considered:

– The justification should be reviewed to ensure that only radiographs that are absolutely necessary are taken, e.g. delay routine periodic checks.
– The patient should be reassured that a minimal dose is being employed and the patient given the option to delay the radiography.

DOSE LIMITATION AND ANNUAL DOSE LIMITS

For the purposes of dose limitation, the ICRP has divided the population into three groups:

- Patients
- Radiation workers (classified and non-classified)
- General public.

Patients

Radiographic investigations involving patients are divided into four subgroups:

- Examinations directly associated with illness
- Systematic examinations (periodic health checks)
- Examinations for occupational, medicolegal or insurance purposes
- Examinations for medical research.

Examinations directly associated with illness

- There are no set dose limits.
- The decision to carry out such an investigation should be based on:
  - A correct assessment of the indications
  - The expected yield
  - The way in which the results are likely to influence the diagnosis and subsequent treatment
  - The clinician having an adequate knowledge of the physical properties and biological effects of ionizing radiation (i.e. *adequately trained*).
- The number, type and frequency of the radiographs requested or taken (selection criteria) are the responsibility of the clinician. Selection criteria recommendations have been published in different countries in recent years to provide guidance in this clinical area of radiation protection. In the UK, the *Selection Criteria in Dental Radiography* 2nd Ed booklet was published in 2004 by the Faculty of General Dental Practice of the Royal College of Surgeons of England and, as stated earlier, should be regarded as essential reading for all dentists. The expert group responsible for this document reviewed the available scientific evidence to formulate evidence-based recommendations as far as was possible. In some areas, where scientific evidence was lacking, their recommendations were based on expert clinical opinion. The overview of their recommendations are reproduced in Table 8.1 together with a summary Table in Chapter 21.

Systematic examinations (periodic health checks)

- There are no set dose limits.
- There should be a high probability of obtaining useful information—see *Selection Criteria* recommendations in Table 8.1.
- The information obtained should be important to the patient's health.

Examinations for occupational, medicolegal or insurance purposes

- There are no set dose limits.
- The benefit is primarily to a third party.
- The patient should at least benefit indirectly.
- The 2001 *Guidance Notes* emphasize that the need for, and the usefulness of, these examinations should be critically examined when assessing whether they are justified. They also recommend that these types of examinations should only be requested by medical/dental practitioners and that the patient's consent should be obtained.

Examinations for medical research

- There are no set dose limits.
- All research projects should be approved on the advice of an appropriate expert group or Ethics Committee and subject to Local Rules and regulations.
- All volunteers should have a full understanding of the risks involved and give their consent.

Radiation workers

Radiation workers are those people who are exposed to radiation during the course of their work. This exposure carries no benefit only risk. The ICRP further divides these workers into two subgroups depending on the level of occupational exposure:

- Classified workers
- Non-classified workers.

The ICRP sets maximum dose limits for each group, based on the principle that the risk to any worker who receives the full dose limit, will be such that the worker will be at no greater risk than a worker in another hazardous, but non-radioactive, environment. The annual dose limits have been revised under the Ionising Radiations Regulations 1999 and these are shown in Table 8.2.

The main features of each group of radiation workers are summarized below:

Classified workers

- Receive high levels of exposure to radiation at work (if *Local Rules* are observed this is highly unlikely in dental practice).
- Require compulsory personal monitoring.
- Require compulsory annual health checks.

Non-classified workers (most dental staff)

- Receive low levels of exposure to radiation at work (as in the dental surgery).
- The annual dose limits are 3/10 of the classified workers' limits. Provided the *Local Rules* are

Table 8.1 *Overview of the recommendations* from the 2004 *Selection Criteria in Dental Radiography* (reproduced with kind permission from the Faculty of General Dental Practice (UK) of the Royal College of Surgeons of England).

Overview of recommendations (No radiographs should be taken without a history and clinical examination having been performed)

Patient category	Dentate individuals				Endentulous
	Child–primary dentition	Child–mixed dentition	Adolescent	Adult	
NEW PATIENT					
Selection criteria					
All new patients, to assess dental diseases, and growth and development	Posterior bitewing examination as indicated after clinical examination	Patient-specific radiographic examination as indicated after clinical assessment	Patient-specific radiographic examination consisting of posterior bitewings and selected periapicals. An extensive intra-oral radiographic examination may be appropriate when the patient presents with clinical evidence of generalized dental disease or a history of extensive dental treatment. Alternatively, a panoramic radiograph may be appropriate in some instances		Periapical radiograph/s of any symptomatic or clinically suspicious areas
Growth and development	Not normally indicated	Patient-specific radiographic indicated after clinical assessment	One-off periapical or panoramic examination to assess development of third molars if symptomatic		Not normally indicated
RECALL PATIENT					
High caries risk	Posterior bitewing examination at six-month intervals* or until no new or progressing carious lesions are evident *Bitewings should not be taken more frequently and it is imperative to reassess caries risk in order to justify using this interval again				Not applicable
Moderate caries risk	Posterior bitewing examination at one-year intervals				Not applicable
Low caries risk	Posterior bitewing examination at 12–18-month intervals	Posterior bitewing examination at two-year intervals. More extended radiographic recall intervals may be employed if there is explicit evidence of continuing low caries risk			Not applicable
Periodontal disease or history of periodontal disease	Patient-specific radiographic examination consisting of selected periapical and/or bitewings for areas where periodontal disease (other than non-specific gingivitis) can be demonstrated clinically				Not applicable

Table 8.2 The previous annual dose limits and those currently in force under the Ionising Radiations Regulations 1999

	Old dose limits	New dose limits (IRR99)
Classified workers	50 mSv	20 mSv
Non-classified workers	15 mSv	6 mSv
General public	5 mSv	1 mSv

observed, all dental staff should receive an annual effective dose of considerably less than the limit of 6 mSv. Hence, the regulations suggest the setting of 'Dose Constraints'. These represent the upper level of individual dose that should not be exceeded in a well-managed practice and for dental radiography the following recommendations are made:

1 mSv	for employees directly involved with the radiography (operators)
0.3 mSv	for employees not directly involved with the radiography and for members of the general public.

In addition to the above dose limits, the legal person must ensure that the dose to the fetus of any pregnant member of staff is unlikely to exceed 1 mSv during the declared term of the pregnancy.

- Personal monitoring (see later) is not compulsory, although it is recommended if the risk assessment indicates that individual doses could exceed 1mSv per year. The 2001 *Guidance Notes* state that in practice this should be considered for those staff whose weekly workload exceeds 100 intraoral or 50 panoramic films, or a pro-rata combination of each type of examination.
- Annual health checks are not required.

The radiation dose to dentists and their staff can come from:

- The primary beam, if they stand in its path
- Scattered radiation from the patient
- Radiation leakage from the tubehead.

The main protective measures to limit the dose that workers might receive are therefore based mainly on a combination of common sense and the knowledge

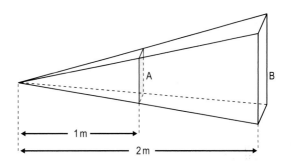

Fig. 8.4 Diagrammatic representation of the inverse square law. Doubling the distance from the source means that the area of B is four times the area of A, thus the radiation per unit area at B is one quarter that at A.

that ionizing radiation is attenuated by distance and obeys the inverse square law (see Fig. 8.4).

The main dose limitation measures relate to:

- Distance from the source of radiation—staff should stand outside the *controlled area* (see Fig. 8.1) and not in the line of the primary beam. If these positions cannot be obtained, appropriate lead screens/barriers should be used
- Safe use of equipment—as summarized in the 2001 *Guidance Notes*
- Radiographic technique—staff should be adequately trained and follow the recommendations summarized in the 2001 *Guidance Notes*
- Monitoring (see later).

General public

This group includes everyone who is not receiving a radiation dose either as a patient or as a radiation worker, but who may be exposed inadvertently, for example, someone in a dental surgery waiting room, in other rooms in the building or passers-by. The annual dose limits for this group have been lowered to 1 mSv, as shown in Table 8.2 although the suggested 'Dose

Constraint' is 0.3 mSv (see earlier). The general public are at risk from the primary beam, so specific consideration should be given to:

- The siting of X-ray equipment to ensure that the primary beam is not aimed directly into occupied rooms or corridors
- The thickness/material of partitioning walls
- Advice from the RPA (see 1999 Regulations) on the siting of all X-ray equipment, surgery design and the placement of radiation warning signs.

MAIN METHODS OF MONITORING AND MEASURING RADIATION DOSE

There are three main devices (shown in Fig. 8.5), for monitoring and measuring radiation dose:

- Film badges
- Thermoluminescent dosemeters (TLD)
  - Badge
  - Extremity monitor
- Ionization chambers.

Film badges

The main features of film badges are:

- They consist of a blue plastic frame containing a variety of different metal filters and a small radiographic film which reacts to radiation
- They are worn on the outside of the clothes, usually at the level of the reproductive organs, for 1–3 months before being processed

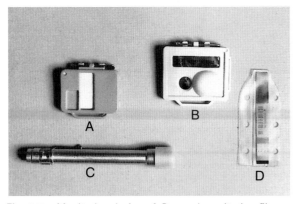

Fig. 8.5 Monitoring devices. **A** Personal monitoring film badge. **B** Personal monitoring TLD badge. **C** Ionization bleeper. **D** TLD extremity monitor.

- They are the most common form of personal monitoring device currently in use.

Advantages
- Provide a permanent record of dose received.
- May be checked and reassessed at a later date.
- Can measure the type and energy of radiation encountered.
- Simple, robust and relatively inexpensive.

Disadvantages
- No immediate indication of exposure — all information is retrospective.
- Processing is required which may lead to errors.
- The badges are prone to filter loss.

Thermoluminescent dosemeters

The main features of TLDs are:

- They are used for personal monitoring of the whole body and/or the extremities, as well as measuring the skin dose from particular investigations
- They contain materials such as lithium fluoride (LiF) which absorb radiation and then release the energy in the form of light when heated
- The intensity of the emitted light is proportional to the radiation energy absorbed originally
- Personal monitors consist of a yellow or orange plastic holder, worn like the film badge for 1–3 months.

Advantages
- The lithium fluoride is re-usable.
- Read-out measurements are easily automated and rapidly produced.
- Suitable for a wide variety of dose measurements.

Disadvantages
- Read-out is destructive, giving no permanent record, results cannot be checked or reassessed.
- Only limited information is provided on the type and energy of the radiation.
- Dose gradients are not detectable.
- Relatively expensive.

Ionization chambers

The main features of ionization chambers are:

- They are used for personal monitoring (thimble chamber) and by physicists (free-air chamber) to measure radiation exposure
- Radiation produces ionization of the air molecules inside the closed chamber, which results in a measurable discharge and hence a direct read-out
- They are available in many different sizes and forms.

Advantages

- The most accurate method of measuring radiation dose.
- Direct read-out gives immediate information.

Disadvantages

- They give no permanent record of exposure.
- No indication of the type or energy of the radiation.
- Personal ionization monitors are not very sensitive to low-energy radiation.
- They are fragile and easily damaged.

PART 4

Radiography

PART CONTENTS

9. Dental radiography – general patient considerations including control of infection   85

10. Periapical radiography   91

11. Bitewing radiography   125

12. Occlusal radiography   135

13. Oblique lateral radiography   141

14. Skull and maxillofacial radiography   149

15. Cephalometric radiography   169

16. Tomography   179

17. Panoramic radiography (dental panoramic tomography)   187

18. The quality of radiographic images and quality assurance   207

19. Alternative and specialized imaging modalities   223

Chapter 9

Dental radiography — general patient considerations including control of infection

This short chapter is designed as a preface to the radiography section. It summarizes the general guidelines relating to patient care, pertinent to all aspects of dental radiography, thus avoiding unnecessary repetition in subsequent chapters. Measures aimed at the control of infection during radiography are also discussed.

GENERAL GUIDELINES ON PATIENT CARE

- For intraoral radiography the patient should be positioned comfortably in the dental chair, ideally with the occlusal plane horizontal and parallel to the floor. For most projections the head should be supported against the chair to minimize unwanted movement. This upright positioning is assumed in subsequent chapters when describing radiographic techniques. However, some clinicians elect to X-ray their patients in the supine position along with most other dental surgery procedures. All techniques need to be modified accordingly, but it can sometimes be more difficult to assess angulations and achieve accurate alignment of film and tubehead with the patient lying down.
- For extraoral views the patient should be reassured about the large, possibly frightening or unfriendly-looking equipment, before being positioned within the machine. This is of particular importance with children.

- The procedure should be explained to the patients in terms they can understand, including warning them not to move during the investigation.
- Spectacles, dentures or orthodontic appliances should be removed. Jewellery including earrings may also need to be removed for certain projections.
- A protective lead thyroid collar, if deemed appropriate for the investigation being carried out, should be placed on the patient (see Ch. 8).
- The exposure factors on the control panel should be selected before positioning the intraoral image receptor and X-ray tubehead, in order to reduce the time of any discomfort associated with the investigation.
- Intraoral image receptor should be positioned carefully to avoid trauma to the soft tissues taking particular care where tissues curve, e.g. the anterior hard palate, lingual to the mandibular incisor teeth and distolingual to the mandibular molars.
- The radiographic investigation should be carried out as accurately and as quickly as possible, to avoid having to retake the radiograph and to lessen patient discomfort.
- The patient should always be watched throughout the exposure to check that he/she has obeyed instructions and has not moved.

SPECIFIC REQUIREMENTS WHEN X-RAYING CHILDREN AND PATIENTS WITH DISABILITIES

These two groups of patients can present particular problems during radiography, including:

- Difficulty in obtaining cooperation
- Anatomical difficulties, such as:
  - large tongue (macroglossia)
  - small mouth (microstomia)
  - tight oral musculature
  - limited neck movement
  - narrow dental arches
  - shallow palate
  - obesity
- Neurological disabilities, such as:
  - communication and learning difficulties
  - tremor
  - palsy.

As a result of these difficulties, the following additional guidelines should be considered:

- Only radiographic investigations appropriate to the limitations imposed by the patient's age, cooperation or disability should be attempted
- Select intraoral image receptor of appropriate size, modifying standard techniques as necessary
- Utilize assistant(s) to help hold the image receptor and/or steady and reassure the patient. This can be accomplished by using an accompanying relative, rather than repeatedly using a member of staff.

NOTE: In the UK, the Ionising Radiations Regulations 1999 require that during an exposure a designated *controlled area* must exist around the X-ray set and theoretically only the patient is allowed in this area (see Ch. 8). Therefore, if assistance is needed and this requirement cannot be fulfilled, the *radiation protection adviser* (RPA)

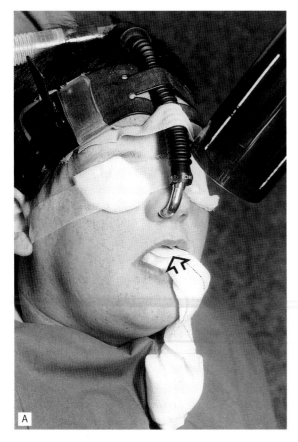

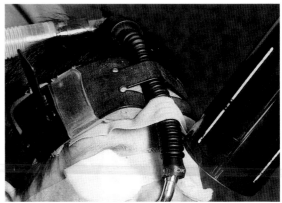

Fig. 9.1 Patient positioning for radiography under general anaesthesia. **A** Periapical radiography of upper incisor teeth. Note the film packet (arrowed) supported in the desired position by a gauze pack. **B** Oblique lateral radiography. Note the tape used to stabilize the cassette and maintain the correct patient position. (Kindly provided by Mr P. Erridge.)

must advise on the appropriate protective measures for the assistant.

- Perform any necessary radiography under general anaesthesia, if an uncooperative patient is having their dental treatment in this manner (see Fig. 9.1). Radiographs taken are usually restricted to oblique laterals and periapicals although bitewings can be taken.
- Avoid dental panoramic radiography because of the need for the patient to remain still for approximately 18 seconds (see Ch. 17). Oblique lateral radiographs should be regarded as the extraoral views of choice.
- Use the paralleling technique, if possible, for periapical radiography because with this technique the relative positions of the image receptor, teeth and X-ray beam are maintained, irrespective of the position of the patient's head (see Ch. 10).

CONTROL OF INFECTION

In the UK, The Health and Safety at Work, Etc, Act of 1974 states that every person working in hospitals or general practice (referred to as *health care workers* or HCWs) has a legal duty to ensure that all necessary steps are taken to prevent cross-infection to protect themselves, their colleagues and the patients. In addition, The Management of Health and Safety Regulations 1992 requires that a risk assessment is carried out for all procedures to reduce the possibility of harm to staff and patients. Effective infection control measures are therefore required in dental radiography even though most investigations are regarded as *non-invasive* or *non-exposure prone procedures*, because they do not involve breaches of the mucosa or skin. The main risk of cross-infection is from one patient to another from salivary contamination of work areas and equipment. HCWs themselves are not at great risk during radiography but there are no grounds for complacency.

Main infections of concern

- *Infective hepatitis caused by hepatitis B (HBV) or hepatitis C (HCV) viruses.* The WHO estimates that of the 2 billion people that have been infected with HBV, more than 350 million have

chronic (lifelong) infections. In the developing world, 8% to 10% of people in the general population become chronically infected. HBV is thought to be 50 to 100 times more infectious than HIV. The WHO estimates that 3% of the world's population has been infected with HCV.
- *Human immunodeficiency virus (HIV disease and AIDS caused by HIV).*
- *Tuberculosis (TB).* The incidence of all forms of TB is rising and now approximately one-third of the world's population is infected. Many of the people with active TB are also infected with HIV.
- *Cold sores caused by herpes simplex virus (HSV).* HCWs are at risk of getting herpetic whitlow, a painful finger infection.
- *Rubella (German measles).*
- *Syphilis.*
- *Diphtheria.*
- *Mumps.*
- *Influenza.*
- *Transmissible spongiform encephalopathies* (TSEs), e.g. Creutzfeldt–Jakob disease (CJD).

A thorough medical history should therefore be obtained from all patients. However, the medical history and examination may not identify asymptomatic carriers of infectious diseases.

It is therefore safer for HCWs to accept that ALL patients may be an infection risk — age or class is no barrier — and universal precautions should be adopted. This means that the same infection control measures should be used for all patients, the only exception being for patients known to have or suspected of having TSEs and the small number of patients in the defined risk groups for TSEs.

Important point to note

If dental clinicians are requesting other HCWs to take their radiographs, either in hospitals or general dental practice, it is their responsibility to ensure that these workers are made aware of any known medical problems or risks, e.g. epilepsy or current infections.

Infection control measures

As mentioned previously, in dental radiography the main concerns arise from salivary contamination of work areas and equipment. Suitable precautions include:

- Training of all staff in infection control procedures and monitoring their compliance.
- All clinical staff should be vaccinated against hepatitis B, have their response to this vaccine checked and maintain this vaccination.
- Open wounds on the hands should be covered with waterproof dressings.
- Protective non-sterile, non-powdered medical gloves (e.g. latex or nitrile) should be worn for all radiographic procedures and changed after every patient.
- Eye protection — either safety glasses or visors (see Fig. 9.2) should be worn but masks are not usually necessary for radiography.
- All required image receptors and holders should be placed on disposable trays to avoid contamination of work surfaces (see Fig. 9.3).
- To prevent salivary contamination of film packets, they should be placed in small barrier envelopes or preferably purchased pre-packed in such envelopes, before use (see Fig. 9.4). After being used in the mouth, the film packet should be emptied out of the barrier envelope onto a clean surface after which it can be handled safely.
- Digital radiography sensors must also be placed inside appropriate barrier envelopes (see Fig. 9.5).
- If barrier envelopes are not used, saliva should be wiped from exposed film packets with disinfectant (e.g. 1% hypochlorite) before handling and processing. This is of particular importance if daylight-loading automatic processors are used because of the risk of salivary contamination of the soft flexible arm sleeves (see Ch. 7 and Fig. 7.3), and if films are collected together during the course of the working day and then processed in batches.
- Film packets must only be introduced into daylight-loading processors using clean hands or washed gloves. Powdered gloves may cause artefacts on the films.
- Contaminated disposable trays, barrier envelopes and image receptor packaging should be discarded directly into suitable clinical waste disposal bags.

- All holders/bite blocks/bite pegs should be rinsed thoroughly to remove saliva, scrubbed in soapy water and autoclaved. Non-autoclavable items such as the aiming ring should be disinfected by soaking in an appropriate solution, e.g. Durr 212 for a minimum of 1 hour.

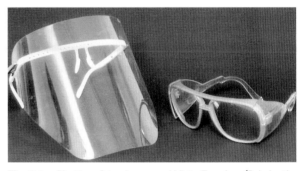

Fig. 9.2 Plastic safety glasses and Vista-Tec visor (Polydentia SA) suitable for eye protection during dental radiography.

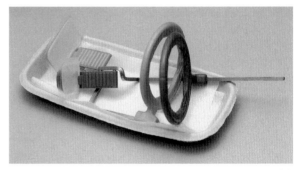

Fig. 9.3 Film holders ready for clinical use on a disposable tray.

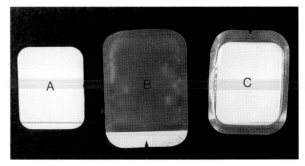

Fig. 9.4A 31 × 41 mm periapical film packet. **B** Plastic barrier envelope to take the periapical film. **C** Pre-packed periapical film packet inside its barrier envelope.

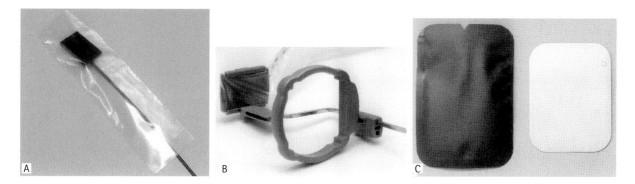

Fig. 9.5A Solid-state digital sensor inside a barrier envelope. **B** Barrier wrapped solid-state sensor inserted into a sensor holder. **C** Barrier envelope for the 31 × 41 mm digital photostimulable phosphor plate shown.

- Disposable holders should be discarded as clinical waste.
- X-ray equipment, including the tubehead, control panel, timer switch and cassettes which have been touched during the radiographic procedure should be wiped after each patient with a suitable surface disinfectant, e.g. Mikrozid®.
- Alternatively, all pieces of equipment can be covered, for example with cling film, which can be replaced after every patient (see Fig. 9.6).

- Soiled gloves and cleaning swabs should be placed in suitable disposal bags and sealed for incineration.

Important points to note
- When X-raying known or suspected TSE patients, extraoral radiographic techniques, that avoid salivary contamination, should be chosen whenever possible (preferably using a technique that does not involve any form of intraoral positioning device) and films should be processed immediately and not left on work surfaces.
- If intraoral techniques are necessary, disposable holders should be used (see Fig. 9.7).
- Infection control measures are of particular importance during sialography when the wearing of an eye protective visor and a mask are recommended (see Ch. 33).

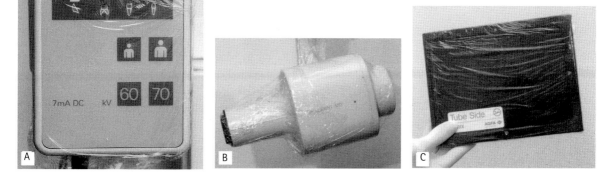

Fig. 9.6 Examples of different pieces of equipment barrier-wrapped in cling film and ready for clinical use **A** a control panel including the exposure button, **B** an X-ray tubehead and **C** a cassette for extraoral use.

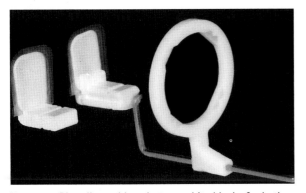

Fig. 9.7 Rinn disposable polystyrene bite blocks for both paralleling and bisected angle technique periapicals.

FOOTNOTE

The importance of effective control of infection measures during dental radiography cannot be over-emphasized. All health care workers should remember that they have a duty of care to do no harm to their patients. Inadequate infection control measures may put other/subsequent patients at risk from infection whether transmitted directly or indirectly.

Chapter 10

Periapical radiography

Periapical radiography describes intraoral techniques designed to show individual teeth and the tissues *around the apices*. Each image usually shows two to four teeth and provides detailed information about the teeth and the surrounding alveolar bone.

MAIN INDICATIONS

The main clinical indications for periapical radiography include:

- Detection of apical infection/inflammation
- Assessment of the periodontal status
- After trauma to the teeth and associated alveolar bone
- Assessment of the presence and position of unerupted teeth
- Assessment of root morphology before extractions
- During endodontics
- Preoperative assessment and postoperative appraisal of apical surgery
- Detailed evaluation of apical cysts and other lesions within the alveolar bone
- Evaluation of implants postoperatively.

IDEAL POSITIONING REQUIREMENTS

The ideal requirements for the position of the image receptor (film packet or digital sensor) and the X-ray beam, relative to a tooth, are shown in Figure 10.1. They include:

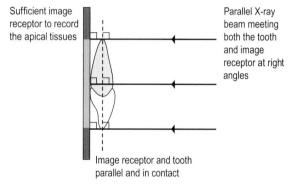

Sufficient image receptor to record the apical tissues

Parallel X-ray beam meeting both the tooth and image receptor at right angles

Image receptor and tooth parallel and in contact

Fig. 10.1 Diagram illustrating the ideal geometrical relationship between image receptor, tooth and X-ray beam.

- The tooth under investigation and the image receptor should be in contact or, if not feasible, as close together as possible
- The tooth and the image receptor should be parallel to one another
- The image receptor should be positioned with its long axis vertically for incisors and canines, and horizontally for premolars and molars with sufficient receptor beyond the apices to record the apical tissues
- The X-ray tubehead should be positioned so that the beam meets the tooth and the image receptor at right angles in both the vertical and the horizontal planes
- The positioning should be reproducible.

RADIOGRAPHIC TECHNIQUES

The anatomy of the oral cavity does not always allow all these ideal positioning requirements to be satisfied. In an attempt to overcome the problems, two techniques for periapical radiography have been developed:

- The paralleling technique
- The bisected angle technique.

Paralleling technique

Theory

1. The image receptor is placed in a holder and positioned in the mouth **parallel** to the long axis of the tooth under investigation.
2. The X-ray tubehead is then aimed at right angles (vertically and horizontally) to both the tooth and the image receptor.
3. By using a film/sensor holder with fixed image receptor and X-ray tubehead positions, the technique is reproducible.

This positioning has the potential to satisfy four of the five ideal requirements mentioned earlier. However, the anatomy of the palate and the shape of the arches mean that the tooth and the image receptor cannot be both parallel and in contact. As shown in Figure 10.2, the image receptor has to be positioned some distance from the tooth.

To prevent the magnification of the image that this separation would cause, an X-ray beam as non-divergent as possible is required (see Fig. 10.3). As explained in Chapter 5, this is achieved by having a **long** *focal spot to skin distance (fsd)*, ideally of 200 mm.

Film packet/sensor holders

A variety of holders has been developed for this technique. The choice of holder is a matter of personal preference and dependent upon the type of image receptor — film packet or digital sensor (solid-state or phosphor plate) — being used. The different holders vary in cost and design, as shown in Figure 10.4, but essentially consist of three basic components:

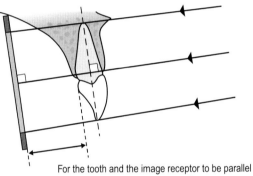

For the tooth and the image receptor to be parallel they have to be positioned some distance apart

Fig. 10.2 Diagram showing the position the image receptor has to occupy in the mouth to be parallel to the long axis of the tooth, because of the slope of the palate.

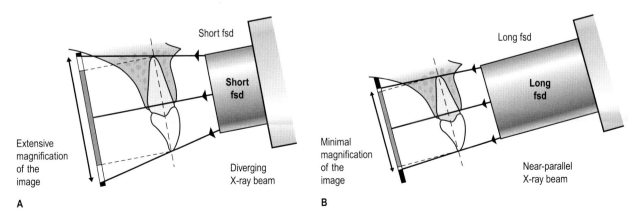

Short fsd · **Short fsd** · Extensive magnification of the image · Diverging X-ray beam

A

Long fsd · **Long fsd** · Minimal magnification of the image · Near-parallel X-ray beam

B

Fig. 10.3 Diagrams showing the magnification of the image that results from using **A** a short focal spot to skin distance (fsd) and a diverging X-ray beam and **B** a long focal spot to skin distance (fsd) and a near-parallel X-ray beam.

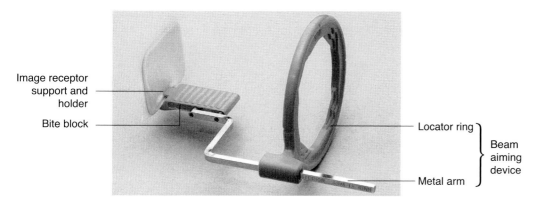

Image receptor support and holder

Bite block

Locator ring ⎤
Beam aiming device ⎬
Metal arm ⎦

Fig. 10.4 Posterior Rinn XCP image receptor holder showing the three basic components common to most holders.

- A mechanism for holding the image receptor parallel to the teeth that also prevents bending of the receptor
- A bite block or platform
- An X-ray beam-aiming device. This may or may not provide additional collimation of the beam.

The different components of the various holders usually need to be assembled together before the holder can be used clinically. The holder design used depends upon whether the tooth under investigation is:

- Anterior or posterior
- In the mandible or maxilla
- On the right or the left hand side of the jaw.

These variables mean that assembling the holder can be confusing, but it must be done correctly. To facilitate this assembly some manufacturers now colour code the various components. Once assembled correctly the entire image receptor should be visible when viewed through the beam-aiming device as shown in Figure 10.5.

The choice of holder is a matter of personal preference and dependent upon the type of image receptor — film packet or digital sensor (solid-state or phosphor plate) — being used. A selection of different holders is shown in Figure 10.6.

Typically, the **same** anterior holder can be used for **right** and **left** maxillary **and** mandibular *incisors and canines* utilizing a small image receptor (22 × 35 mm) with its long axis vertical. Four images in the maxilla and three images in the mandible are usually required to cover the right and left incisors and canines as shown in Figure 10.7.

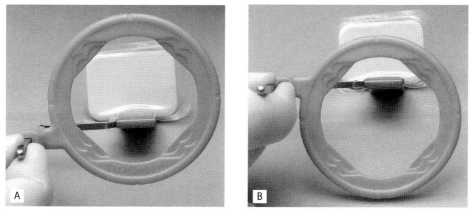

A

B

Fig. 10.5A The appearance of the film packet when viewed through the locator ring of a *correctly* assembled Rinn XCP holder. **B** The appearance when the film holder has been assembled *incorrectly*.

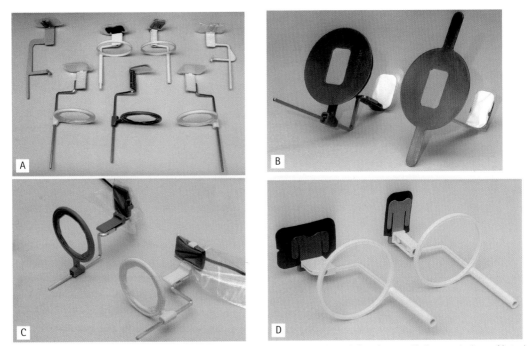

Fig. 10.6A   A selection of film packet and digital phosphor plate holders designed for the paralleling technique. Note how some manufactuters use colour coding to identifiy holders for differenct parts of the mouth. **B** Holders incorporating additional rectangular collimation – the Masel Precision all-in-one metal holder and the Rinn XCP holder with the metal collimator attached to the locator ring. **C** Blue anterior and yellow posterior Rinn XCP-DS solid-state digital sensor holders. **D** Green/yellow anterior and red/yellow posterior Hawe-Neos holders suitable for film packets and digital phosphor plates (shown here).

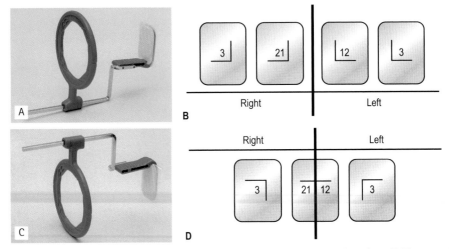

Fig. 10.7A   The anterior Rinn XCP holder suitable for imaging the maxillary incisors and canines. **B** Diagram showing the *four* small image receptors required to image the right and left maxillary incisors and canines. **C** The anterior Rinn XCP holder suitable for imaging the mandibular incisors and canines. **D** Diagram showing the **three** small image receptors required to image the right and left mandibular incisors and canines

Typically **different** holders are required for the **right** and **left** *premolar and molar* maxillary and mandibular posterior teeth. The different designs allow the holders to hook around the cheek and corner of the mouth. A large image receptor (31 × 41 mm) is ideally utilized with its long axis horizontal. Two images are usually required to cover the premolar and molar teeth in each quadrant as shown is Figure 10.8.

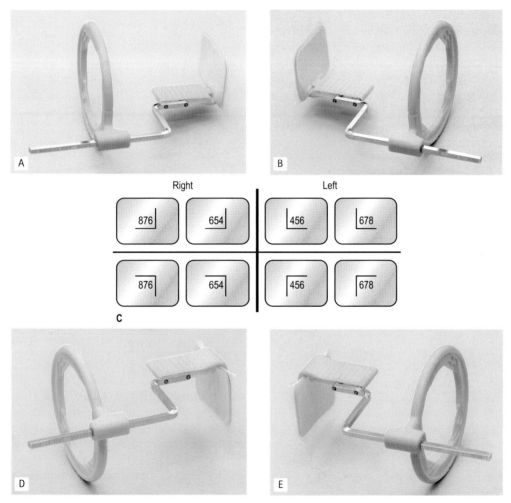

Fig. 10.8A   The posterior Rinn XCP holder assembled for imaging the RIGHT maxillary premolars and molars. **B** The posterior Rinn XCP holder assembled for imaging the LEFT maxillary premolars and molars. **C** Diagram showing the *two* large image receptors required to image the right and left premolars and molars in each quadrant. **D** The posterior Rinn XCP holder assembled for imaging the RIGHT mandibular premolars and molars. **E** The posterior Rinn XCP holder assembled for imaging the LEFT mandibular premolars and molars.

Positioning techniques

The radiographic techniques for the permanent dentition can be summarized as follows:

1. The patient is positioned with the head supported and with the occlusal plane horizontal.
2. The holder and image receptor are placed in the mouth as follows:
   a. *Maxillary incisors and canines* — the image receptor is positioned sufficiently posteriorly to enable its height to be accommodated in the vault of the palate
   b. *Mandibular incisors and canines* — the image receptor is positioned in the floor of the mouth, approximately in line with the lower canines or first premolars
   c. *Maxillary premolars and molars* — the image receptor is placed in the midline of the palate, again to accommodate its height in the vault of the palate
   d. *Mandibular premolars and molars* — the image receptor is placed in the lingual sulcus next to the appropriate teeth.
3. The holder is rotated so that the teeth under investigation are touching the bite block.
4. A cottonwool roll is placed on the reverse side of the bite block. This often helps to keep the tooth and image receptor parallel and may make the holder less uncomfortable.
5. The patient is requested to bite **gently** together, to stabilize the holder in position.
6. The locator ring is moved down the indicator rod until it is just in contact with the patient's face. This ensures the correct focal spot to film distance (fsd).
7. The spacer cone is aligned with the locator ring. This automatically sets the vertical and horizontal angles and centres the X-ray beam on the image receptor
8. The exposure is made.

Positioning clinically using film packets and digital phosphor plates is shown in Figures 10.9–10.16 for the following different areas of the mouth:

Maxillary central incisor (Fig. 10.9)

Maxillary canine (Fig. 10.10)

Maxillary premolars (Fig. 10.11)

Maxillary molars (Fig. 10.12)

Mandibular incisors (Fig. 10.13)

Mandibular canine (Fig. 10.14)

Mandibular premolars (Fig. 10.15)

Mandibular molars (Fig. 10.16)

Note:
1. *Full mouth survey* is the terminology used to describe the full collection of 15 periapical radiographs (seven anterior and eight posterior) showing the full dentition.
2. When using film packets and digital phosphor plates the end of the receptor with the orientation dot should be placed opposite the crowns of the teeth to avoid subsequent superimposition of the dot over an apex.

Positioning using solid-state digital sensors

Clinical positioning of holders for the paralleling technique when using solid-state digital sensors can be more difficult because of the bulk and absolute rigidity of the sensor. Those systems employing cables also require extra care with regard to the position of the cable to avoid damaging it. Once the holder is inserted into the mouth, the positioning of the tubehead is the same as described previously when using other types of image receptors and is shown in Figure 10.17 for different parts of the mouth.

Maxillary incisors

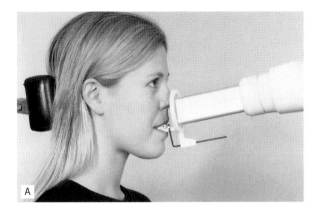

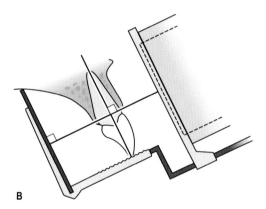

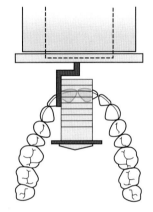

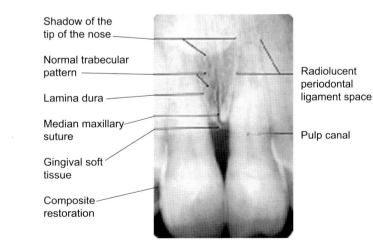

Shadow of the
tip of the nose

Normal trabecular
pattern

Lamina dura

Median maxillary
suture

Gingival soft
tissue

Composite
restoration

Radiolucent
periodontal
ligament space

Pulp canal

D

Fig. 10.9A   Patient positioning (maxillary central incisor). B Diagram of the positioning. C Plan view of the positioning.
D Resultant radiograph with the main radiographic features indicated.

Maxillary canine

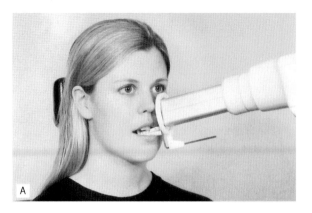

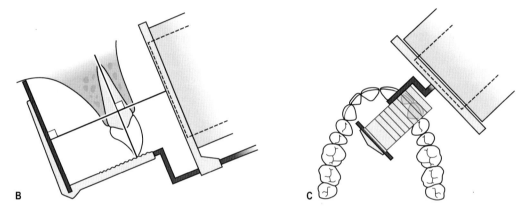

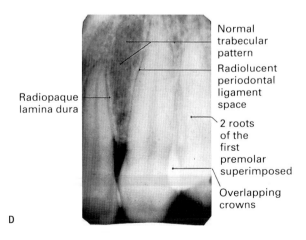

Radiopaque lamina dura

Normal trabecular pattern

Radiolucent periodontal ligament space

2 roots of the first premolar superimposed

Overlapping crowns

Fig. 10.10A Patient positioning (maxillary canine). **B** Diagram of the positioning. **C** Plan view of the positioning. **D** Resultant radiograph with the main radiographic features indicated.

Maxillary premolars

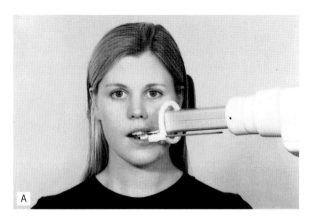

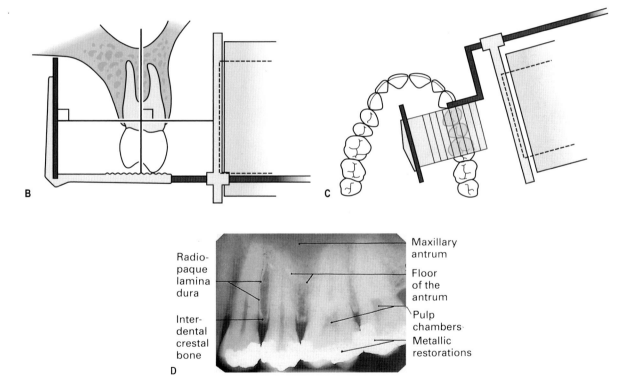

Radio-
paque
lamina
dura

Inter-
dental
crestal
bone

Maxillary
antrum

Floor
of the
antrum

Pulp
chambers

Metallic
restorations

Fig. 10.11A Patient positioning (maxillary premolars). **B** Diagram of the positioning. **C** Plan view of the positioning. **D** Resultant radiograph with the main radiographic features indicated.

Maxillary molars

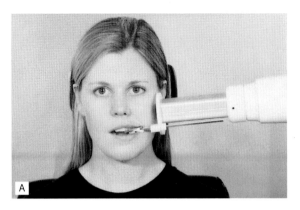

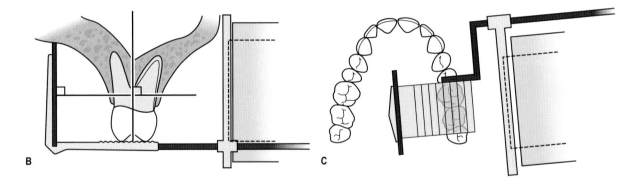

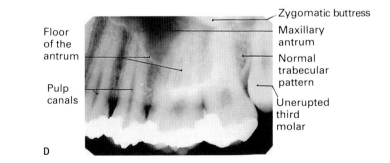

Fig. 10.12A   Patient positioning (maxillary molars). **B** Diagram of the positioning. **C** Plan view of the positioning.
D Resultant radiograph with the main radiographic features indicated.

Mandibular incisors

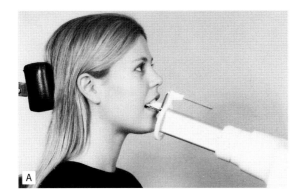

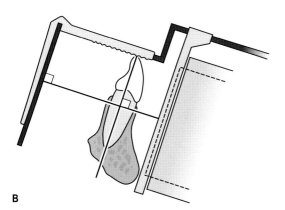

B

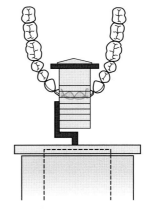

C

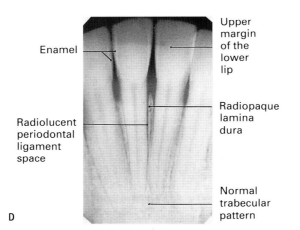

Enamel

Radiolucent periodontal ligament space

Upper margin of the lower lip

Radiopaque lamina dura

Normal trabecular pattern

D

Fig. 10.13A Patient positioning (mandibular incisors). **B** Diagram of the positioning. **C** Plan view of the positioning. **D** Resultant radiograph with the main radiographic features indicated.

Mandibular canine

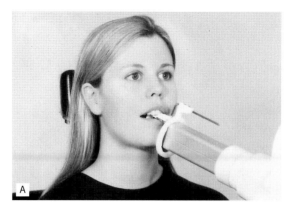

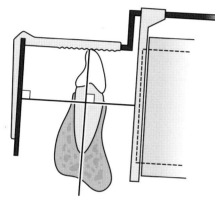

B

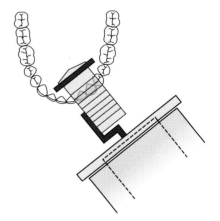

C

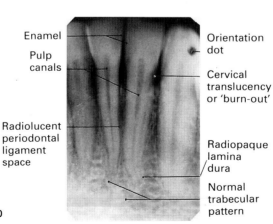

Enamel

Pulp canals

Radiolucent periodontal ligament space

Orientation dot

Cervical translucency or 'burn-out'

Radiopaque lamina dura

Normal trabecular pattern

D

Fig. 10.14A Patient positioning (mandibular lateral and canine). **B** Diagram of the positioning. **C** Plan view of the positioning. **D** Resultant radiograph with the main radiographic features indicated.

Mandibular premolars

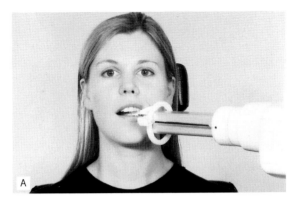

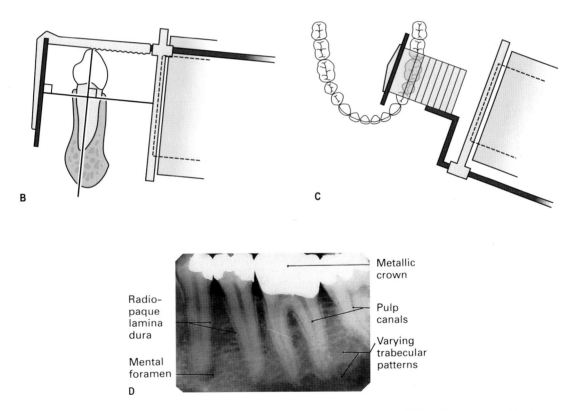

Fig. 10.15A   Patient positioning (mandibular premolars). B Diagram of the positioning. C Plan view of the positioning.
D Resultant radiograph with the main radiographic features indicated.

Mandibular molars

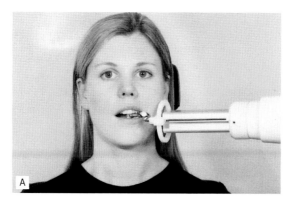

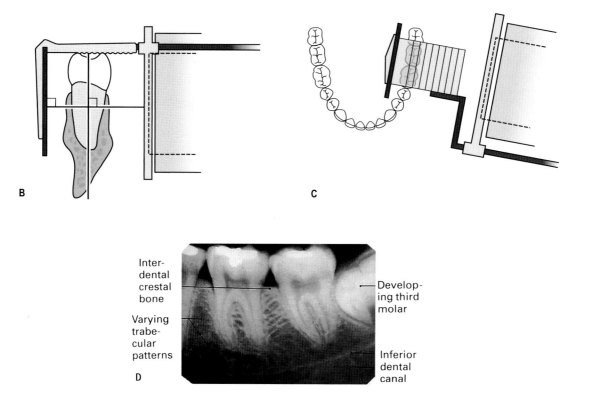

Fig. 10.16A   Patient positioning (mandibular molars). B Diagram of the positioning. C Plan view of the positioning. D Resultant radiograph with the main radiographic features indicated.

Solid-state digital sensor positioning

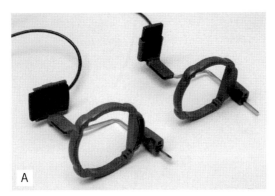

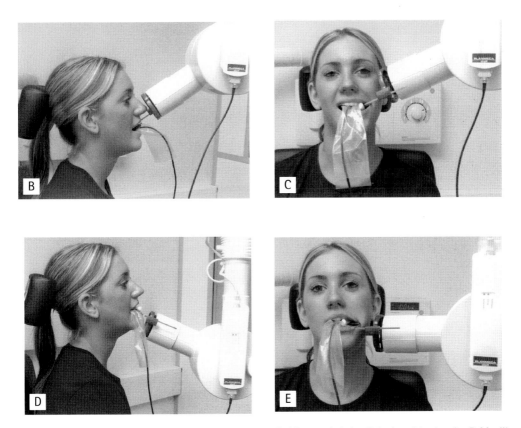

Fig. 10.17A   Anterior and posterior Planmeca solid-state sensor holders and their clinical positioning for **B** Maxillary incisors. **C** Maxillary molars, **D** Mandibular incisors and **E** Mandibular molars.

Bisected angle technique

Theory

The theoretical basis of the bisected angle technique is shown in Figure 10.18 and can be summarized as follows:

1. The image receptor is placed as close to the tooth under investigation as possible without bending the packet.
2. The angle formed between the long axis of the tooth and the long axis of the image receptor is assessed and mentally bisected.
3. The X-ray tubehead is positioned at right angles to this bisecting line with the central ray of the X-ray beam aimed through the tooth apex.
4. Using the geometrical principle of similar triangles, the actual length of the tooth in the mouth will be equal to the length of the tooth on the image.

Vertical angulation of the X-ray tubehead

The angle formed by continuing the line of the central ray until it meets the occlusal plane determines the *vertical angulation* of the X-ray beam to the occlusal plane (see Fig. 10.18).

Note: Vertical angles are often quoted but inevitably they are only approximate. Patient differences including head position, and individual tooth position and inclination mean that each positioning should be assessed independently. The vertical angulations suggested should be taken only as a general guide.

Horizontal angulation of the X-ray tubehead

In the horizontal plane, the central ray should be aimed through the interproximal contact areas, to avoid overlapping the teeth. The *horizontal angulation* is therefore determined by the shape of the arch and the position of the teeth (see Fig. 10.19).

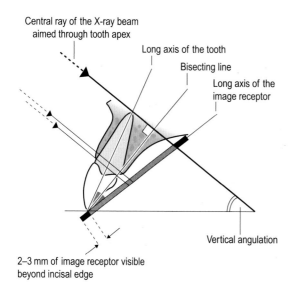

Central ray of the X-ray beam aimed through tooth apex

Long axis of the tooth

Bisecting line

Long axis of the image receptor

Vertical angulation

2–3 mm of image receptor visible beyond incisal edge

Fig. 10.18 Theoretical basis of the bisected angle technique. The angle between the long axes of the tooth and image receptor is bisected and X-ray beam aimed at right angles to this line, through the apex of the tooth. With this geometrical arrangement, the length of the tooth in the mouth is equal to the length of the image of the tooth on the image receptor, but, as shown, the periodontal bone levels will not be represented accurately.

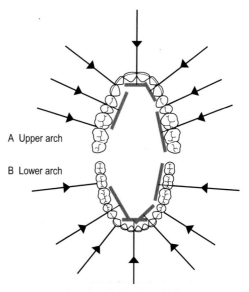

A Upper arch

B Lower arch

Fig. 10.19 Diagram of A the upper arch and B the lower arch. The various horizontal angulations of the X-ray beam are shown.

Positioning techniques

The bisected angle technique can be performed either by using an image receptor holder to support the image receptor in the patient's mouth or by asking the patient to support the image receptor **gently** using either an index finger or thumb. Both techniques are described.

Note: the 2001 *Guidance Notes* recommend that the image receptor should only be held by the patient when it cannot otherwise be kept in position.

Using film packet/digital sensor holders

Various holders are available, a selection of which are shown in Figure 10.20. The Rinn Bisected Angle Instruments (BAI) closely resemble the paralleling technique holders and consist of the same three basic components — image receptor holding mechanism, bite block and an X-ray beam-aiming device — but the image receptor is not held parallel to the teeth. The more simple holders and the disposable bite blocks hold the image receptor in the desired position but the X-ray tubehead then has to be aligned independently. In summary:

1. The image receptor is pushed securely into the chosen holder. Either a large or small size of image receptor is used so that the particular tooth being examined is in the middle of the receptor, as shown in Figure 10.21. When using a film packet the white surface faces the X-ray tubehead and the film orientation dot is opposite the crown.
2. The X-ray tubehead is positioned using the beam-aiming device if available OR the operator has to assess the *vertical* and *horizontal angulations* by observation and then position the tubehead without a guide.
3. The exposure is made.

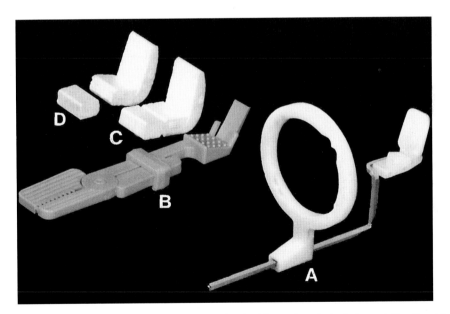

Fig. 10.20 A selection of film packet/phosphor plate holders for the bisected angle technique. **A** The Rinn bisected angle instrument (BAI). **B** The Emmenix® film holder. **C** The Rinn Greene Stabe® bite block. **D** The Rinn Greene Stabe® bite block reduced in size for easier positioning and for use in children.

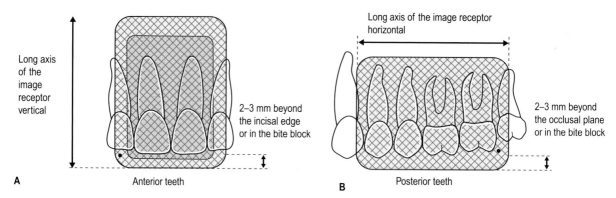

Fig. 10.21   Diagrams showing the general requirements of the image receptor position for **A** anterior and **B** posterior teeth.

Using the patient's finger

1. The appropriate sized image receptor is positioned and orientated in the mouth as shown in Figure 10.18 with about 2 mm extending beyond the incisal or occlusal edges, to ensure that all of the tooth will appear on the image. The patient is then asked to gently support the image receptor using either an index finger or thumb.

2. The operator then assesses the *vertical* and *horizontal angulations* by observation and positions the tubehead without a guide. The effects of incorrect tubehead position are shown in Figure 10.22.

3. The exposure is made.

The specific positioning for different areas of the mouth, using both simple holders and the patient's finger to support the image receptor, is shown in Figures 10.23–10.30.

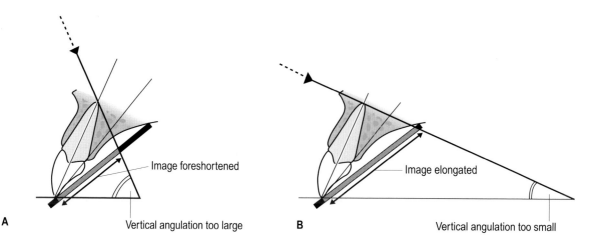

Fig. 10.22   Diagrams showing the effects of incorrect vertical tubehead positioning. **A** Foreshortening of the image. **B** Elongation of the image.

Positioning using film packets and digital phosphor plates

Maxillary central incisors

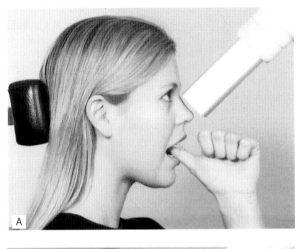

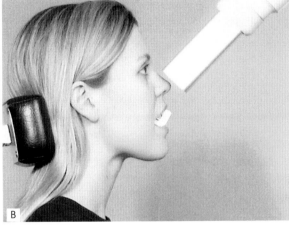

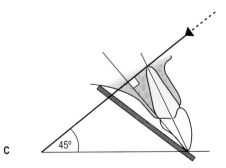

Fig. 10.23   Patient positioning with the patient
A supporting the image receptor with the ball of the left
thumb and B using the Rinn Greene Stabe® bite block.
C Diagram of the relative positions of image receptor,
incisor and X-ray beam.

Maxillary canine

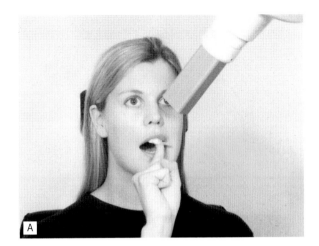

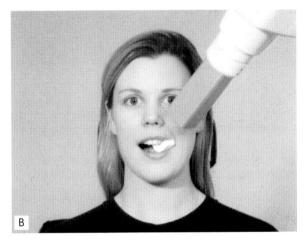

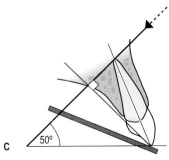

Fig. 10.24   Patient positioning with the patient
A supporting image receptor with the ball of the right index
finger and B using the Rinn Greene Stabe® bite block.
C Diagram of the relative positions of image receptor,
canine and X-ray beam.

Maxillary premolars

Maxillary molars

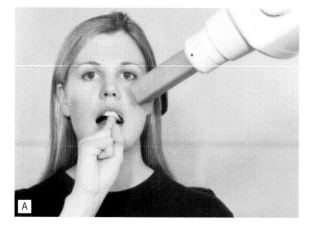

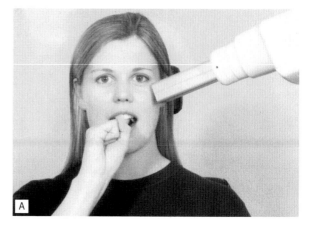

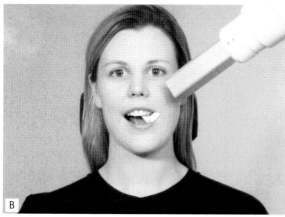

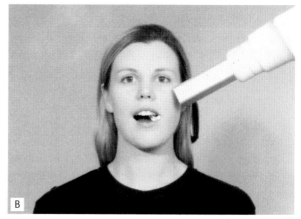

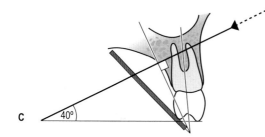

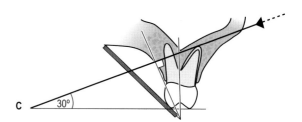

Fig. 10.25 Patient positioning with the patient **A** supporting the image receptor and **B** using the Rinn Greene Stabe® bite block. **C** Diagram of the relative positions of image receptor, premolar and X-ray beam.

Fig. 10.26 Patient positioning with the patient **A** supporting the image receptor and **B** using the Rinn Greene Stabe® bite block. **C** Diagram of the relative positions of image receptor, molar and X-ray beam.

Mandibular incisors

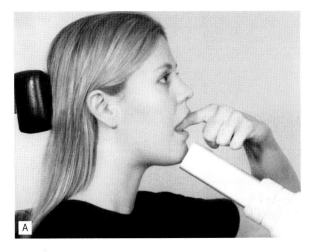

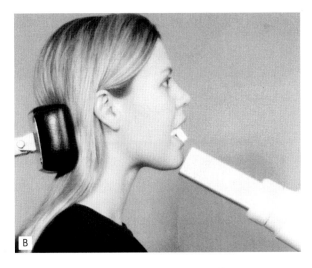

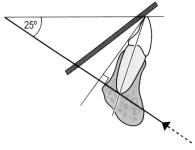

Fig. 10.27 Patient positioning with **A** the patient's index finger on the upper edge of the image receptor, supporting and depressing it into the floor of the mouth and **B** using the Rinn Greene Stabe® bite block. **C** Diagram of the relative positions of image receptor, incisor and X-ray beam.

Mandibular canine

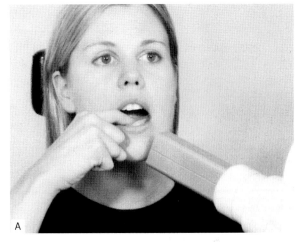

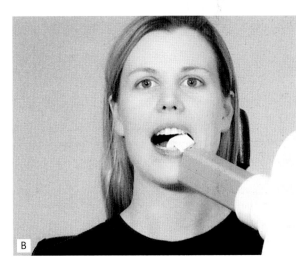

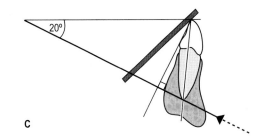

Fig. 10.28 Patient positioning with the patient **A** supporting and depressing the upper edge of the image receptor and **B** using the Rinn Greene Stabe® bite block. **C** Diagram of the relative positions of image receptor, canine and X-ray beam.

Mandibular premolars

Mandibular molars

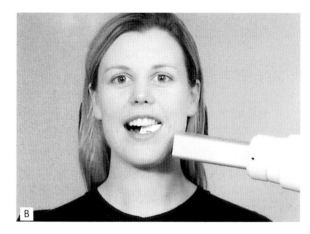

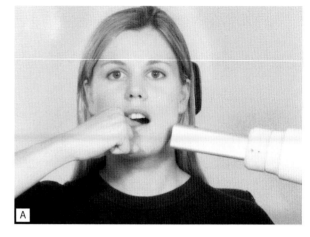

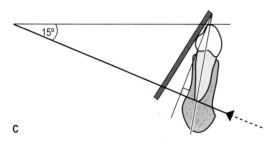

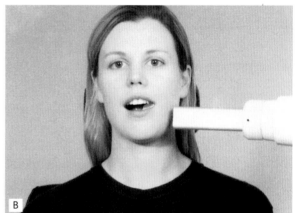

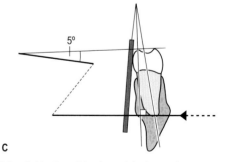

Fig. 10.29   Patient positioning with the patient
A supporting the image receptor and B using the Rinn
Greene Stabe® bite block. C Diagram of the relative
positions of image receptor, premolar and X-ray beam.

Fig. 10.30   Patient positioning with the patient
A supporting the image receptor and B using the Rinn
Greene Stabe® bite block. C Diagram of the relative
positions of image receptor, molar and X-ray beam.

Comparison of the paralleling and bisected angle techniques

The advantages and disadvantages of the two techniques can be summarized as follows:

Advantages of the paralleling technique

- Geometrically accurate images are produced with little magnification.
- The shadow of the zygomatic buttress appears **above** the apices of the molar teeth.
- The periodontal bone levels are well represented.
- The periapical tissues are accurately shown with minimal foreshortning or elongation.
- The crowns of the teeth are well shown enabling the detection of approximal caries.
- The horizontal and vertical angulations of the X-ray tubehead are automatically determined by the positioning devices if placed correctly.
- The X-ray beam is aimed accurately at the centre of the image receptor — all areas of the image receptor are irradiated and there is no *coning off* or *cone cutting*.
- Reproducible radiographs are possible at different visits and with different operators.
- The relative positions of the image receptor, teeth and X-ray beam are always maintained, irrespective of the position of the patient's head. This is useful for some patients with disabilities.

Disadvantages of the paralleling technique

- Positioning of the image receptor can be very uncomfortable for the patient, particularly for posterior teeth, often causing gagging.
- Positioning the holders within the mouth can be difficult for inexperienced operators particularly when using solid-state digital sensors.
- The anatomy of the mouth sometimes makes the technique impossible, e.g. a shallow, flat palate.
- The apices of the teeth can sometimes appear very near the edge of the image.
- Positioning the holders in the lower third molar regions can be very difficult.
- The technique cannot be performed satisfactorily using a short focal spot to skin distance (i.e. a short spacer cone) because of the resultant magnification.
- The holders need to be autoclavable or disposable.

Advantages of the bisected angle technique

- Positioning of the image receptor is reasonably comfortable for the patient in all areas of the mouth.
- Positioning is relatively simple and quick.
- If all angulations are assessed correctly, the image of the tooth will be the same length as the tooth itself and should be *adequate* (but not ideal) for most diagnostic purposes.

Disadvantages of the bisected angle technique

- The many variables involved in the technique often result in the image being badly distorted.
- Incorrect vertical tube head angulation will result in foreshortening or elongation of the image.
- The periodontal bone levels are poorly shown.
- The shadow of the zygomatic buttress frequently overlies the roots of the upper molars.
- The horizontal and vertical angles have to be assessed by observation for every patient and considerable skill is required.
- It is not possible to obtain reproducible views.
- *Coning off* or *cone cutting* may result if the central ray is not aimed at the centre of the image receptor, particularly if using rectangular collimation.
- Incorrect horizontal tube head angulation will result in overlapping of the crowns and roots.
- The crowns of the teeth are often distorted, thus preventing the detection of approximal caries.
- The buccal roots of the maxillary premolars and molars are foreshortened.

A visual comparison between the two techniques, showing how dramatic the variation in image quality and reproductibility can be, is shown in Figures 10.31 and 10.32.

A   B

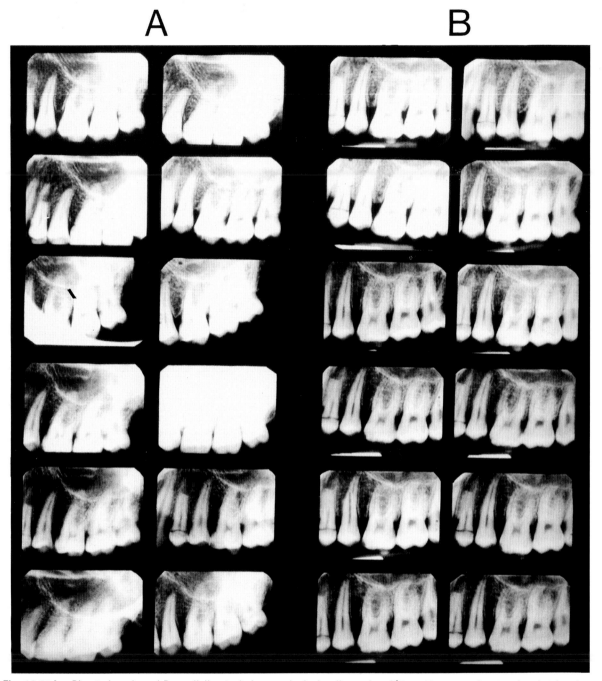

Fig. 10.31A   Bisected angle and **B** paralleling technique periapical radiographs of |6, on the *same* phantom head, taken by 12 *different* experienced operators. The obvious reproducibility and accurate imaging show why the paralleling technique should be regarded as the technique of choice.

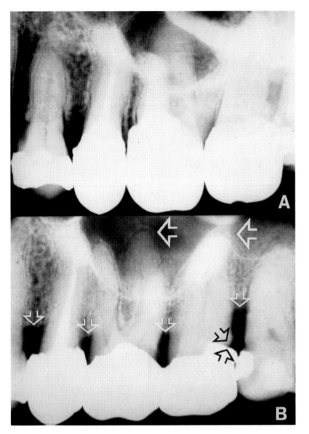

Fig. 10.32A Bisected angle and **B** paralleling technique periapicals of the ⌊45678 taken on the *same* patient, by the *same* operator, on the *same* day. Note the difference in the periodontal bone levels (small white open arrows), the restoration in ⌊7 (black open arrows) and the apical tissues ⌊67 (large white open arrows).

Conclusion

The diagnostic advantages of the accurate, reproducible images produced by the paralleling technique using image receptor holders and beam-aiming devices ensure that this technique should be regarded as the technique of choice for periapical radiography. The 2001 *Guidance Notes* recommend that whenever practicable, techniques using image receptor holders with beam aiming devices should be adopted (see Ch. 8).

POSITIONING DIFFICULTIES OFTEN ENCOUNTERED IN PERIAPICAL RADIOGRAPHY

Placing the image receptor intraorally in the *textbook-described* positions is not always possible. The radiographic techniques described earlier often need to be modified. The main difficulties encountered involve:

- Mandibular third molars
- Gagging
- Endodontics
- Edentulous alveolar ridges
- Children
- Patients with disabilities (see Ch. 9).

Problems posed by mandibular third molars

The main difficulty is placement of the image receptor sufficiently posteriorly to record the entire third mandibular molar (particularly when it is horizontally impacted) **and** the surrounding tissues, including the inferior dental canal (see Fig. 10.33).

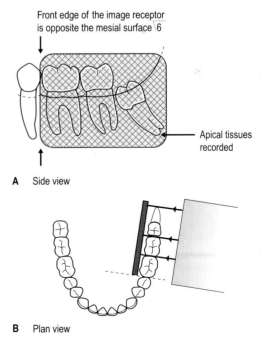

A Side view

B Plan view

Fig. 10.33A Side view and **B** plan view diagrams showing the ideal image receptor position for mandibular third molars to ensure the tooth and apical tissues are recorded.

Possible solutions

These include:

- Using specially designed or adapted holders as shown in Figure 10.34 to hold and position the image receptor in the mouth, as follows:
    1. The holder is clipped securely on to the top edge of the image receptor.
    2. With the mouth open, the image receptor is positioned gently in the lingual sulcus as far posteriorly as possible.
    3. The patient is asked to close the mouth (so relaxing the tissues of the floor of the mouth) and at the same time the image receptor is eased further back into the mouth, if required, until its front edge is opposite the mesial surface of the mandibular first molar.
    4. The patient is asked to bite on the holder and to support it in position.

5. The X-ray tubehead is positioned at right angles to the third molar and the image receptor and centred 1 cm up from the lower border of the mandible, on a vertical line dropped from the outer corner of the eye (see Fig. 10.34).

- Taking two radiographs of the third molar using two different horizontal tubehead angulations, as follows:
    1. The image receptor is positioned as posteriorly as possible (using the technique described with the holders)
    2. The X-ray tubehead is aimed with the *ideal* horizontal angulation so the X-ray beam passes between the second and third molars. (With horizontally impacted third molars, the apex may not be recorded using this positioning, as shown in Figure 10.35).

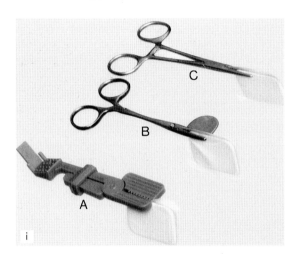

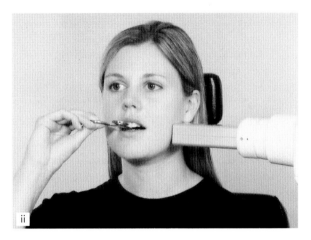

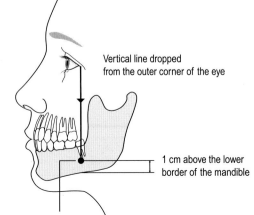

Fig. 10.34 (i) A selection of film packet/phosphor plate holders for mandibular third molars: **A** Emmenix® film holder. **B** Worth film holder and **C** a conventional pair of artery forceps. (ii) Patient positioning — having closed the mouth, the patient is stabilizing the image receptor holder with a hand. (iii) Diagram indicating the external centring point for the X-ray beam.

Vertical line dropped from the outer corner of the eye

1 cm above the lower border of the mandible

(iii)   External centring point

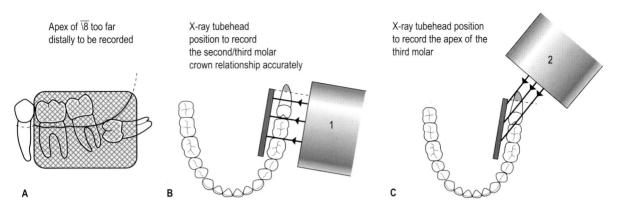

Apex of ⎯|8̄ too far distally to be recorded

X-ray tubehead position to record the second/third molar crown relationship accurately

X-ray tubehead position to record the apex of the third molar

A **B** **C**

Fig. 10.35   The problem of the horizontal third molar. **A** Side view showing the often achievable image receptor position. **B** Plan view showing X-ray tubehead position 1. **C** Plan view showing X-ray tubehead position 2.

3. A *second* image receptor is placed in the same position as before, but the X-ray tubehead is positioned further posteriorly aiming forwards to project the apex of the third molar on to the receptor. (With this positioning, the crowns of the second and third molars will be overlapped, as shown in Figure 10.35.)

Note: The vertical angulation of the X-ray tubehead is the same for both projections.

Problems of gagging

The gag reflex is particularly strong in some patients. This makes the placement of the image receptor in the desired position particularly difficult, especially in the upper and lower molar regions.

Possible solutions

These include:

- Patient sucking a local anaesthetic lozenge before attempting to position the image receptor
- Asking the patient to concentrate on breathing deeply while the image receptor is in the mouth

- Placing the image receptor flat in the mouth (in the occlusal plane) so it does not touch the palate, and applying the principles of the bisected angle technique — the long axes of the tooth and image receptor are assessed by observation and the X-ray tubehead's position modified accordingly, as shown in Figure 10.36.

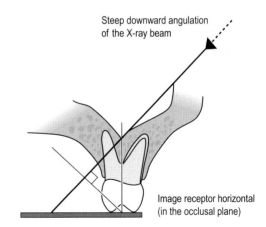

Steep downward angulation of the X-ray beam

Image receptor horizontal (in the occlusal plane)

Fig. 10.36   Diagram showing the relative position of the X-ray beam to the maxillary molar and receptor, when the image receptor is placed in the occlusal plane. Note: The length of the image of the tooth on the radiograph should again equal the length of the tooth in the mouth. However, there will be considerable distortion of the surrounding tissues.

Problems encountered during endodontics

The main difficulties involve:

- Image receptor placement and stabilization when endodontic instruments, rubber dam and rubber dam clamps are in position
- Identification and separation of root canals
- Assessing root canal lengths from foreshortened or elongated radiographs.

Possible solutions

These include:

- The problem of image receptor placement and stabilization can be solved by:
  - Using a simple image receptor holder such as the Rinn Eezee-Grip®, as shown in Figure 10.37. This is positioned in the mouth and then held in place by the patient.
  - Using one of the special endodontic image receptor holders that have been developed. These incorporate a modified bite platform area, to accommodate the handles of the endodontic instruments, while still allowing the image receptor and the tooth to be parallel. (See Fig. 10.38.)
- The problem of identifying and separating the root canals can be solved by taking at least two radiographs, using different horizontal X-ray tubehead positions, as shown in Figure 10.39.

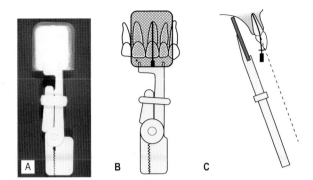

Fig. 10.37A The Rinn Eezee–Grip® film/phosphor plate holder. **B** and **C** Diagrams showing its use in endodontics. (**Note:** Rubber dam not shown.)

- The problems of assessing root canal length can be solved by:
  - Taking an accurate paralleling technique periapical preoperatively and measuring the lengths of the root(s) directly from the radiograph before beginning the endodontic treatment. The amount of distortion on subsequent films can then be assessed.
  - Calculating mathematically the actual length of a root canal from a distorted bisected angle technique periapical taken with the diagnostic instrument within the root canal at the clinically assessed apical *stop*.

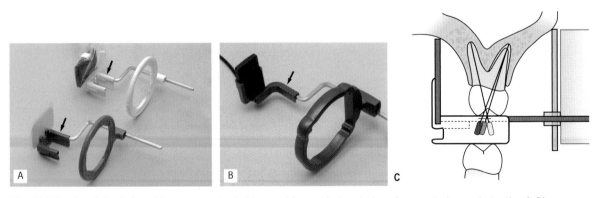

Fig. 10.38 Specially designed image receptor holders and beam aiming devices for use during endodontics **A** Rinn Endoray® suitable for film packets and digital phosphor plates (green) and solid-state digital sensors (white) **B** Anterior Planmeca solid-state digital sensor holder. Note the modified designs of the biteblocks (arrowed) to accommodate the handles of the endodontic instruments. Colour coding of instruments by some manufacturers is now used to facilitate clinical use. **C** Diagram of the Rinn Endoray® in place.

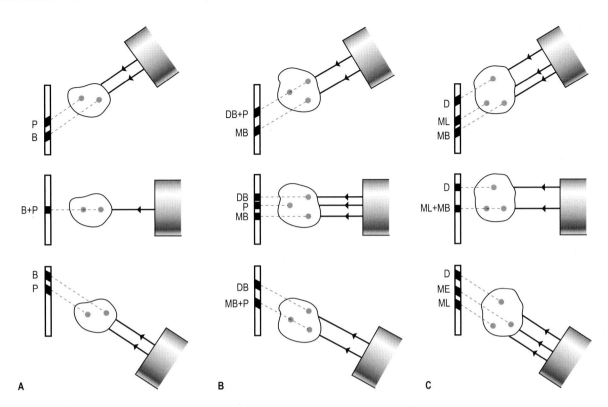

Fig. 10.39 Diagrams showing the effect of different horizontal X-ray tubehead positions on root separation for **A** maxillary premolars, **B** maxillary first molars and **C** mandibular first molars. (The images of the canals are designated: P = palatal, B = buccal, MB = mesiobuccal, DB = distobuccal, ML = mesiolingual and D = distal.)

The calculation is done as follows (see Fig. 10.40):

1. Measure:
   a. The *radiographic tooth length*
   b. The *radiographic instrument length*
   c. The *actual instrument length*
2. Substitute the measurements into the formula:

$$\text{Actual tooth length} = \frac{\text{Radiographic tooth length} \times \text{Actual instrument length}}{\text{Radiographic instrument length}}$$

3. Calculate the *actual tooth length* and adjust the working length of the instrument as necessary.

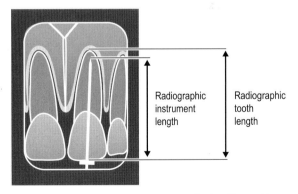

Fig. 10.40 Diagram showing the required radiographic measurements in endodontics to calculate the actual tooth length.

Problems of the edentulous ridge

The main difficulty in the edentulous and partially dentate patient is again image receptor placement.

Possible solutions

These include:

- In edentulous patients, the lack of height in the palate, or loss of lingual sulcus depth, contraindicates the paralleling technique and all periapical radiographs should be taken using a modified bisected angle technique. The long axes of the image receptor and the alveolar ridge are assessed by observation and the X-ray tubehead position adjusted accordingly as shown in Figure 10.41.
- In partially dentate patients, the paralleling technique can usually be used. If the edentulous area causes the image receptor holder to be displaced, the deficiency can be built up by using cottonwool rolls, as shown in Figure 10.42.

Problems encountered in children

Once again the main technical problem (as opposed to management problems) encountered in children is the size of their mouths and the difficulty in placing the image receptor intraorally. The paralleling technique is not possible in very small children, but can often be used (and is recommended) anteriorly, for investigating traumatized permanent incisors. The reproducibility afforded by this technique is invaluable for future comparative purposes.

A modified bisected angle technique is possible in most children, with the image receptor placed flat in the mouth (in the occlusal plane) and the position of the X-ray tubehead adjusted accordingly, as shown in Figure 10.43.

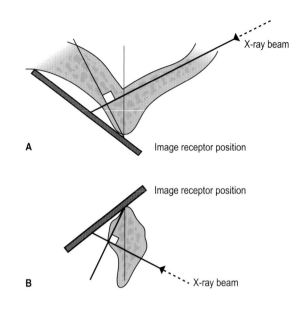

Fig. 10.41 Diagrams showing the relative position of the image receptor and X-ray beam. **A** For the molar region of an edentulous maxillary ridge. **B** For the molar region of an edentulous mandibular ridge.

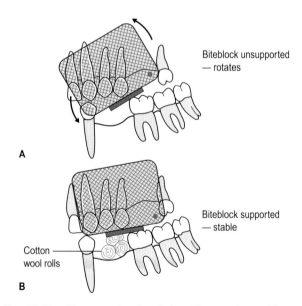

Fig. 10.42 Diagrams showing **A** the effect on the position of the image receptor and holder created by an edentulous area, and **B** how the problem can be solved using cottonwool rolls to rebuild the edentulous area, thus supporting the bite block.

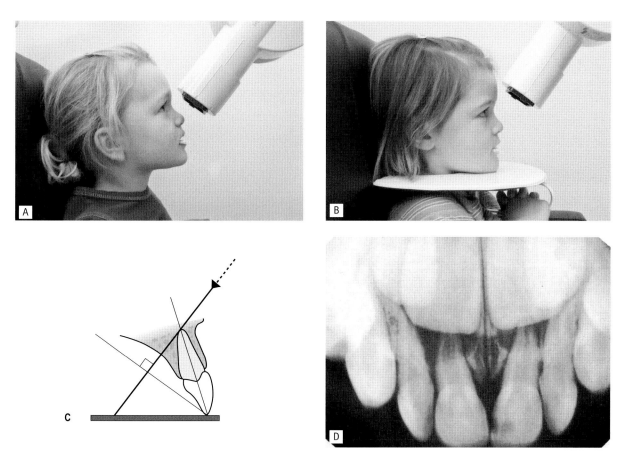

Fig. 10.43   Positioning for a child's maxillary incisors **A** in 3-year-old and **B** in a 6-year-old showing the use of a thyroid shield. **C** Diagram showing the relative positions of the image receptor, in the occlusal plane, and the X-ray beam. **D** An example of the resultant radiograph.

Assessment of image quality

Assessment of the quality of **all** radiographic images should be regarded as a routine part of any quality assurance (QA) programme (see Ch. 18). Essentially image quality assessment involves three separate stages, namely:

- Comparison of the image against ideal quality criteria
- Subjective rating of image quality using published standards
- Detailed assessment of rejected films to determine the sources of error.

Ideal quality criteria

Irrespective of the type of image receptor or technique being used, typical quality criteria for a periapical radiograph should include:

- The image should have acceptable definition with no distortion or blurring.
- The image should include the correct anatomical area together with the apices of the tooth/teeth under investigation with at least 3–4 mm of surrounding bone.
- There should be no overlap of the approximal surfaces of the teeth.

- The desired density and contrast for film-captured images will depend on the clinical reasons for taking the radiograph, e.g.
  - to assess *caries, restorations and the periapical tissues* films should be well exposed and show good contrast to allow differentiation between enamel and dentine and between the periodontal ligament space, the lamina dura and trabecullar bone.
  - to assess the *periodontal status* films should be under-exposed to avoid *burnout* of the thin alveolar crestal bone. (see Ch. 23)
- The images should be free of *coning off* or *cone-cutting* and other film handling errors.
- The images should be comparable with previous periapical images both geometrically and in density and contrast.

Subjective rating of image quality

A simple three-point subjective rating scale for all intra-oral and extra-oral film-captured radiographs was published in the UK in 2001 in the *Guidance Notes for Dental Practitioners on the Safe Use of X-ray Equipment*. A summary is shown in Table 10.1, and is repeated in Chapters 11 and 17. Image quality is discussed in detail, together with the errors associated with exposure factors and chemical processing, in Chapter 18. Patient preparation and positioning errors in periapical radiography are described below.

Assessment of rejected films and determination of errors

Patient preparation and positioning (radiographic technique) errors (Fig. 10.44)
These can include:

- Failure to remove dentures or orthodontic appliances
- Failure to position the image receptor correctly to capture the area of interest, thereby failing to image the apices and periapical tissues
- Failure to position the image receptor correctly causing it to bend (if flexible) creating geometrical distortion
- Failure to orientate the image receptor correctly and using it back-to-front
- Failure to align the X-ray tubehead correctly in the horizontal plane, either
  - Too far anteriorly or posteriorly (*coning off* or *cone cutting*)
  - Not aimed through the contact areas at right angles to the teeth and the image receptor causing overlapping of the contact areas
- Failure to align the X-ray tubehead correctly in the vertical plane, either
  - Too far superiorly or inferiorly (*coning off* or *cone cutting*)
  - Too steep an angle causing foreshortening and geometrical distortion
  - Too shallow an angle causing elongation and geometrical distortion
- Failure to instruct the patient to remain still during the exposure with subsequent movement resulting in blurring
- Failure to set correct exposure settings (see Ch. 18)
- Careless inadvertent use of the image receptor twice.

Note: Many of these technique errors can be avoided by using the paralleling technique utilizing image receptor holders with beam-aiming devices.

Table 10.1 Subjective quality rating criteria for film-captured images published in the 2001 *Guidance Notes for Dental Practitioners on the Safe Use of X-ray Equipment*

Rating	Quality	Basis
1	Excellent	No errors of patient preparation, exposure, positioning, processing or film handling
2	Diagnostically acceptable	Some errors of patient preparation, exposure, positioning, processing or film handling, but which do not detract from the diagnostic utility of the radiograph
3	Unacceptable	Errors of patient preparation, exposure, positioning, processing or film handling, which render the radiograph diagnostically unacceptable

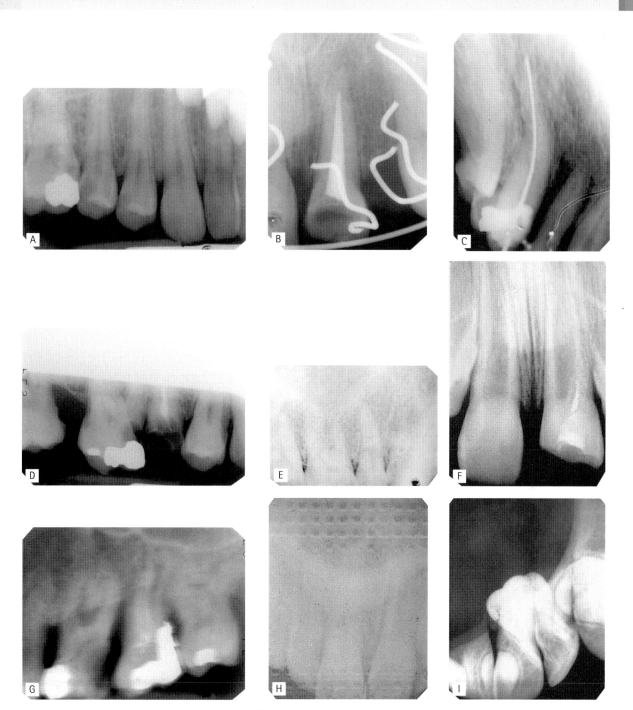

Fig. 10.44   A selection of patient preparation and positioning (radiographic technique) errors.

A Image receptor not positioned sufficiently apically to cover the area of interest — apices and periapical tissues not shown.

B Failure to remove an orthodontic appliance.

C Image receptor positioned incorrectly and bent during exposure — image geometically distorted.

D Failure to align the X-ray tubehead correctly in the vertical plane — *coning off* of the superior part of the image.

E X-ray tubehead positioned at too steep an angle in the vertical plane — foreshortening and geometrical distortion of the image.

F X-ray tubehead positioned at too shallow an angle in the vertical plane — elongation and geometrical distortion of the image.

G Failure to instruct the patient to remain still — image blurred as a result of movement.

H Image receptor (film packet) incorrectly placed back to front — pattern of the lead foil is evident.

I Image receptor (film packet) inadvertently used twice — double exposure.

Chapter 11

Bitewing radiography

Bitewing radiographs take their name from the original technique which required the patient to *bite* on a small *wing* attached to an intraoral film packet (see Fig. 11.1). Modern techniques use holders, as shown later, which have eliminated the need for the wing (now termed a *tab*), and digital image receptors (solid-state or phosphor plate) can be used instead of film, but the terminology and clinical indications have remained the same. An individual image is designed to show the crowns of the premolar and molar teeth on one side of the jaws.

MAIN INDICATIONS

These include:

- Detection of lesions of caries
- Monitoring the progression of dental caries

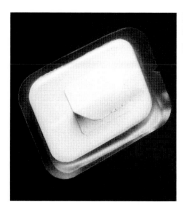

Fig.11.1 An intraoral barrier-wrapped film packet with a *wing* or *tab* attached.

- Assessment of existing restorations
- Assessment of the periodontal status.

IDEAL TECHNIQUE REQUIREMENTS

These include:

- An appropriate image receptor holder with beam aiming device should be used and is recommended in the UK in the 2001 *Guidance Notes for Dental Practitioners on the Safe Use of X-ray Equipment.*
- The image receptor should be positioned centrally within the holder with the upper and lower edges of the image receptor parallel to the bite-platform.
- The image receptor should be positioned with its long axis horizontally for a *horizontal bitewing* or vertically for a *vertical bitewing* (Fig. 11.2).
- The posterior teeth and the image receptor should be in contact or as close together as possible.
- The posterior teeth and the image receptor should be parallel — the shape of the dental arch may necessitate two separate image receptor positions to achieve this requirement for both the premolar and the molar teeth (Fig. 11.3).
- The beam aiming device should ensure that in the horizontal plane, the X-ray tubehead is aimed so that the beam meets the teeth and the image receptor at right angles, and passes directly through **all** the contact areas (Fig. 11.3).
- The beam aiming device should ensure that in the vertical plane, the X-ray tubehead is aimed

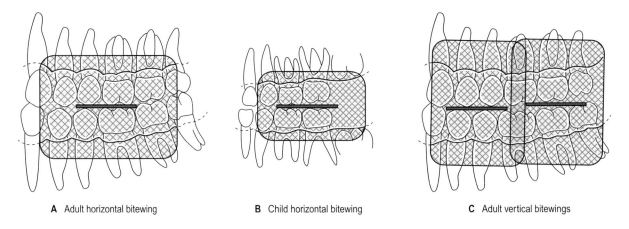

A Adult horizontal bitewing   **B** Child horizontal bitewing   **C** Adult vertical bitewings

Fig. 11.2 Diagrams showing the ideal image receptor positions for different types of bitewings.

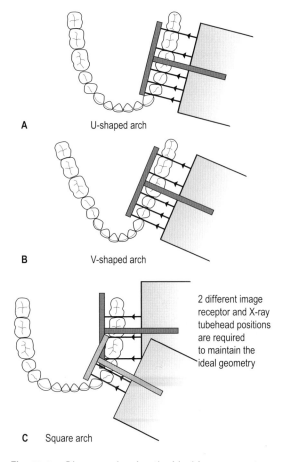

A   U-shaped arch

B   V-shaped arch

2 different image receptor and X-ray tubehead positions are required to maintain the ideal geometry

C   Square arch

Fig. 11.3 Diagrams showing the ideal image receptor and X-ray tubehead positions (determined by the beam aiming device) for different arch shapes.

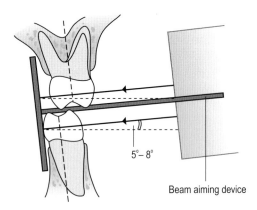

5°– 8°

Beam aiming device

Fig. 11.4 Diagram showing the ideal image receptor position and the approximate 5°– 8° downward vertical angulation of the X-ray beam (determined by the beam aiming device) compensating for the curve of Monson.

downwards (approximately 5°–8° to the horizontal) to compensate for the upwardly rising curve of Monson (Fig. 11.4).

● The positioning should be reproducible.

It is sometimes not possible to use an image receptor holder (with beam aiming device) and achieve these ideal technical requirements — particularly in children. Clinicians therefore still need to be aware of the original technique of using a tab attached to the film packet or phosphor plate and aligning the X-ray tubehead by eye.

POSITIONING TECHNIQUES

Using image receptor holders with beam aiming devices

Several image receptor holders with different beam aiming devices have been produced for use with film packets or digital phosphor plates and with digital solid state sensors, held either horizontally or vertically. A selection of different holders is shown in Figure 11.5. As in periapical radiography, the choice of holder is a matter of personal preference and dependent upon the type of image receptors being employed. The various holders vary in cost and design but essentially

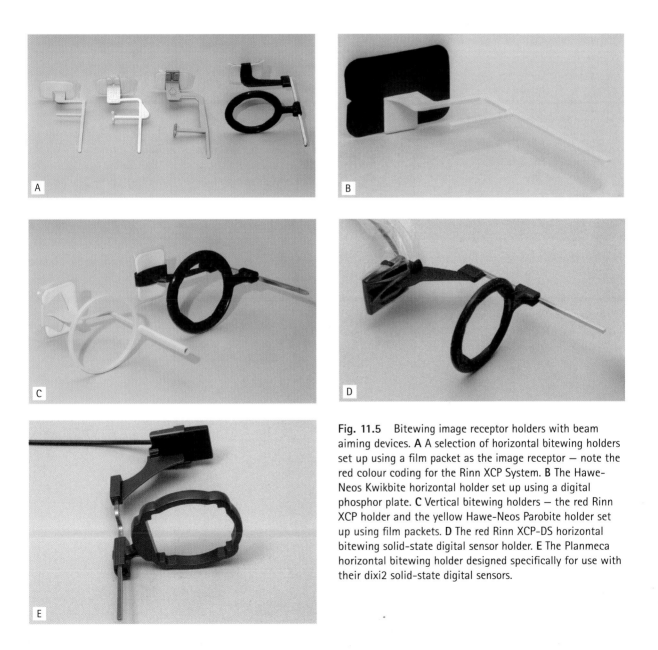

Fig. 11.5 Bitewing image receptor holders with beam aiming devices. **A** A selection of horizontal bitewing holders set up using a film packet as the image receptor — note the red colour coding for the Rinn XCP System. **B** The Hawe-Neos Kwikbite horizontal holder set up using a digital phosphor plate. **C** Vertical bitewing holders — the red Rinn XCP holder and the yellow Hawe-Neos Parobite holder set up using film packets. **D** The red Rinn XCP-DS horizontal bitewing solid-state digital sensor holder. **E** The Planmeca horizontal bitewing holder designed specifically for use with their dixi2 solid-state digital sensors.

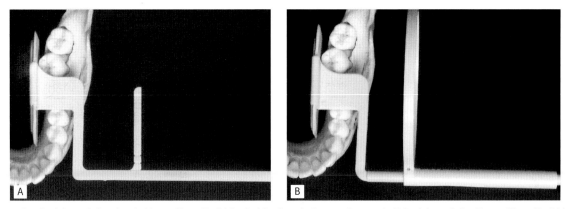

Fig. 11.6A Position of the simple Hawe-Neos Kwikbite holder in relation to the teeth. **B** Position of the Hawe-Neos Kwikbite holder (with circular beam-aiming device) in relation to the teeth.

consist of the same three basic components that make up periapical holders (see Ch. 10), namely:

- A mechanism for holding the image receptor parallel to the teeth
- A bite-platform that replaces the original *wing*
- An X-ray beam-aiming device.

The radiographic technique can be summarized as follows:

1. The desired holder is selected together with an appropriate sized image receptor — typically a 31 × 41 mm film packet or phosphor plate or the equivalent sized solid-state sensor.
2. The patient is positioned with the head supported and with the occlusal plane horizontal.
3. The holder is inserted carefully into the lingual sulcus opposite the posterior teeth.

4. The anterior edge of the image receptor should be positioned opposite the distal aspect of the lower canine — in this position the image receptor extends usually just beyond the mesial aspect of the lower third molar (see Fig. 11.6).
5. The patient is asked to close the teeth firmly together onto the bite platform. (Note: Extra care needs to be taken of solid state sensor cables.)
6. The X-ray tubehead is aligned accurately using the beam aiming device to achieve optimal horizontal and vertical angulations (see Fig. 11.7).
7. The exposure is made.
8. If required, the procedure is repeated for the premolar teeth with a new image receptor and X-ray tubehead position.

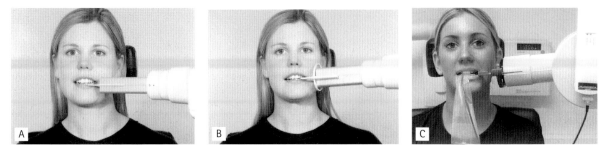

Fig 11.7 Clinical positioning for **A** Simple Hawe-Neos Kwikbite holder using a film packet or digital phosphor plate, **B** Hawe-Neos holder (with circular beam aiming device) using a film packet or digital phosphor plate and **C** Planmeca holder using a solid-state digital sensor.

Advantages
- Relatively simple and straightforward.
- Image receptor is held firmly in position and cannot be displaced by the tongue.
- Position of X-ray tubehead is determined by the beaming device so assisting the operator in ensuring that the X-ray beam is always at right angles to the image receptor.
- Avoids *coning off* or *cone cutting* of the anterior part of the image receptor.
- Holders are autoclavable or disposable.

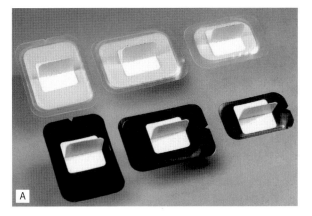

Disadvantages
- Position of the holder in the mouth is operator-dependent, therefore images are not 100% reproducible, so still not ideal for monitoring progression of caries.
- Positioning of the film holder and image receptor can be uncomfortable for the patient particularly when using solid-state digital sensors.
- Some holders are relatively expensive.
- Holders not usually suitable for children.

Using a tab attached to the image receptor

The traditional bitewing technique is particularly suitable when using film packets or digital phosphor plates as the image receptor. Although, as explained below, the technique is very operator-dependent and not recommended for adults, it is still widely used for children.

The radiographic technique can be summarized as follows:

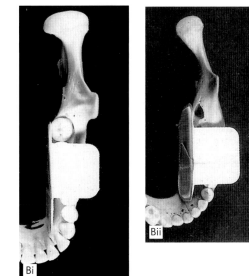

Fig. 11.8A Film packets and phosphor plates with tabs attached suitable for adult *vertical* bitewings, adult *horizontal* bitewings and child's *horizontal* bitewings. **B** The ideal bitewing and film packet position in relation to the teeth for **(i)** an adult and **(ii)** a child.

1. The appropriate sized barrier-wrapped film packet or phosphor plate is selected and the tab attached, orientated appropriately for *horizontal* or *vertical* projections, as shown in Figure 11.8A:
   - Large film packets/phosphor plates (31 × 41 mm) for adults
   - Small film packets/phosphor plates (22 × 35 mm) for children under 12 years. Once the second permanent molars have erupted the adult size is required
   - Occasionally a long film packet/phosphor plate (53 × 26 mm) is used for adults.

2. The patient is positioned with the head supported and with the occlusal plane horizontal.
3. The shape of the dental arch and the number of films required are assessed.
4. The operator holds the tab between thumb and forefinger and inserts the image receptor into the lingual sulcus opposite the posterior teeth.

5. The anterior edge of the image receptor should again be positioned opposite the distal aspect of the lower canine — in this position, the posterior edge of the film packet extends usually just beyond the mesial aspect of the lower third molar (see Fig. 11.8B).

6. The tab is placed on to the occlusal surfaces of the lower teeth.

7. The patient is asked to close the teeth firmly together on the tab.

8. As the patient closes the teeth, the operator pulls the tab firmly between the teeth to ensure that the image receptor and teeth are in contact.

9. The operator releases the tab.

10. The operator assesses the horizontal and vertical angulations and positions the X-ray tubehead so that the X-ray beam is aimed directly through the contact areas, at right angles to the teeth and the image receptor, with an approximately 5°–8° downward vertical angulation (see Fig. 11.9A and B).

11. The exposure is made.

12. If required, the procedure is repeated for the premolar teeth with a new image receptor and X-ray tubehead position.

Note: When positioning the X-ray tubehead, after the patient has closed the mouth, the film can no longer be seen. To ensure that the anterior part of the image receptor is exposed and to avoid *coning off* and *cone cutting*, a simple guide to remember is that the front edge of the open-ended spacer cone should be positioned adjacent to the corner of the mouth.

Advantages
- Simple.
- Inexpensive.
- The tabs are disposable, so no extra cross-infection control procedures required.
- Can be used easily in children.

Disadvantages
- Arbitrary, operator-dependent assessment of horizontal and vertical angulations of the X-ray tubehead.

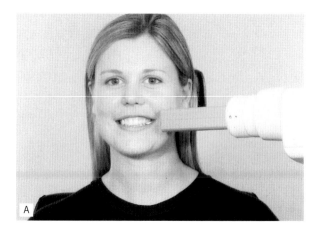

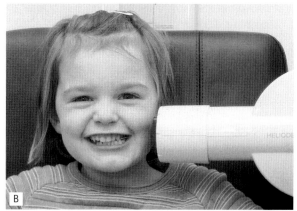

Fig. 11.9A   Adult patient and X-ray tubehead positioning for a left bitewing. **B** Positioning for a child.

- Images not accurately reproducible, so not ideal for monitoring the progression of caries.
- *Coning off* or *cone cutting* of anterior part of image receptor is common,
- Not compatible with using solid-state digital sensors.
- The tongue can easily displace the image receptor.

RESULTANT RADIOGRAPHS

Whichever radiographic technique is used, the resultant radiographic images and the anatomical structures they show are very similar — it is their accuracy that varies. Examples are shown in Figure 11.10–11.12.

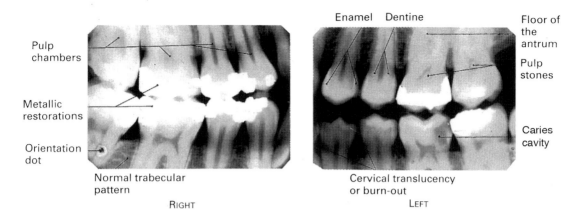

Enamel   Dentine

Pulp
chambers

Metallic
restorations

Orientation
dot

Normal trabecular
pattern

RIGHT

Floor of
the
antrum

Pulp
stones

Caries
cavity

Cervical translucency
or burn-out

LEFT

Fig. 11.10 Examples of typical RIGHT and LEFT horizontal adult bitewing radiographs, suitable for the assessment of caries and restorations, with the main radiographic features indicated.

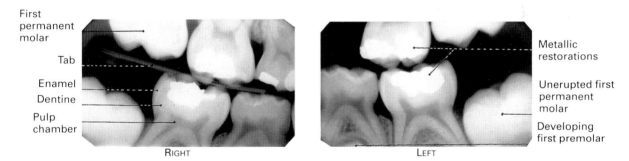

First
permanent
molar

Tab

Enamel

Dentine

Pulp
chamber

RIGHT

Metallic
restorations

Unerupted first
permanent
molar

Developing
first premolar

LEFT

Fig. 11.11 Examples of typical RIGHT and LEFT bitewing radiographs of a child with the main radiographic features indicated.

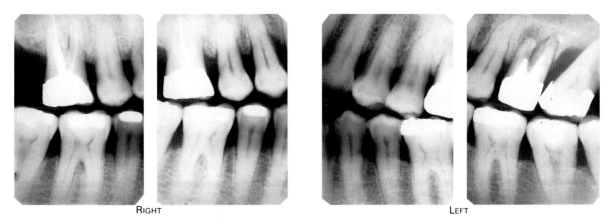

RIGHT   LEFT

Fig. 11.12 Example of typical RIGHT and LEFT vertical adult bitewing radiographs. Note that two films are used on each side to image both the premolars and molars.

Assessment of image quality

As described in Chapter 10, image quality assessment essentially involves three separate stages, namely:

- Comparison of the image against ideal quality criteria
- Subjective rating of image quality using published standards
- Detailed assessment of rejected films to determine the source of error.

Ideal quality criteria

Irrespective of the type of image receptor being used, typical quality criteria for a bitewing radiograph should include:

- The image should have acceptable definition with no distortion or blurring.
- The image should include from the mesial surface of the first premolar to the distal surface of the second molar — if the third molars are erupted then the 7/8 contact should be included.
- The occlusal plane/bite-platform should be in the middle of the image so that the crowns and coronal parts of the roots of the maxillary teeth are shown in the upper half of the image and the crowns and coronal parts of the roots of the mandibular teeth are shown in the lower half of the image, and the buccal and lingual cusps should be superimposed.
- The maxillary and mandibular alveolar crests should be shown.
- There should be no overlap of the approximal surfaces of the teeth.
- The desired density and contrast for film-captured images will depend on the clinical reasons for taking the radiograph, e.g.
  - to assess *caries and restorations* films should be well exposed and show good contrast to allow differentiation between enamel and dentine and to allow the enamel–dentine junction (EDJ) to be seen.
  - to assess the *periodontal status* films should be under-exposed to avoid *burn-out* of the thin alveolar crestal bone (See Ch. 21).
- The image should be free of *coning off* or *cone-cutting* and other film handling errors.

Table 11.1 Subjective quality rating criteria for film-captured images published in the 2001 *Guidance Notes for Dental Practitioners on the Safe Use of X-ray Equipment*

Rating	Quality	Basis
1	Excellent	No errors of patient preparation, exposure, positioning, processing or film handling
2	Diagnostically acceptable	Some errors of patient preparation, exposure, positioning, processing or film handling, but which do not detract from the diagnostic utility of the radiograph
3	Unacceptable	Errors of patient preparation, exposure, positioning, processing or film handling, which render the radiograph diagnostically unacceptable

- The image should be comparable with previous bitewing images both geometrically and in density and contrast.

Subjective rating of image quality

The simple three-point subjective rating scale published in the 2001 *Guidance Notes* was introduced in Chapter 10 and is discussed in detail, together with the errors associated with exposure factors and chemical processing, in Chapter 18. A summary is shown again in Table 11.1. Patient preparation and positioning errors in bitewing radiography are described below.

Assessment of rejected films and determination of errors

Patient preparation and positioning (radiographic technique) errors (Fig. 11.13)
These can include:

- Positioning the image receptor too far posteriorly in the mouth thereby failing to image the premolar teeth.
- Failure to insert image receptor correctly into the lingual sulcus between the tongue and posterior teeth allowing the tongue to displace the film.

- Failure to align the X-ray tubehead correctly in the horizontal plane, either
  - Too far posteriorly (*coning off* or *cone cutting*)
  - Too far anteriorly — rarely (*coning off* or *cone cutting*)
  - Not aimed through the contact areas at right angles to the line of the arch and the image receptor causing overlapping of the contact areas.
- Failure to align the X-ray tubehead correctly in the vertical plane thereby not superimposing the buccal and lingual cusps.

- Failure to set correct exposure settings.
- Failure to instruct the patient to remain still during the exposure with subsequent movement resulting in blurring.

Note: Many of these positioning errors can be avoided by using image receptor holders with beam-aiming devices but are relatively common when not using a holder and aligning and positioning the X-ray tubehead without a guide.

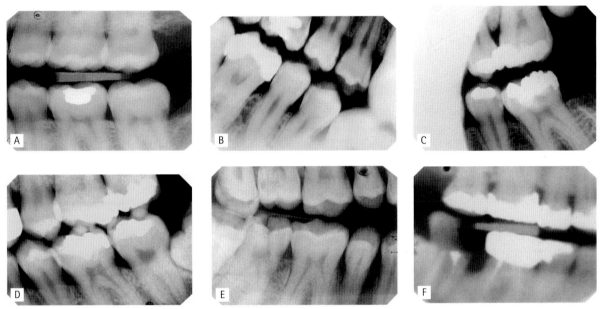

Fig. 11.13   A selection of bitewings showing patient preparation and positioning errors.
A Image receptor positioned too far posteriorly — the edentulous area distal to the lower second is imaged but not the premolar teeth.
B Image receptor displaced by tongue — occlusal plane not horizontal.
C Failure to align the X-ray tubehead correctly in the horizontal plane — *coning off* of the anterior part of the image.
D Failure to align the X-ray tubehead correctly in the horizontal plane — overlapping of the contact areas.
E Failure to align the X-ray tubehead correctly in the vertical plane — buccal and lingual cusps not superimposed and distortion of the teeth.
F Failure to instruct the patient to remain still — image blurred as a result of movement.

Chapter **12**

Occlusal radiography

Occlusal radiography is defined as those intraoral radiographic techniques taken using a dental X-ray set where the image receptor (film packet or digital phosphor plate — 5.7 × 7.6 cm) is placed in the occlusal plane. Suitable sized solid-state digital sensors are not currently available.

TERMINOLOGY AND CLASSIFICATION

The terminology used in occlusal radiography is very confusing. The British Standards Glossary of Dental Terms (BS 4492: 1983) is inadequate in defining the various occlusal projections and in differentiating between them. The result is that there is still little uniformity in terminology.

The terminology used here is based broadly on the British Standards terms, shown in parentheses, but they have been modified in an attempt to make them more explicit, straightforward and practical so that often the name of the view indicates how it is taken.

Maxillary occlusal projections

- *Upper standard occlusal* (standard occlusal)
- *Upper oblique occlusal* (oblique occlusal)
- *Vertex occlusal* (vertex occlusal) — no longer used.

Mandibular occlusal projections

- *Lower 90° occlusal* (true occlusal)
- *Lower 45° (or anterior) occlusal* (standard occlusal)
- *Lower oblique occlusal* (oblique occlusal).

Upper standard (or anterior) occlusal

This projection shows the anterior part of the maxilla and the upper anterior teeth.

Main clinical indications

- Periapical assessment of the upper anterior teeth, especially in children but also in adults unable to tolerate periapical holders
- Detecting the presence of unerupted canines, supernumeraries and odontomes
- As the midline view, when using the parallax method for determining the bucco/palatal position of unerupted canines (see Ch. 25)
- Evaluation of the size and extent of lesions such as cysts or tumours in the anterior maxilla
- Assessment of fractures of the anterior teeth and alveolar bone. It is especially useful in children following trauma because image receptor placement is straightforward.

Technique and positioning

1. The patient is seated with the head supported and with the occlusal plane horizontal and parallel to the floor and is asked to support a protective thyroid shield.
2. The image receptor, suitably barrier wrapped, is placed flat into the mouth on to the occlusal surfaces of the lower teeth. The patient is asked to bite together gently. The image receptor is placed centrally in the mouth with its long axis crossways in adults and antero-posteriorly in children.

3. The X-ray tubehead is positioned above the patient in the midline, aiming downwards through the bridge of the nose at an angle of 65°–70° to the image receptor (see Fig. 12.1).

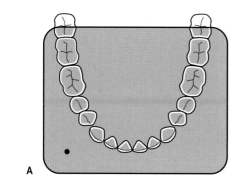

A

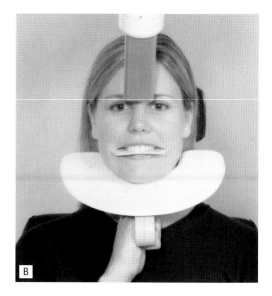

B

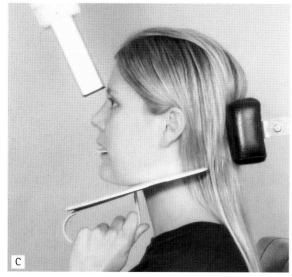

C

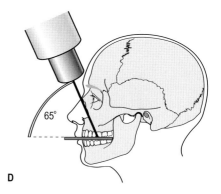

D

Fig. 12.1A   Diagram showing the position of the image receptor in relation to the lower arch. **B** Positioning from the front; note the use of the protective thyroid shield. **C** Positioning from the side. **D** Diagram showing the positioning from the side.

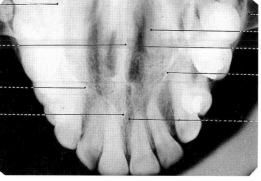

Naso-lacrimal canal

Nasal septum

Lateral wall of the nasal fossa

Anterior nasal spine

Maxillary antrum

Inferior turbinate

Nasal fossa

Lateral wall of the nasal fossa

Nasopalatine foramen

Fig. 12.2   An example of an upper standard occlusal radiograph with the main anatomical features indicated.

Upper oblique occlusal

This projection shows the posterior part of the maxilla and the upper posterior teeth on one side.

Main clinical indications

- Periapical assessment of the upper posterior teeth, especially in adults unable to tolerate periapical image receptor holders
- Evaluation of the size and extent of lesions such as cysts, tumours or other bone lesions affecting the posterior maxilla
- Assessment of the condition of the antral floor
- As an aid to determining the position of roots displaced inadvertently into the antrum during attempted extraction of upper posterior teeth
- Assessment of fractures of the posterior teeth and associated alveolar bone including the tuberosity.

Technique and positioning

1. The patient is seated with the head supported and with the occlusal plane horizontal and parallel to the floor.
2. The image receptor, suitably barrier wrapped, is inserted into the mouth on to the occlusal surfaces of the lower teeth, with its long axis anteroposteriorly. It is placed to the side of the mouth under investigation, and the patient is asked to bite together gently.
3. The X-ray tubehead is positioned to the side of the patient's face, aiming downwards through the cheek at an angle of 65°–70° to the image receptor, centring on the region of interest (see Fig. 12.3).

Note: If the X-ray tubehead is positioned too far posteriorly, the shadow cast by the body of the zygoma will obscure the posterior teeth.

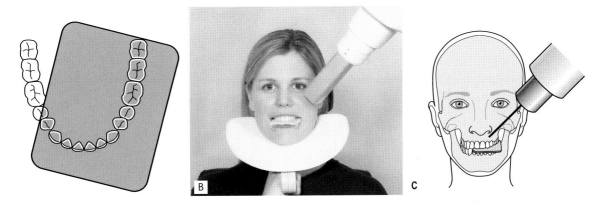

Fig. 12.3A Diagram showing the position of the image receptor in relation to the lower arch for a LEFT upper oblique occlusal. **B** Positioning for the LEFT upper oblique occlusal from the front; note the use of the protective thyroid shield. **C** Diagram showing the positioning from the front.

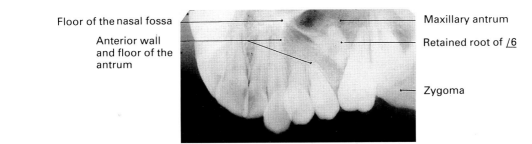

Floor of the nasal fossa

Anterior wall and floor of the antrum

Maxillary antrum

Retained root of /6

Zygoma

Fig. 12.4 An example of an upper left oblique occlusal radiograph with the main anatomical features indicated.

Lower 90° occlusal

This projection shows a plan view of the tooth-bearing portion of the mandible and the floor of the mouth. A minor variation of the technique is also used to show unilateral lesions.

Main clinical indications

- Detection of the presence and position of radiopaque calculi in the submandibular salivary ducts
- Assessment of the bucco-lingual position of unerupted mandibular teeth
- Evaluation of the bucco-lingual expansion of the body of the mandible by cysts, tumours or other bone lesions
- Assessment of displacement fractures of the anterior body of the mandible in the horizontal plane.

Technique and positioning

1. The image receptor, suitably barrier wrapped and facing downwards, is placed centrally into the mouth, on to the occlusal surfaces of the lower teeth, with its long axis crossways. The patient is asked to bite together gently.
2. The patient *then* leans forwards and *then* tips the head backwards as far as is comfortable, where it is supported.
3. The X-ray tubehead, with circular collimator fitted, is placed below the patient's chin, in the midline, centring on an imaginary line joining the first molars, at an angle of 90° to the image receptor (see Fig. 12.5).

Variation of technique. To show a particular part of the mandible, the image receptor is placed in the mouth with its long axis anteroposteriorly over the area of interest. The X-ray tubehead, still aimed at 90° to the film, is centred below the body of the mandible in that area.

Note: The lower 90° occlusal is mounted as if the examiner were looking into the patient's mouth. The radiographic film is therefore mounted with the embossed dot pointing *away* from the examiner.

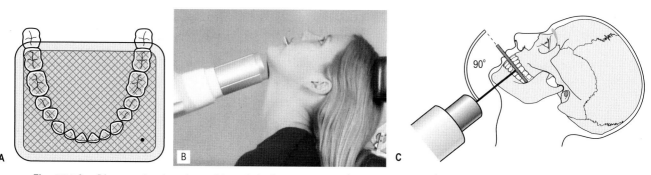

Fig. 12.5A Diagram showing the position of the image receptor (facing downwards) in relation to the lower arch. **B** Positioning for the lower 90° occlusal from the side. **C** Diagram showing the positioning from the side.

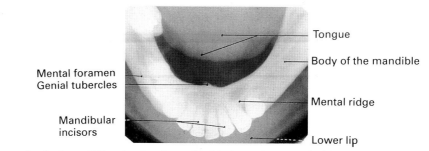

Tongue
Body of the mandible
Mental foramen
Genial tubercles
Mental ridge
Mandibular incisors
Lower lip

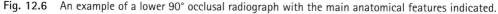

Fig. 12.6 An example of a lower 90° occlusal radiograph with the main anatomical features indicated.

Lower 45° (or anterior) occlusal

This projection is taken to show the lower anterior teeth and the anterior part of the mandible. The resultant radiograph resembles a large bisected angle technique periapical of this region.

Main clinical indication

- Periapical assessment of the lower incisor teeth, especially useful in adults and children unable to tolerate periapical image receptor holders
- Evaluation of the size and extent of lesions such as cysts or tumours affecting the anterior part of the mandible

- Assessment of displacement fractures of the anterior mandible in the vertical plane.

Technique and positioning

1. The patient is seated with the head supported and with the occlusal plane horizontal and parallel to the floor.
2. The image receptor, suitably barrier wrapped and facing downwards, is placed centrally into the mouth, on to the occlusal surfaces of the lower teeth, with its long axis anteroposteriorly, and the patient is asked to bite gently together.
3. The X-ray tubehead is positioned in the midline, centring through the chin point, at an angle of 45° to the image receptor (see Fig. 12.7).

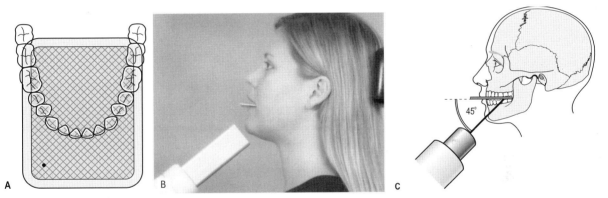

Fig. 12.7A   Diagram showing the position of the image receptor (facing downwards) in relation to the lower arch. **B** Positioning for the lower 45° occlusal from the side. **C** Diagram showing the positioning from the side.

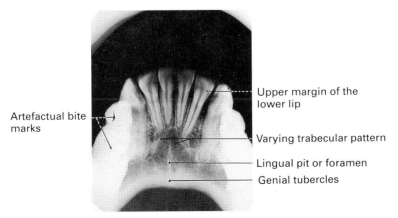

Fig. 12.8   An example of a lower 45° occlusal radiograph with the main anatomical features indicated.

Lower oblique occlusal

This projection is designed to allow the image of the submandibular salivary gland, on the side of interest, to be projected on to the film. However, because the X-ray beam is oblique, all the anatomical tissues shown are distorted.

Main clinical indications

- Detection of radiopaque calculi in the submandibular salivary gland of interest
- Assessment of the bucco-lingual position of unerupted lower wisdom teeth
- Evaluation of the extent and expansion of cysts, tumours or other bone lesions in the posterior part of the body and angle of the mandible.

Technique and positioning

1. The image receptor, suitably barrier wrapped, and facing downwards, is inserted into the mouth, on to the occlusal surfaces of the lower teeth, over to the side under investigation, with its long axis anteroposteriorly. The patient is asked to bite together gently.
2. The patient's head is supported, then rotated away from the side under investigation and the chin is raised. This rotated positioning allows the subsequent positioning of the X-ray tubehead.
3. The X-ray tubehead with circular collimator is aimed upwards and forwards towards the image receptor, from below and behind the angle of the mandible and parallel to the lingual surface of the mandible (see Fig. 12.9).

Note: The lower oblique occlusal radiographic film is also mounted with the embossed dot pointing *away* from the examiner.

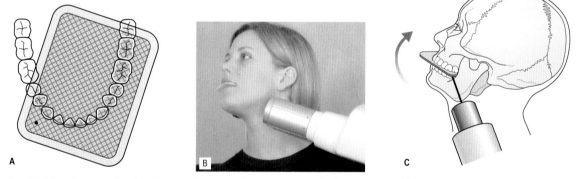

Fig. 12.9A   Diagram showing the position of the image receptor (facing downwards) in relation to the lower arch for the LEFT lower oblique occlusal. **B** Positioning for the LEFT lower oblique occlusal from the side. **C** Diagram showing the positioning from the side and indicating that the patient's chin is raised and that the head is rotated AWAY from the side under investigation.

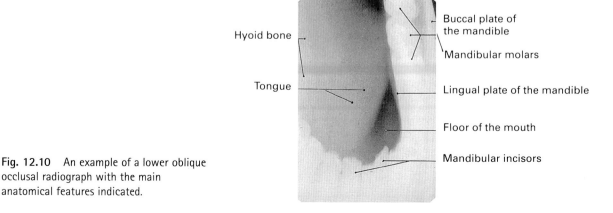

Hyoid bone

Tongue

Buccal plate of the mandible

Mandibular molars

Lingual plate of the mandible

Floor of the mouth

Mandibular incisors

Fig. 12.10   An example of a lower oblique occlusal radiograph with the main anatomical features indicated.

Chapter 13

Oblique lateral radiography

INTRODUCTION

Oblique lateral radiographs are extraoral views of the jaws that can be taken using a dental X-ray set (see Fig. 13.1). Before the development of dental panoramic equipment they were the routine extraoral radiographs used both in hospitals and in general practice. In recent years, their popularity has waned, but the limitations of panoramic radiographs (see Ch. 17) have ensured that oblique lateral radiographs still have an important role.

TERMINOLOGY

Lateral radiographs of the head and jaws are divided into:

- True laterals
- Oblique laterals
- Bimolars (two oblique laterals on one film).

The differentiating adjectives *true* and *oblique* are used to indicate the relationship of the image receptor, patient and X-ray beam, as shown in Figure 13.2.

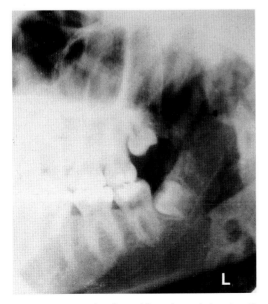

Fig. 13.1 An example of an oblique lateral showing the left molars.

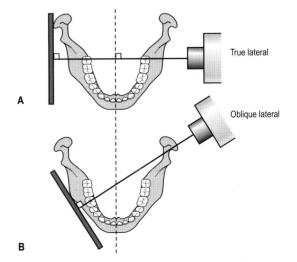

Fig. 13.2 Diagrams showing what is meant by the terms *true* and *oblique* lateral.

True lateral positioning

The image receptor and the sagittal plane of the patient's head are parallel and the X-ray beam is perpendicular to both of them. This is the positioning for the *true lateral skull radiograph* taken in a cephalostat unit described in Chapter 15.

Oblique lateral positioning

The image receptor and the sagittal plane of the patient's head are **not** parallel. The X-ray beam is aimed perpendicular to the image receptor but is *oblique* to the sagittal plane of the patient. A variety of different *oblique lateral* projections is possible with different head and X-ray beam positions.

MAIN INDICATIONS

The main clinical indications for oblique lateral radiographs include:

- Assessment of the presence and/or position of unerupted teeth
- Detection of fractures of the mandible
- Evaluation of lesions or conditions affecting the jaws including cysts, tumours, giant cell lesions, and other bone lesions
- As an alternative when intraoral views are unobtainable because of severe gagging or if the patient is unable to open the mouth or is unconscious (see Ch. 9, Fig. 9.1)
- As specific views of the salivary glands or temporomandibular joints.

EQUIPMENT REQUIRED

This includes (see Fig. 13.3):

- A dental X-ray set
- An extraoral cassette containing film and intensifying screens or a digital phosphor plate (usually 13 × 18 cm)
- A lead shield to cover half the cassette when taking bimolar views.

Specially constructed angle boards as shown in Figure 13.3B can be used to facilitate positioning, but are not considered necessary by the author.

BASIC TECHNIQUE PRINCIPLES

As stated, a wide range of different oblique lateral projections of the jaws are possible. However, all the variations rely on the same basic principles regarding the position of:

- The cassette (image receptor)
- The patient's head
- The X-ray tubehead.

Cassette position

The cassette is held by the patient against the side of the face overlying the area of the jaws under investigation. The exact position of the cassette is determined by the area of interest.

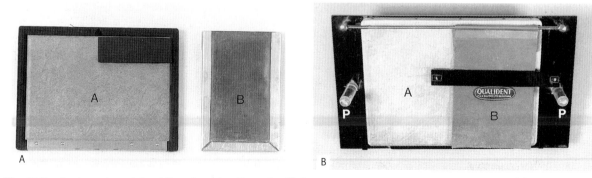

Fig. 13.3   Equipment used for oblique lateral radiography. (i) An 13 × 18 cm cassette **A** and lead shield **B**. (ii) An example of an angle board showing the cassette **A**, lead shield **B** and the plastic earpieces **P** for patient positioning.

Patient's head position

The patient is normally seated upright in the dental chair and is then instructed to:

1. *Rotate the head to the side of interest.* This is done to bring the contra-lateral ramus forwards, avoiding its superimposition and to increase the space available between the neck and shoulder in which to position the X-ray set.
2. *Raise the chin.* This is done to increase the triangular space between the back of the ramus and the cervical spine (the so-called *radiographic keyhole*, see Fig. 13.4) through which the X-ray beam will pass.

X-ray tubehead position

The X-ray tubehead is positioned on the opposite side of the patient's head to the cassette. There are two basic positions, depending on the area of the jaws under investigation:

- *Behind the ramus aiming through the radiographic keyhole.* The X-ray tubehead is positioned along the line of the occlusal plane, just below the ear, behind the ramus aiming through the radiographic keyhole at the particular maxillary **and** mandibular teeth under investigation. The view from this position is illustrated in Figure 13.4A. As shown, the X-ray beam will not pass directly between the contact areas of the posterior teeth. This may result in some overlapping of the crowns.
- *Beneath the lower border of the mandible.* The X-ray tubehead is positioned beneath the lower border of the contra-lateral body of the mandible, directly opposite the particular mandibular teeth under investigation, aiming slightly upwards. The view from this position is illustrated in Figure 13.4B. As shown, the X-ray beam will now pass between the contact areas of the teeth. However, there will still be some distortion of the image in the vertical plane owing to the upward angulation of the X-ray beam. In addition, the shadow of the body of the mandible will be superimposed over the maxillary teeth.

Once these principles are understood, the technique becomes straightforward and can be modified readily for different anatomical regions and clinical situations.

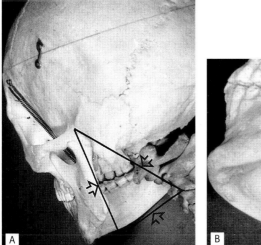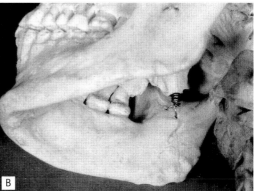

Fig. 13.4A The view through the *radiographic keyhole* (arrowed) showing the right mandibular and maxillary posterior teeth. Note the anterior teeth are obscured by the left ramus of the mandible. **B** The view from underneath the left body of the mandible showing the right mandible and right posterior mandibular teeth. Note the right maxillary teeth are obscured by the left body of the mandible.

POSITIONING EXAMPLES FOR VARIOUS OBLIQUE LATERAL RADIOGRAPHS

Examples of the required positioning for different oblique laterals and the resultant radiographs are shown in Figures 13.5–13.8. Illustrations show the positioning for both adults and children.

Important points to note

- For stability, a small child is usually rotated through 90° in the chair, so the shoulder is supported and the cassette and head can be rested on the headrest.
- The area under investigation determines the position of the cassette and the X-ray tubehead.
- An X-ray request for an oblique lateral must specify the **exact** region of the jaws required.

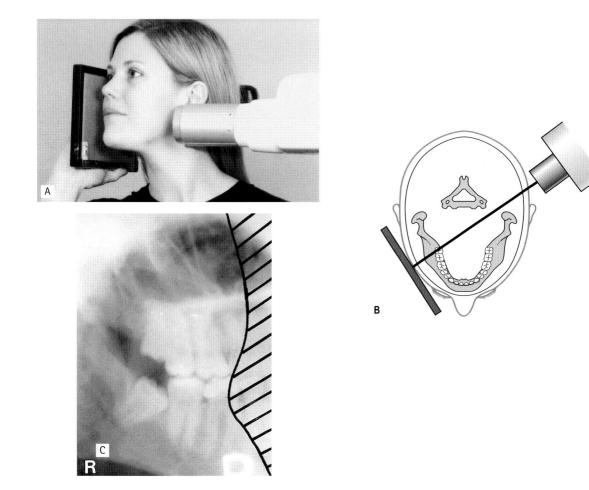

Fig. 13.5A Cassette and X-ray tubehead positions for the RIGHT mandibular **and** maxillary molars on an adult. **B** Diagram of the positioning from above showing the cassette overlying the molar teeth and the X-ray beam passing between the cervical spine and mandibular ramus. **C** A typical resultant radiograph. The shadow of the superimposed left ramus, overlying the premolars, has been drawn in to emphasize its position. Compare with Figure 13.4A. Note the radiograph is mounted and viewed as if the observer is looking at the patient's right side.

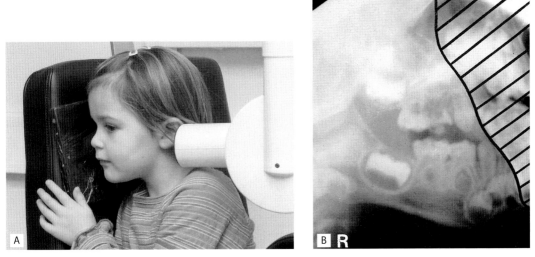

Fig. 13.6A   Positioning of a child, cassette and X-ray tubehead for the RIGHT deciduous maxillary and mandibular molars.
B A typical resultant radiograph. The shadow of the superimposed left ramus has been drawn in.

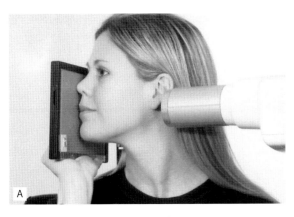

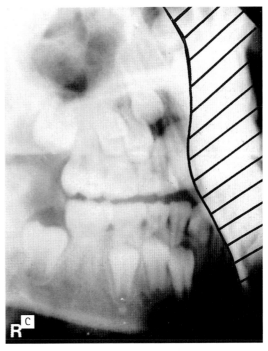

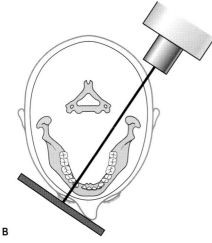

Fig. 13.7A   Cassette and X-ray tubehead positions for the RIGHT mandibular and maxillary canines. Note the displacement of the nose needed to achieve the desired position for the cassette. B Diagram of the positioning from above, showing the cassette overlying the canine teeth and the X-ray tubehead aimed through the *radiographic keyhole*. C A typical resultant radiograph of a patient in the mixed dentition. The shadow of the superimposed left ramus has been drawn in—it now overlies the lateral incisors. Again note the orientation of the radiograph and how it is viewed.

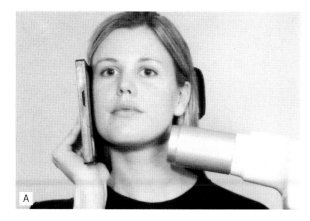

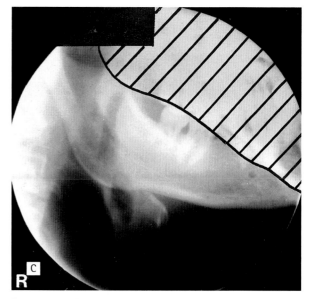

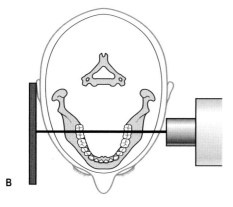

Fig. 13.8A Cassette and X-ray tubehead position for the RIGHT mandibular molars. Note the upward angulation of the X-ray tubehead and its position beneath the left body of the mandible. **B** Diagram of the positioning from above. Note the position of the X-ray tubehead and compare with Figure 13.5B. **C** A typical resultant radiograph showing the right mandibular molars. The superimposed shadow of the left mandibular body has been drawn in overlying the maxillary molars. Compare with Figure 13.4B.

BIMOLAR TECHNIQUE

As mentioned earlier, *bimolar* is the term used for the radiographic projection showing oblique lateral views of the right and left sides of the jaws on the different halves of the **same** radiograph as shown in Figure 13.9.

The technique can be summarized as follows:

1. The patient is positioned with one side of the face in the middle of one half of the cassette, with the nose towards the midline. The precise positioning depends on which teeth or area of the jaws are being examined (like any other oblique lateral).

2. The other half of the cassette is covered by a lead shield to prevent exposure of this side of the image receptor.
3. The X-ray tubehead is positioned to show the desired area, and the exposure is made.
4. The lead shield is then placed over the other side of the cassette to protect the part of the film already exposed.
5. The patient is then positioned in a similar manner with the cassette held on the other side of the face.
6. The X-ray tubehead is re-positioned and a second exposure made.

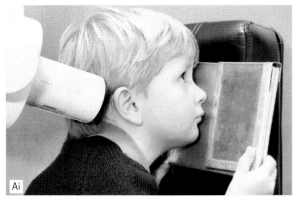

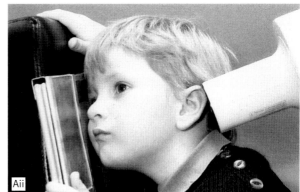

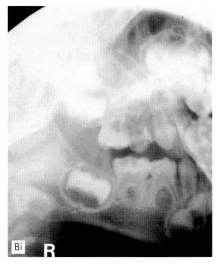

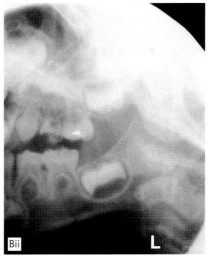

Fig. 13.9A   (i) Position of a child, cassette and X-ray tubehead for the LEFT side of the jaws and (ii) positioning for the RIGHT side. Note the lead shield covering the half of the cassette not being used. **B** An example of a child's bimolar.

Chapter 14

Skull and maxillofacial radiography

Radiographs of the whole head may be required for a variety of purposes. However, the complexity of the structure of the maxillofacial skeleton, the base of the skull and the temporomandibular joint (TMJ) means that many different projections have had to be devised. They are gradually being replaced by cone beam (CT) (see Ch. 19) as this equipment becomes more widely available.

MAIN INDICATIONS

The main clinical indications requiring radiographs of the skull and maxillofacial skeleton include:

- Fractures of the maxillofacial skeleton
- Fractures of the skull
- Investigation of the antra
- Diseases affecting the skull base and vault
- TMJ disorders.

EQUIPMENT

Most skull radiographs are taken using either an *isocentric* skull unit such as the Orbix®, often with the patient lying down, or using a conventional skull unit such as the Craniotome® with the patient sitting up as shown in Figure 14.1.

The image receptor is commonly a cassette (18 × 24 cm) containing either conventional intensifying screens and indirect-action film or an appropriately sized digital phosphor plate (see Ch. 6)

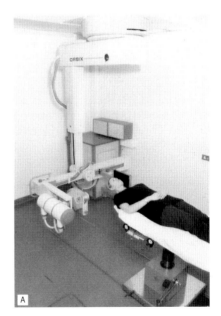

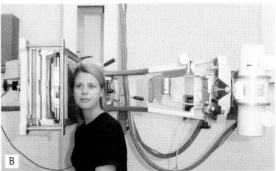

Fig. 14.1A Patient supine in the Orbix® skull unit and **B** erect in the Craniotome®. In both X-ray units, the patient is positioned to produce a lateral view of the skull.

The basic components of the Craniotome® shown in Figure 14.2 include:

- *X-ray generating apparatus* that is:
  - Capable of producing a high-intensity (about 200 mA), and highly penetrating X-ray beam (60–100 kV). As shown in Figure 14.2, the step-up transformer is independent of the tubehead, thus requiring heavy insulated high-tension cables (a totally different design from dental X-ray equipment as described in Ch. 5)
  - Movable in the vertical plane
  - Capable of adjustable X-ray beam collimation
- *Counter balance*, to allow easy positioning of the very heavy tubehead
- *Degree scale*, so the X-ray tubehead can be set at specific vertical angulations for different projections
- *Cassette holder*
- *Anti-scatter grid*, designed originally to be used with **film-based radiography** to stop the photons scattered within the patient from reaching the film (see Ch. 2). These scattered photons would degrade the final overall image quality. The design and function of the anti-scatter grid is shown in Figure 14.3. As some of the photons are absorbed by the lead strips in the grid, a higher dose of radiation is required to ensure sufficient photons reach the film. There are two types of grid:
  - *Fixed* or *stationary* — however the very fine grid lines are evident on the final radiograph

- *Moving* — these oscillate very rapidly from side to side during the exposure thus excluding the grid lines.

When using **digital phosphor plates** as the image receptor and similar exposure factors, insufficient photons penetrate the grid for an acceptable image to be obtained. Either the exposure factors (kV) have to be increased or the grid has to be removed.

PATIENT POSITIONING

The positioning of the patient for skull radiography depends on the general condition of the patient, particularly following trauma, and the equipment available. With the *isocentric* Orbix®, the patient simply remains supine and the equipment is rotated around the head to produce the required projections as shown in Figure 14.4A and B. Using the Craniotome®, as described in this chapter, the patient's head **and** the equipment are moved into different positions.

Positioning the head is facilitated by the *radiographic baseline* — a line representing the base of the skull. It extends from the outer canthus of the eye to the external auditory meatus and is sometimes referred to as the *orbitomeatal line* (see Fig. 14.4C).

In the photographs and diagrams of the positioning techniques, the *radiographic baseline* has been drawn on the patient's face so it can be seen clearly.

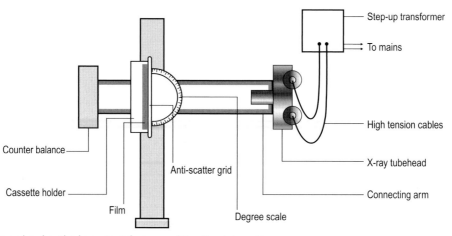

Fig. 14.2 Diagram showing the important features of the Craniotome®.

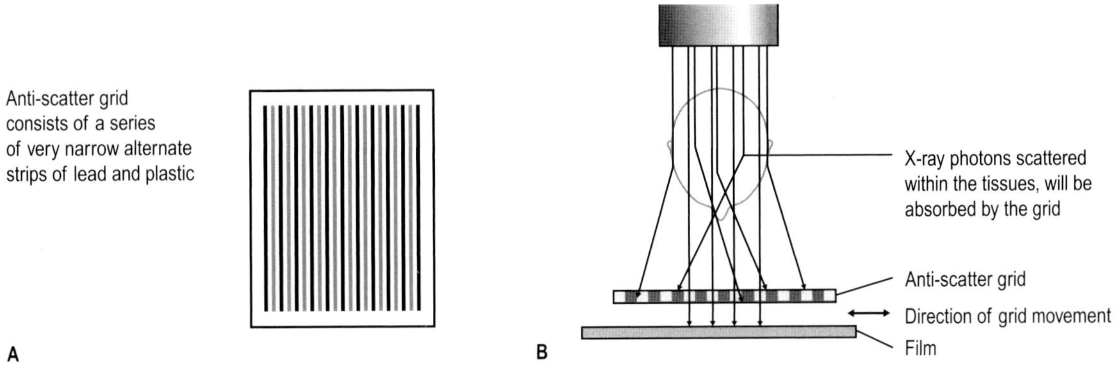

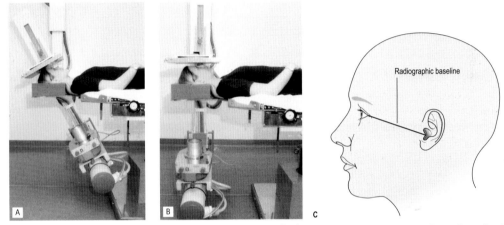

Anti-scatter grid consists of a series of very narrow alternate strips of lead and plastic

X-ray photons scattered within the tissues, will be absorbed by the grid

Anti-scatter grid

Direction of grid movement

Film

A

B

Fig. 14.3 Diagrams showing **A** the design and **B** the function of anti-scatter grids.

Radiographic baseline

A

B

C

Fig. 14.4 Patient positioned in the Orbix® for **A** a posteroanterior (PA) projection and **B** a reverse Towne's projection. **C** Diagram showing the radiographic baseline extending from the outer canthus of the eye to the external auditory meatus.

MAIN MAXILLOFACIAL/SKULL PROJECTIONS

- Standard occipitomental (0° OM)
- 30° occipitomental (30° OM)
- Posteroanterior of the skull (PA skull) sometimes referred to as occipitofrontal (OF)
- Posteroanterior of the jaws (PA jaws)
- Reverse Towne's
- Rotated posteroanterior (rotated PA)
- True lateral skull
- Submentovertex (SMV)
- Transpharyngeal.

This terminology complies with the British Standards Glossary of Dental Terminology (BS 4492: 1983). It may seem confusing, but most of the views are named according to the *direction the X-ray beam is travelling*, e.g. for *occipitomental* (OM) views the X-ray beam is travelling *from the occipital region to the mental region*, for *transpharyngeal* views the X-ray beam is travelling *across the pharynx*.

Each of these projections will now be described in detail, except for the *transpharyngeal* which is used specifically for the TMJ and is discussed in Chapter 31.

Once again the format used is based on the essential knowledge required by clinicians, namely:

- *WHY* each projection is taken
- *HOW* the projection is taken
- *WHAT* the resultant radiograph should look like and which normal anatomical features it shows.

Standard occipitomental (0° OM)

This projection shows the facial skeleton and maxillary antra, and avoids superimposition of the dense bones of the base of the skull.

Main indications

The main clinical indications include:
- Investigation of the maxillary antra
- Detecting the following middle third facial fractures:
  – Le Fort I
  – Le Fort II
  – Le Fort III
  – Zygomatic complex
  – Naso-ethmoidal complex
  – Orbital blow-out
- Coronoid process fractures
- Investigation of the frontal and ethmoidal sinuses

- Investigation of the sphenoidal sinus (projection needs to be taken with the patient's mouth open).

Technique and positioning

This can be summarized as follows:

1. The patient is positioned facing the image receptor with the head tipped back so the radiographic baseline is at 45° to the image receptor, the so-called *nose–chin* position. This positioning drops the dense bones of the base of the skull downwards and raises the facial bones so they can be seen.
2. The X-ray tubehead is positioned with the central ray horizontal (0°) centred through the occiput (see Fig. 14.5B).

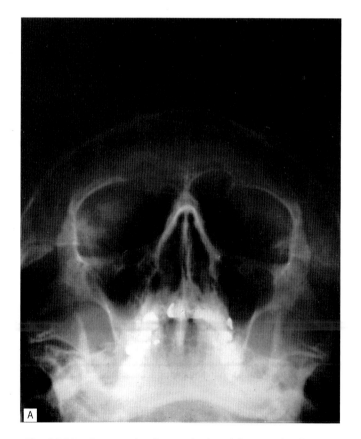

Fig. 14.6A   An example of a standard occipitomental radiograph.

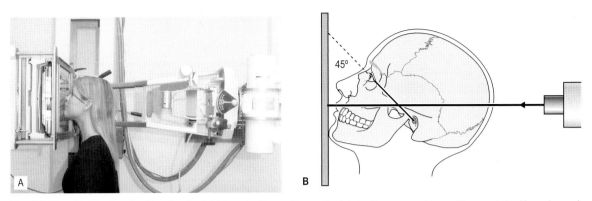

Fig. 14.5A Positioning for the standard OM projection — the patient is in the *nose–chin* position and the X-ray beam is horizontal. **B** Diagram of the positioning — the radiographic baseline is at 45° to the image receptor, and the X-ray beam is horizontal.

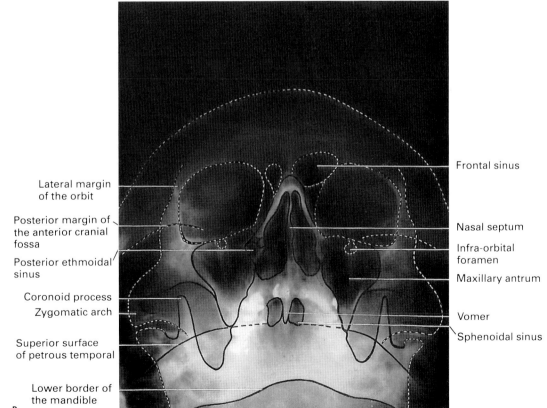

Fig. 14.6B The same radiograph with the major anatomical features drawn in.

30° occipitomental (30° OM)

This projection also shows the facial skeleton, but from a different angle from the 0° OM, enabling certain bony displacements to be detected.

Main indications

The main clinical indications include:
- Detecting the following middle third facial fractures:
  - Le Fort I
  - Le Fort II
  - Le Fort III
- Coronoid process fractures.

Note: Ideally for fracture diagnosis two views at right angles are required (see Ch. 30), but the 0° OM and 30° OM provide two views of the facial bones at two different angles — therefore in cases of suspected facial fracture **both** views are needed.

Technique and positioning

This can be summarized as follows:

1. The patient is in exactly the same position as for the 0° OM, i.e. the head tipped back, radiographic baseline at 45° to the image receptor, in the *nose–chin* position.
2. The X-ray tubehead is aimed downwards from above the head, with the central ray at 30° to the horizontal, centred through the lower border of the orbit (see Fig. 14.7).

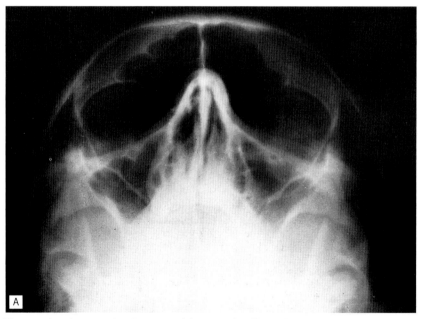

Fig. 14.8A   An example of a 30° occipitomental radiograph.

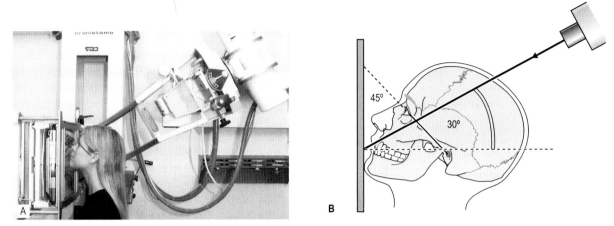

Fig. 14.7A   Positioning for the 30° OM projection – the patient is in the *nose–chin* position and the X-ray beam is aimed downwards at 30°. **B** Diagram of the positioning – the radiographic baseline is at 45° to the image receptor, and the X-ray beam is aimed downwards at 30°.

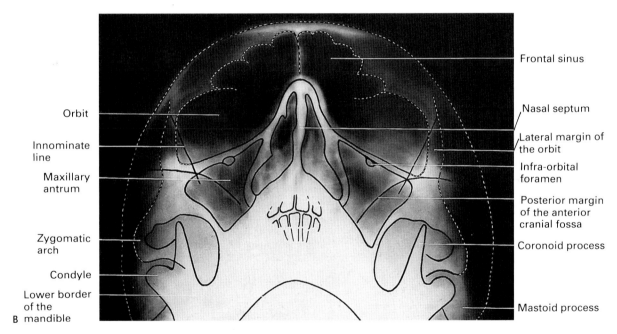

Frontal sinus

Orbit

Innominate line

Maxillary antrum

Nasal septum

Lateral margin of the orbit

Infra-orbital foramen

Posterior margin of the anterior cranial fossa

Zygomatic arch

Condyle

Lower border of the
B mandible

Coronoid process

Mastoid process

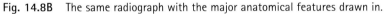

Fig. 14.8B   The same radiograph with the major anatomical features drawn in.

Posteroanterior of the skull (PA skull)

This projection shows the skull vault, primarily the frontal bones and the jaws.

Main indications

The main clinical indications include:

- Fractures of the skull vault
- Investigation of the frontal sinuses
- Conditions affecting the cranium, particularly:
  - Paget's disease of bone
  - multiple myeloma
  - hyperparathyroidism
- Intracranial calcification.

Technique and positioning

This can be summarized as follows:

1. The patient is positioned facing the image receptor with the head tipped forwards so that the forehead and tip of the nose touch the image receptor — the so-called *forehead–nose* position. The radiographic baseline is horizontal and at right angles to the image receptor. This positioning levels off the base of the skull and allows the vault of the skull to be seen without superimposition.
2. The X-ray tubehead is positioned with the central ray horizontal (0°) centred through the occiput (see Fig. 14.9).

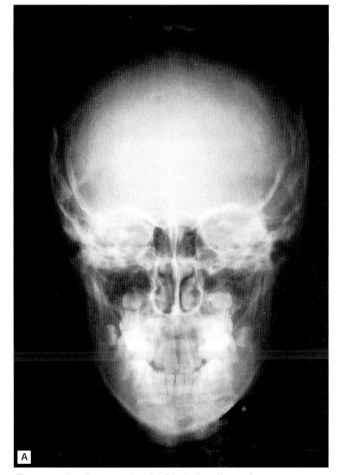

Fig. 14.10A   An example of a PA skull radiograph.

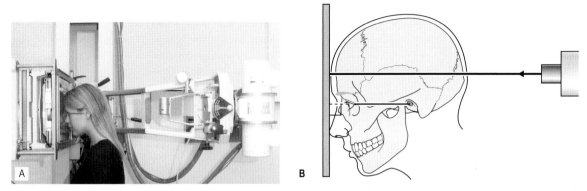

Fig. 14.9A Positioning for the PA skull projection — the patient is in the *forehead–nose* position and the X-ray beam is horizontal. **B** Diagram of the positioning — the radiographic baseline is horizontal and perpendicular to the image receptor, and the X-ray beam is also horizontal.

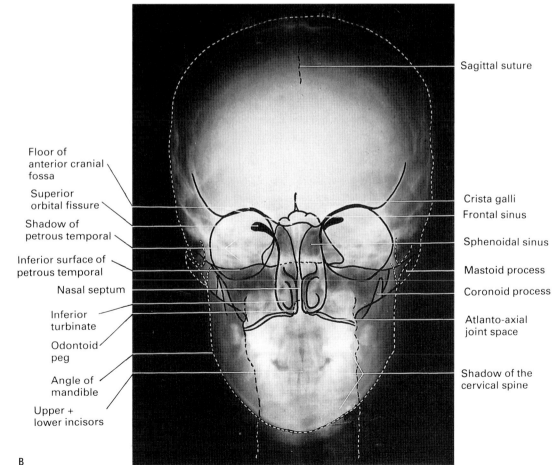

B

Fig. 14.10B The same radiograph with the major anatomical features drawn in.

Posteroanterior of the jaws (PA jaws/PA mandible)

This projection shows the posterior parts of the mandible. It is not suitable for showing the facial skeleton because of superimposition of the base of the skull and the nasal bones.

Main indications

The main clinical indications include:

- Fractures of the mandible involving the following sites:
  - Posterior third of the body
  - Angles
  - Rami
  - Low condylar necks
- Lesions such as cysts or tumours in the posterior third of the body or rami to note any mediolateral expansion
- Mandibular hypoplasia or hyperplasia
- Maxillofacial deformities.

Technique and positioning

This can be summarized as follows:

1. The patient is in exactly the same position as for the PA skull, i.e. the head tipped forward, the radiographic baseline horizontal and perpendicular to the image receptor in the *forehead–nose* position.
2. The X-ray tubehead is again horizontal (0°), but now the central ray is centred through the cervical spine at the level of the rami of the mandible (see Fig. 14.11).

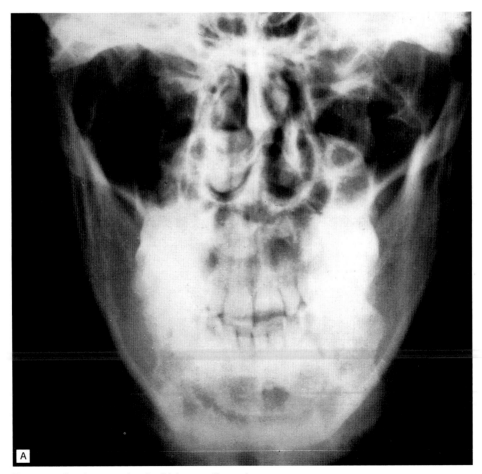

Fig. 14.12A   An example of a PA jaws radiograph.

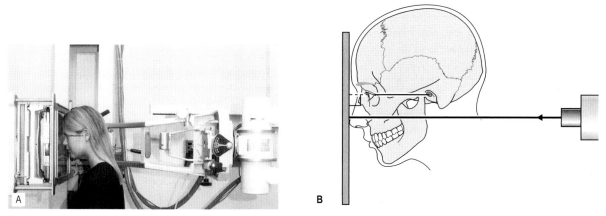

Fig. 14.11A Positioning for the PA jaws/PA mandible projection — the patient is in the *forehead–nose* position and the X-ray beam is horizontal centred through the rami. **B** Diagram of the positioning — the radiographic baseline is horizontal and perpendicular to the image receptor, and the X-ray beam is also horizontal.

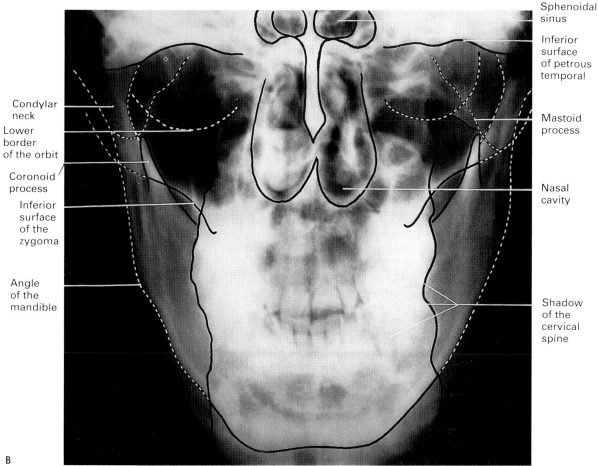

Condylar neck

Lower border of the orbit

Coronoid process

Inferior surface of the zygoma

Angle of the mandible

Sphenoidal sinus

Inferior surface of petrous temporal

Mastoid process

Nasal cavity

Shadow of the cervical spine

B

Fig. 14.12B The same radiograph with the major anatomical features drawn in.

Reverse Towne's

This projection shows the condylar heads and necks. The original Towne's view (an AP projection) was designed to show the occipital region, but also showed the condyles. However, since all skull views used in dentistry are taken conventionally in the posterior-anterior direction, the *reverse Towne's* (a PA projection) is used.

Main indications

The main clinical indications include:

- High fractures of the condylar necks
- Intracapsular fractures of the TMJ
- Investigation of the quality of the articular surfaces of the condylar heads in TMJ disorders
- Condylar hypoplasia or hyperplasia.

Technique and positioning

This can be summarized as follows:

1. The patient is in the PA position, i.e. the head tipped forwards in the *forehead–nose* position, but in addition the mouth is **open**. The radiographic baseline is horizontal and at right angles to the image receptor. Opening the mouth takes the condylar heads out of the glenoid fossae so they can be seen.
2. The X-ray tubehead is aimed upwards from below the occiput, with the central ray at 30° to the horizontal, centred through the condyles (see Fig. 14.13).

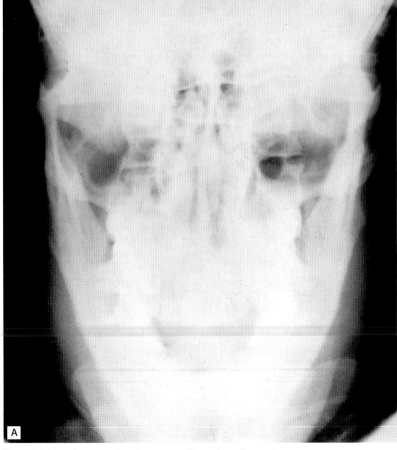

Fig. 14.14A An example of a reverse Towne's radiograph.

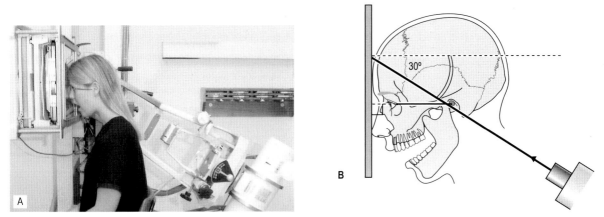

Fig. 14.13A Positioning for the reverse Towne's projection — the patient is in the *forehead–nose* position with the mouth open and the X-ray beam is aimed upwards at 30°. **B** Diagram of the positioning — the radiographic baseline is horizontal and perpendicular to the image receptor, the mouth is open and the X-ray beam is aimed upwards at 30°.

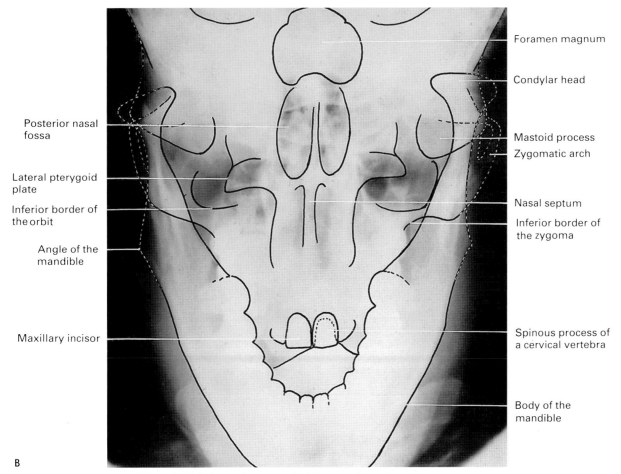

B

Fig. 14.14B The same radiograph with the major anatomical features drawn in.

Rotated posteroanterior (rotated PA)

This projection shows the tissues of one side of the face and is used to investigate the parotid gland and the ramus of the mandible.

Main indications

The main clinical indications include:

- Stones/calculi in the parotid glands
- Lesions such as cysts or tumours in the ramus to note any medio-lateral expansion
- Submasseteric infection — to note new bone formation.

Technique and positioning

This can be summarized as follows:

1. The patient is positioned facing the image receptor, with the occlusal plane horizontal and the tip of the nose touching the image receptor in the so-called *normal head* position.
2. The head is then rotated 10° to the side of interest. This positioning rotates the bones of the back of the skull away from the side of the face under investigation.
3. The X-ray tubehead is positioned with the central ray horizontal (0°), aimed down the side of the face (see Fig. 14.15).

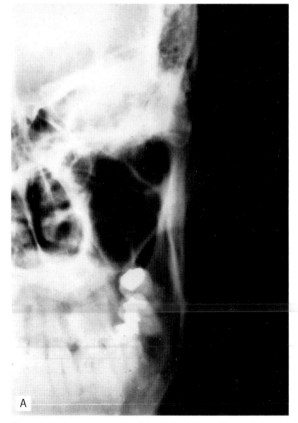

A

Fig. 14.16A An example of a rotated PA radiograph.

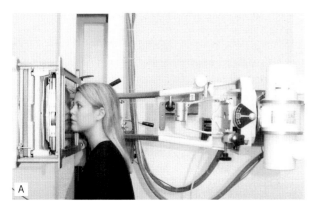

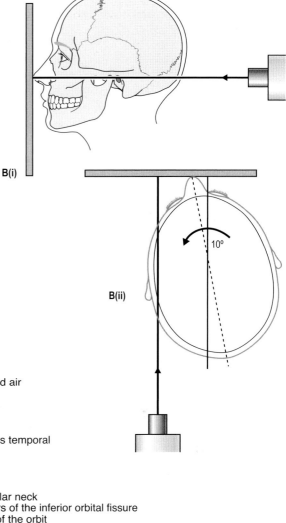

B(i)

B(ii)

10°

Fig. 14.15A Positioning for the rotated PA projection — the patient is in the *normal head* position and rotated to the side of interest and the X-ray beam is horizontal.
B Diagrams of the positioning (i) from the side, **normal head** position and the X-ray beam horizontal, (ii) from above, 10° rotation of the head to the side of interest and the X-ray beam aimed along the side of the face.

Mastoid air cells

Petrous temporal

Condylar neck
Borders of the inferior orbital fissure
Floor of the orbit
Zygomatic arch

Maxillary antrum

Angle of the mandible

Fig. 14.16B The same radiograph with the major anatomical features drawn in.

True lateral skull

This projection shows the skull vault and facial skeleton from the lateral aspect. The main difference between the *true lateral skull* and the *true cephalometric lateral skull* taken on the cephalostat (see Ch. 15) is that the *true lateral skull* is not standardized or reproducible. This view is used when a single lateral view of the skull is required but not in orthodontics or growth studies.

Main indications

The main clinical indications include:

- Fractures of the cranium and the cranial base
- Middle third facial fractures, to show possible downward and backward displacement of the maxillae
- Investigation of the frontal, sphenoidal and maxillary sinuses

- Conditions affecting the skull vault, particularly:
    - Paget's diseaseof bone
    - multiple myeloma
    - hyperparathyroidism
- Conditions affecting the sella turcica, such as:
    - tumour of the pituitary gland in acromegaly.

Technique and positioning

This can be summarized as follows:

1. The patient is positioned with the head turned through 90°, so the side of the face touches the image receptor. In this position, the sagittal plane of the head is parallel to the image receptor.
2. The X-ray tubehead is positioned with the central ray horizontal (0°) and perpendicular to the sagittal plane and the image receptor, centred through the external auditory meatus (see Fig. 14.17).

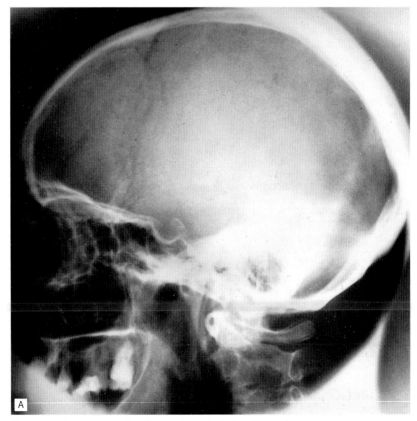

Fig. 14.18A An example of a true lateral skull radiograph.

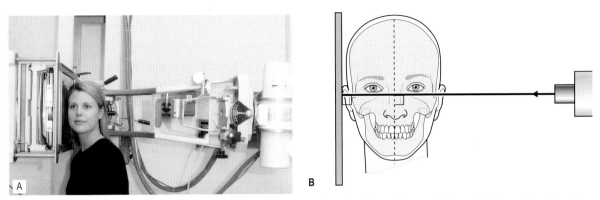

Fig. 14.17A   Positioning for the true lateral skull projection — the patient's head is turned through 90°, and the X-ray beam is horizontal. **B** Diagram of the positioning — the sagittal plane of the head is parallel to the image receptor and the X-ray beam is horizontal and perpendicular to the sagittal plane and the image receptor.

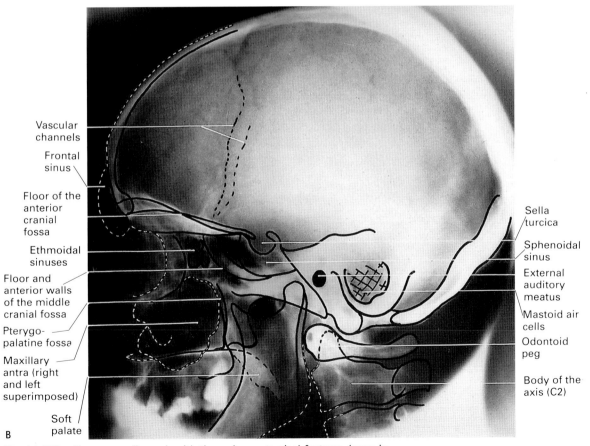

Vascular channels

Frontal sinus

Floor of the anterior cranial fossa

Ethmoidal sinuses

Floor and anterior walls of the middle cranial fossa

Pterygo-palatine fossa

Maxillary antra (right and left superimposed)

Soft palate

Sella turcica

Sphenoidal sinus

External auditory meatus

Mastoid air cells

Odontoid peg

Body of the axis (C2)

B

Fig. 14.18B   The same radiograph with the major anatomical features drawn in.

Submentovertex (SMV)

This projection shows the base of the skull, sphenoidal sinuses and facial skeleton from below.

Main indications

The main clinical indications include:

- Destructive/expansive lesions affecting the palate, pterygoid region or base of skull
- Investigation of the sphenoidal sinus
- Assessment of the thickness (mediolateral) of the posterior part of the mandible before osteotomy
- Fracture of the zygomatic arches — to show these thin bones the SMV is taken with reduced exposure factors.

Technique and positioning

This can be summarized as follows:

1. The patient is positioned facing away from the image receptor. The head is tipped backwards as far as is possible, so the vertex of the skull touches the image receptor. In this position, the radiographic baseline is vertical and parallel to the image receptor.
2. The X-ray tubehead is aimed upwards from below the chin, with the central ray at 5° to the horizontal, centred on an imaginary line joining the lower first molars (see Fig. 14.19).

Note: The head positioning required for this projection means it is **contraindicated** in patients with suspected neck injuries, especially suspected fracture of the odontoid peg.

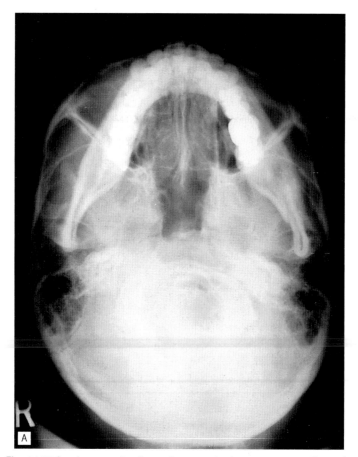

Fig. 14.20A An example of a well-exposed submentovertex radiograph.

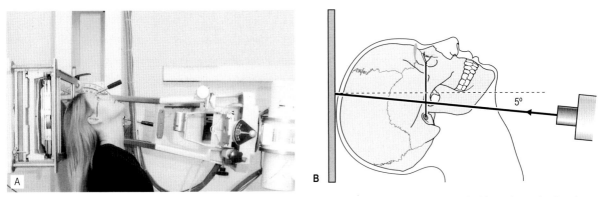

Fig. 14.19A   Positioning for the SMV projection — the patient's head is tipped backwards and the X-ray beam is aimed upwards at 5° to the horizontal. **B** Diagram of the positioning — the radiographic baseline is vertical and parallel to the image receptor and the X-ray beam is aimed upwards at 5° to the horizontal.

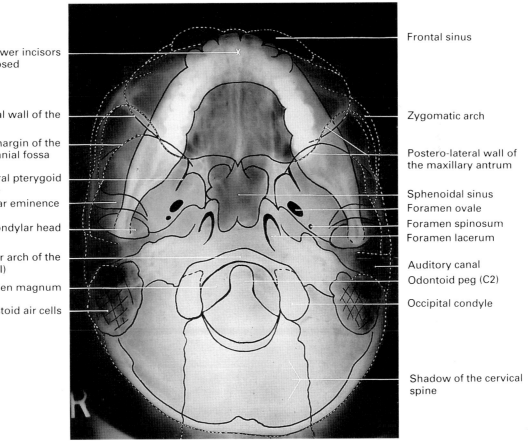

Upper + lower incisors superimposed

Lateral wall of the orbit

Anterior margin of the middle cranial fossa

Lateral pterygoid plate
Articular eminence

Condylar head

Anterior arch of the atlas (CI)

Foramen magnum

Mastoid air cells

Frontal sinus

Zygomatic arch

Postero-lateral wall of the maxillary antrum

Sphenoidal sinus
Foramen ovale
Foramen spinosum
Foramen lacerum

Auditory canal
Odontoid peg (C2)

Occipital condyle

Shadow of the cervical spine

B

Fig. 14.20B   The same radiograph with the major anatomical features drawn in.

Chapter 15

Cephalometric radiography

Cephalometric radiography is a standardized and reproducible form of skull radiography used extensively in orthodontics to assess the relationships of the teeth to the jaws and the jaws to the rest of the facial skeleton. Standardization was essential for the development of *cephalometry* — the measurement and comparison of specific points, distances and lines within the facial skeleton, which is now an integral part of orthodontic assessment. The greatest value is probably obtained from these radiographs if they are traced or digitized and this is essential when they are being used for the monitoring of treatment progress.

MAIN INDICATIONS

The main clinical indications can be considered under two major headings — orthodontics and orthognathic surgery.

Orthodontics

- Initial diagnosis — confirmation of the underlying skeletal and/or soft tissue abnormalities
- Treatment planning
- Monitoring treatment progress, e.g. to assess anchorage requirements and incisor inclination
- Appraisal of treatment results, e.g. 1 or 2 months before the completion of active treatment to ensure that treatment targets have been met and to allow planning of retention.

When considering these indications, it should be remembered that all radiographs must be clinically justified under current legislation (see Ch. 8). In the UK, indications and selection criteria for cephalometric radiographs are clearly identified in the British Orthodontic Society's 2001 booklet *Orthodontic Radiographs – Guidelines for the Use of Radiographs in Clinical Orthodontics* and in the Faculty of General Dental Practice (UK)'s 2004 booklet *Selection Criteria in Dental Radiography*. These guidelines are designed to assist in the *justification* process so as to avoid the use of unnecessary radiographs.

Orthognathic surgery

- Preoperative evaluation of skeletal and soft tissue patterns
- To assist in treatment planning
- Postoperative appraisal of the results of surgery and long-term follow-up studies.

EQUIPMENT

Several different types of equipment are available for cephalometric radiography, either as separate units, or as additional attachments to panoramic units. In some equipment the patients are seated, while in others they remain standing. Traditional equipment was designed to use indirect-action radiographic film in an extra-oral cassette as the image receptor. The advent of

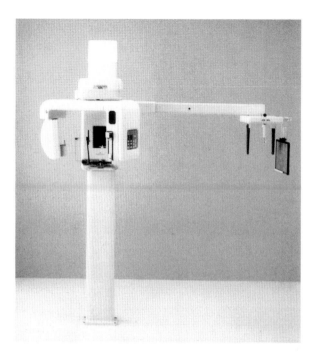

Fig. 15.1 An example of a traditional combined panoramic and cephalostat unit suitable for film-based or phosphor plate imaging.

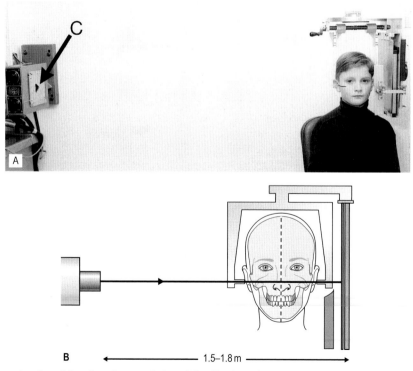

Fig. 15.2A An example of traditional equipment designed for film-based cephalometric radiography showing the cephalostat and X-ray tubehead in fixed positions. The triangular collimator (C) is indicated by the arrow.
B Diagram showing the fixed relationship between X-ray tubehead and film, separated by 1.5–1.8 m. The patient is immobilized in the cephalostat with the mid-sagittal plane of the head parallel to the film.

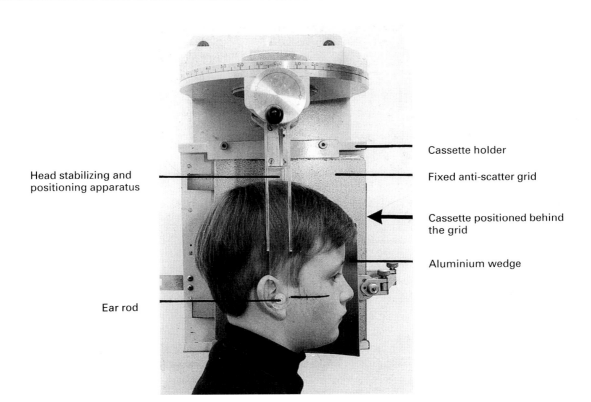

Fig. 15.3   A traditional cephalostat (craniostat) designed for film-based imaging. A fixed anti-scatter grid is included and the aluminium wedge filter positioned between the patient and the grid. The Frankfort plane is marked on the patient's face.

digital imaging, using phosphor plates and solid-state sensors, has seen the development of new dedicated digital equipment. The basic components of these different types of equipment are described below.

Traditional film-based equipment

This either consists of an additional attachment to a panoramic unit as shown in Figure 15.1, or as a completely separate dedicated unit as shown in Figure 15.2. The basic components include:

- *X-ray generating apparatus* that should:
  - Be in a fixed position relative to the cephalostat and film so that successive radiographs are reproducible and comparable. To minimize the effect of magnification the focus-to-film distance should be greater than 1 m and ideally in the range 1.5–1.8 m (see Fig. 15.2).
  - Include a light beam diaphragm to facilitate the collimation. The beam should be colli-

mated to an approximately triangular shape to restrict the area of the patient irradiated to the required cranial base and facial skeleton, so avoiding the skull vault and cervical spine and thyroid gland (see Fig. 15.2).
  - Be capable of producing an X-ray beam that is sufficiently penetrating to reach the film and parallel in nature.
- *Cephalostat* (or *craniostat*) (see Fig. 15.3) comprising:
  - Head positioning and stabilizing apparatus with ear rods to ensure a standardized patient position. Additional positioning guides can include forehead supports and infraobrbital guide rods.
  - Cassette holder.
  - Optional fixed anti-scatter grid to stop photons scattered within the patient reaching the film and degrading the image (see Ch. 14). This is not usually included in combined panoramic/cephalostat units.

- *Cassette* (usually 18 × 24 cm) containing rare-earth intensifying screens and indirect action film.
- *Aluminium wedge filter* designed to attenuate the X-ray beam selectively in the region of the facial soft tissues to enable the soft tissue profile to be seen on the final radiograph. This is either attached to the tubehead, covering the anterior part of the beam (the preferred position) or it is included as part of the cephalostat and positioned between the patient and the anterior part of the cassette.

Digital equipment

Equipment variations exist depending on the type of digital image receptor chosen.

Using phosphor plates

Equipment **not** incorporating anti-scatter grids, such as combined panoramic/cephalostat units can be converted to digital by simply replacing the film and intensifying screens in the cassette with a suitably sized phosphor plate. As explained in Chapter 14, the grid prevents sufficient photons from reaching the phosphor plate to create an acceptable image. Either the exposure factors (kV) have to be increased or the grid removed.

Using solid-state sensors

Several manufacturers have developed combined panoramic/cephalostat units utilizing specially designed solid-state sensors. An example is shown in Figure 15.4. Sensor design was discussed in Chapter 6 and illustrated in Figure 6.18.

The sensor is obviously not the same size as an 18 × 24 cm cassette and the image cannot be captured in the same way. During the exposure, the X-ray beam and sensor **move** either *horizontally* or *vertically* to scan the patient, as shown in Figure 15.5. The final image therefore takes a few seconds to build up. To ensure that the X-ray beam is the same shape as the CCD array in

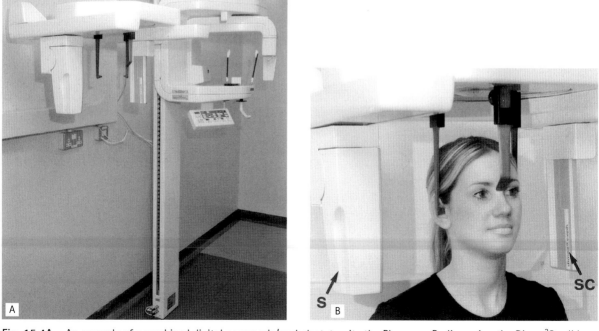

Fig. 15.4A   An example of a combined digital panoramic/cephalostat unit—the Planmeca Proline using the Dimax³® solid-state sensor. **B** Patient positioned and immobilized within the cephalostat unit. Note the solid-state sensor (S) and the secondary collimator (SC) (arrowed).

the sensor and that they are aligned exactly, the beam passes through a *secondary collimator*, which also moves throughout the exposure, as shown in Figure 15.5.

Other features to note include:

- An aluminium wedge filter is not usually included. Soft tissue profile is enhanced by using computer software.
- Triangular beam collimation to avoid the skull vault and cervical spine and thyroid gland is not usually included.
- There is no anti-scatter grid.

MAIN RADIOGRAPHIC PROJECTIONS

These include:

- True cephalometric lateral skull
- Cephalometric posteroanterior of the jaws (PA jaws).

True cephalometric lateral skull

As stated in Chapter 13, the terminology used to describe lateral skull projections is somewhat confusing, the adjective *true*, as opposed to *oblique*, being used to describe lateral skull projections when:

- The image receptor is parallel to the sagittal plane of the patient's head

- The X-ray beam is perpendicular to image receptor and sagittal plane.

In addition, the word *cephalometric* should be included when describing the *true lateral skull* radiograph taken in the cephalostat. This enables differentiation from the non-standardized *true lateral skull* projection taken in a skull unit, as described in Chapter 14. It is now an accepted convention to view orthodontic lateral skull radiographs with the patient facing to the *right*, as shown in Figure 15.6.

Technique and positioning

This can be summarized as follows:

1. The patient is positioned within the cephalostat, with the sagittal plane of the head vertical and parallel to the image receptor and with the Frankfort plane horizontal. The teeth should generally be in maximum intercuspation.
2. The head is immobilized carefully within the apparatus with the plastic ear rods being inserted gradually into the external auditory meati.
3. The aluminium wedge if used, is positioned to cover the anterior part of the image receptor.
4. The equipment is designed to ensure that when the patient is positioned correctly, the X-ray beam is horizontal and centred on the ear rods, (see Fig. 15.6).

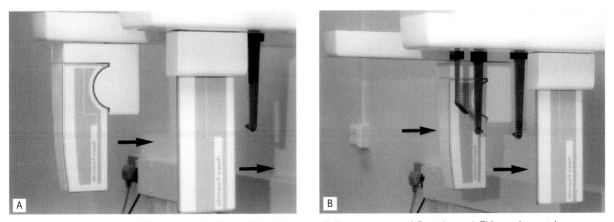

Fig. 15.5   Close up of the Planmeca cephalostat. **A** At the start of the exposure and **B** at the end. This equipment is designed to scan the patient *horizontally* with the X-ray beam, secondary collimator and sensor moving horizontally throughout the exposure (arrowed).

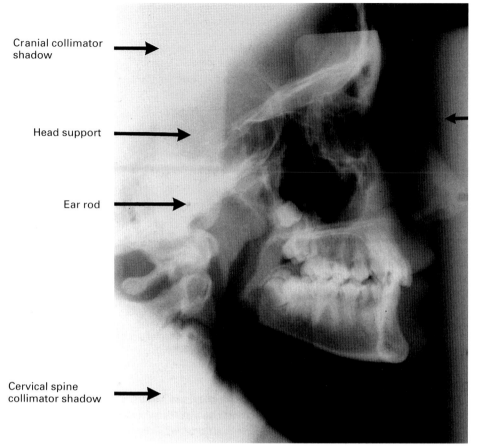

Cranial collimator shadow

Head support

Ear rod

Aluminium wedge filter

Cervical spine collimator shadow

Fig. 15.6 An example of a film-captured true cephalometric lateral skull radiograph. Note the images of the ear rods should ideally appear superimposed on one another. The various shadows of the cephalostat equipment and the collimator are indicated.

Cephalometric tracing / digitizing

This produces a diagrammatic representation of certain anatomical points or landmarks evident on the lateral skull radiograph (see Fig. 15.7). These points are traced on to an overlying sheet of paper or acetate or digitally recorded. Either method allows precise measurements to be made. As a basic system these could include:

- The outline and inclination of the anterior teeth
- The positional relationship of the mandibular and maxillary dental bases to the cranial base
- The positional relationship of the dental bases to one another, i.e. the skeletal patterns
- The relationship between the bones of the skull and the soft tissues of the face.

Main cephalometric points

The definitions of the main cephalometric points (as indicated in a clockwise direction on the tracing shown in Fig. 15.7) include:

Sella (S). The centre of the sella turcica, (determined by inspection).

Orbitale (Or). The lowest point on the infraorbital margin.

Nasion (N). The most anterior point on the frontonasal suture.

Anterior nasal spine (ANS). The tip of the anterior nasal spine.

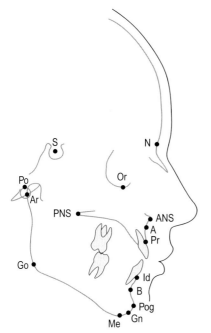

Fig. 15.7   A cephalometric tracing of a lateral skull radiograph showing the main cephalometric points.

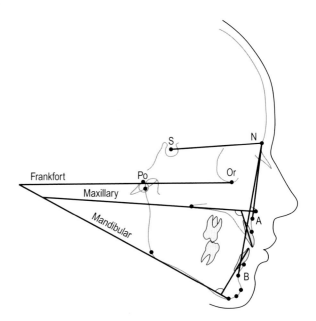

Fig. 15.8   A cephalometric tracing of a lateral skull radiograph showing the main cephalometric planes and angles.

Subspinale or point A.   The deepest midline point between the anterior nasal spine and prosthion.

Prosthion (Pr).   The most anterior point of the alveolar crest in the premaxilla, usually between the upper central incisors.

Infradentale (Id).   The most anterior point of the alveolar crest, situated between the lower central incisors.

Supramentale or point B.   The deepest point in the bony outline between the infradentale and the pogonion.

Pogonion (Pog).   The most anterior point of the bony chin.

Gnathion (Gn).   The most anterior and inferior point on the bony outline of the chin, situated equidistant from pogonion and menton.

Menton (Me).   The lowest point on the bony outline of the mandibular symphysis.

Gonion (Go).   The most lateral external point at the junction of the horizontal and ascending rami of the mandible.

Note: The gonion is found by bisecting the angle formed by tangents to the posterior and inferior borders of the mandible.

Posterior nasal spine (PNS).   The tip of the posterior spine of the palatine bone in the hard palate.

Articulare (Ar).   The point of intersection of the dorsal contours of the posterior border of the mandible and temporal bone.

Porion (Po).   The uppermost point of the bony external auditory meatus, usually regarded as coincidental with the uppermost point of the ear rods of the cephalostat.

Main cephalometric planes and angles

The definitions of the main cephalometric planes and angles shown in Figure 15.8 include:

Frankfort plane.   A transverse plane through the skull represented by the line joining porion and orbitale.

Mandibular plane.   A transverse plane through the skull representing the lower border of the horizontal ramus of the mandible.

There are several definitions:

- A tangent to the lower border of the mandible
- A line joining gnathion and gonion
- A line joining menton and gonion.

Maxillary plane. A transverse plane through the skull represented by a joining of the anterior and posterior nasal spines.

SN plane. A transverse plane through the skull represented by the line joining sella and nasion.

SNA. Relates the anteroposterior position of the maxilla, as represented by the A point, to the cranial base.

SNB. Relates the anteroposterior position of the mandible, as represented by the B point, to the cranial base.

ANB. Relates the anteroposterior position of the maxilla to the mandible, i.e. indicates the antero-posterior skeletal pattern — Class I, II or III.

Maxillary incisal inclination. The angle between the long axis of the maxillary incisors and the maxillary plane.

Mandibular incisal inclination. The angle between the long axis of the mandibular incisors and the mandibular plane.

All the definitions are those specified in The British Standards Glossary of Dental Terms (BS4492: 1983).

CEPHALOMETRIC POSTEROANTERIOR OF THE JAWS (PA JAWS)

This projection is identical to the PA view of the jaws described in Chapter 14, except that it is standardized and reproducible. This makes it suitable for the assessment of facial asymmetries and for preoperative and postoperative comparisons in orthognathic surgery involving the mandible.

Technique and positioning (Fig. 15.9)

This can be summarized as follows:

1. The head-stabilizing apparatus of the cephalostat is rotated through 90°.

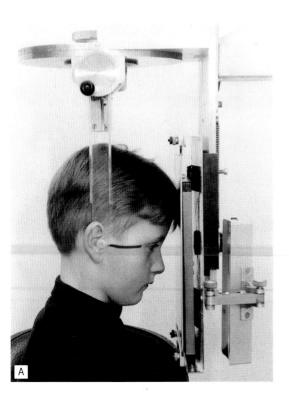

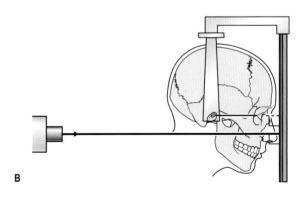

B

Fig. 15.9A Positioning for the cephalometric PA jaws projection. The patient is in the *forehead–nose* position, with the radiographic baseline (marked on the face) horizontal and perpendicular to the image receptor.
B Diagram of the patient positioning and showing the X-ray beam horizontal and centred through the rami.

2. The patient is positioned in the apparatus with the head tipped forwards and with the radiographic baseline horizontal and perpendicular to the film, i.e. in the *forehead–nose* position.

3. The head is immobilized within the apparatus by inserting the plastic ear rods into the external auditory meati.

4. The fixed X-ray beam is horizontal with the central ray centred through the cervical spine at the level of the rami of the mandible (see Figs. 15.9 and 15.10).

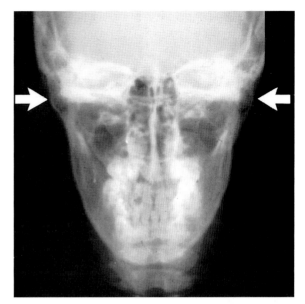

Fig. 15.10   An example of a cephalometric PA jaws radiograph. The arrows indicate the position of the ear rods.

Chapter 16

Tomography

INTRODUCTION

Tomography is a specialized technique for producing radiographs showing only a *section* or *slice* of a patient. A useful analogy is to regard the technique as dividing up the patient like a loaf of sliced bread (see Fig. 16.1). Each *tomograph* (or slice of bread) shows the tissues within that section sharply defined and in focus. The section is thus referred to as the *focal plane* or *focal trough*. Structures outside the section (i.e. the rest of the loaf) are blurred and out of focus. By taking multiple slices, three-dimensional information about the whole patient can be obtained.

Production of each conventional tomographic slice requires controlled, accurate **movement** of both the X-ray tubehead and the film during the exposure, thereby differing from all the techniques described in previous chapters. Originally sections were obtained in either the sagittal or coronal planes (see Fig. 16.2), but modern equipment now allows tomography in other planes as well.

Conventional tomography has essentially been superseded in medical radiography by the development of computed tomography (CT). It is however still important in dentistry, forming the basis of dental panoramic tomography (see Ch. 17) and multifunctional dental and maxillo-facial tomographic machines, such as the Scanora®, or the Tomax® Ultrascan.

The concept of *slice* or *sectional images* is also important to appreciate because it forms the basis of many of the modern imaging modalities, described in Chapter 19, that are being used increasingly in dentistry particularly cone beam CT (CBCT).

ORIGINAL INDICATIONS

The original clinical indications for conventional tomographic sectional images in dentistry include:

- Assessment of jaw height, thickness and texture before inserting implants (see Ch. 24)
- Postoperative evaluation of implants
- Assessment of the antra including the position of displaced teeth and foreign bodies

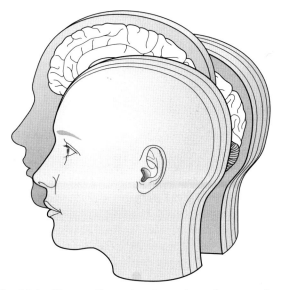

Fig. 16.1 Diagram illustrating the analogy of tomography dividing the patient up like a loaf of sliced bread.

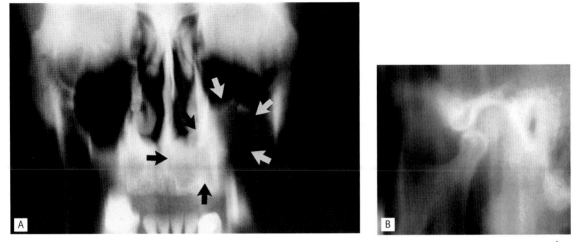

Fig. 16.2A A linear tomograph in the coronal plane of the antrum and facial skeleton showing an antral tumour (arrowed). **B** A linear tomograph in the sagittal plane of the left TMJ. In both examples, the tissues imaged in the tomographic sections are sharply defined and in focus, while the unwanted structures are blurred out. Note the vertical straight-line blurring on both images.

- Evaluation of grossly comminuted facial fractures to determine all the fracture sites
- Assessment of the extent of orbital blow-out fractures
- As an additional investigation of the TMJ and condylar head — particularly useful if patients were unable to open their mouths, since most other radiographs of the TMJ require the mouth to be open (see Ch. 31)
- In conjunction with arthrography of the TMJ.

THEORY

Tomographic movement

As stated, tomography requires controlled, accurate **movement** of both the X-ray tubehead and the film. They are therefore linked together. During the exposure, the X-ray tubehead moves in one direction around the patient while the film moves in the opposite direction, as shown in Figure 16.3. The point (O) at the centre of this rotating movement will appear in focus on the resultant radiograph, since its shadow will appear in the same place on the film throughout the exposure. All other structures will appear blurred or out of focus.

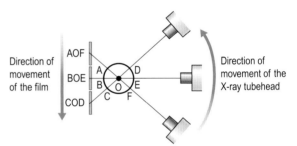

Fig. 16.3 Diagram illustrating the principle of tomographic movement. The X-ray tubehead moves in one direction while the film moves in the opposite direction. Points A,B,C,D,E and F will all appear on different parts of the film and thus will be blurred out, while point O, the centre of rotation, will appear in the same place on the film throughout the exposure and will therefore be sharply defined.

Types of tomographic movement

During tomography, equipment has been designed to move in one of five ways, as shown in Figure 16.4:

- Linear
- Circular
- Elliptical
- Spiral
- Hypocycloidal.

In each case the centre of rotation remains the same, it is only the movement of the equipment

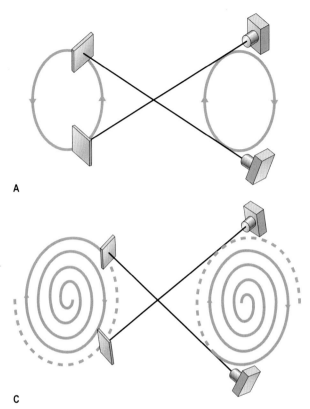

A

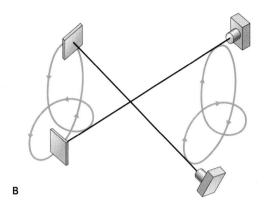

B

C

Fig. 16.4   Diagrams showing various types of tomographic movement. **A** Circular or elliptical. **B** Hypocycloidal. **C** Spiral. Note that the centre of rotation remains the same in each case; it is only the movement of the equipment that becomes more complicated.

that becomes more complicated. *Linear* movement is the simplest and easiest to illustrate and is described later. Its main disadvantage is that it produces straight-line blurred shadows of unwanted structures (see Fig. 16.2). The other types of equipment movement have been developed to produce tomographs of better definition with more blurring of unwanted structures making them less obvious on the final film.

BROAD–BEAM LINEAR TOMOGRAPHY

The principle of tomography illustrated in Figure 16.3 shows a very thin X-ray beam producing one point (O) — the centre of rotation — in focus on the film. To produce a *section* or *slice* of the patient in focus, a broad X-ray beam is used. For each part of the beam, there is a separate centre of rotation, all of which lie in the same *focal plane*. The resultant tomograph will therefore show all these points sharply defined. The principle of broadbeam tomography is illustrated in Figure 16.5.

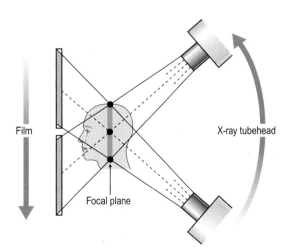

Fig. 16.5   Diagram showing the principle of broad–beam tomography. Using a broad beam there will be multiple centres of rotation (three are indicated: ●) all of which will lie in the shaded zone. As all the centres of rotation will be *in focus*, this zone represents the *focal plane* or section of the patient that will appear sharply defined on the resultant tomograph.

Width/thickness of the focal plane

The thickness of the focal plane is determined by the amount of movement, or angle of swing, of the equipment. As shown in Figure 16.6, the larger the angle of swing, the thinner the section in focus, while the smaller the angle of swing the thicker the section.

Equipment (Fig. 16.7)

Linear tomography of the skull can be performed using the *Craniotome®*, described in Chapter 14, with the following modifications:

1. A rigid connecting bar is inserted to join the X-ray tubehead and the cassette holder (see Fig. 16.7).
2. The brake on the film–tubehead assembly is released. This frees the assembly, enabling it to move in the vertical plane during the exposure.
3. The position of the fulcrum or pivot of the connecting bar can be adjusted accurately. This alters the centre of rotation and thus the section of the patient to be imaged.

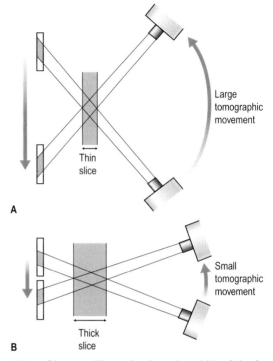

Fig. 16.6 Diagrams illustrating how the width of the focal plane is governed by the amount of movement by the equipment. **A** A large tomographic movement produces a thin slice. **B** A small tomographic movement produces a thick slice.

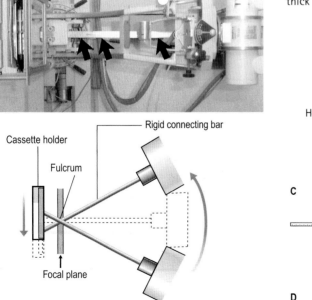

Fig. 16.7A The Craniotome® with rigid tomographic bar attached (black arrows). **B** Diagram showing the fulcrum and the relative movements of the linked X-ray tubehead and cassette holder. **C** Diagram showing the fulcrum and measurement scale for selecting different sections. **D** Diagram showing the fulcrum positioned in line with the different sections of the patient to be imaged.

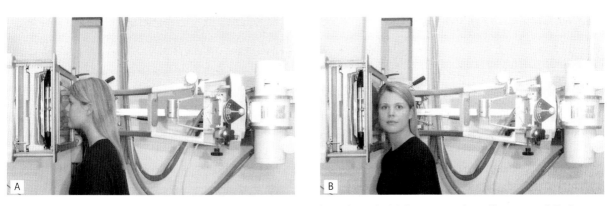

Fig. 16.8A   Patient positioning for coronal plane tomography to investigate facial fractures and maxillary antra. **B** Patient positioning for sagittal plane tomography to investigate the right TMJ.

Patient positioning

The patient is positioned within the skull unit. The exact positioning of the patient's head in either the coronal or sagittal planes depends on the precise area under investigation. Examples are shown in Figure 16.8.

Specialized tomographic units

As mentioned earlier, several specialized dental tomographic units have been developed in recent years. One example is Soredex's Scanora® unit, which is described below. It is a multifunctional unit enabling tomographs of the dental and maxillofacial region to be obtained in many different planes. The equipment (see Fig. 16.9) consists of patient chair, vertical control panel, and tubehead and cassette-carriage assembly linked together and positioned at either ends of a C-arm and placed in a rotating unit. This arrangement allows the freedom for a large number of dental and maxillofacial imaging procedures and projections to be selected, all of which are computer controlled and automatically executed. The resultant images, produced using complex broad beam **spiral** tomography (see

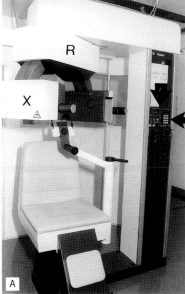

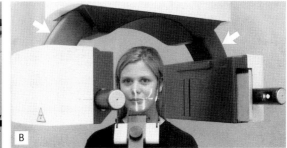

Fig. 16.9A   The original film-based Scanora tomographic unit. The X-ray tubehead (X), cassette-carriage assembly (C) and rotating unit (R) are all indicated. **B** Patient positioned in the unit; note the light-markers on the face. The linking C-arm is arrowed.

Fig. 16.4), have better definition and higher resolution than simple linear tomographs.

Recent developments have seen the Scanora® upgraded for digital imaging using phosphor plate technology. Following exposure the plate is *read* (see Ch. 7) in situ and the information relayed to the computer for visual display on the monitor.

Range of investigations

The full range of investigations possible using the Scanora® (at present over 600), and the other specialized units available, is beyond the scope of this book. However, some of the more useful applications include:

- Conventional dental panoramic tomographs (see Fig. 16.10 and Ch. 17)

- Mid-facial panoramic tomographs to assess the antrum and fractures of the inferior orbital rim
- Cross-sectional (transverse) tomographic sections of the mandible or maxilla to:
  - Assess the jaw height, thickness and texture, and the position of the inferior dental nerve and/or antrum before inserting implants (see Figs 16.10 and 16.11 and Chs 24 and 29)
  - Assess the site, size and extent of cysts, tumours and other pathological lesions
- Cross-sectional (transverse) and tangential tomographic sections of teeth to localize root defects and assess the location of any associated disease (see Fig. 16.12)
- Stereoscopic views to localize unerupted structures
- Corrected sagittal and coronal tomographic sections of the TMJ (see Ch. 31).

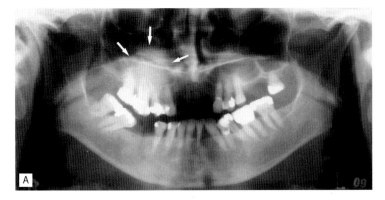

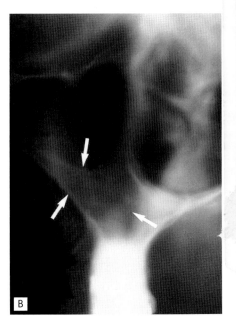

Fig. 16.10A Scanora® dental panoramic tomograph showing a poorly defined zone of opacity in the right maxilla (arrowed) in the area of the antrum. **B** Cross-sectional (transverse) tomographic image through the right maxilla showing the opacity to be caused by an increased bone thickness in the base of the antrum and lateral margin (arrowed). The patient had had previous surgery in this area.

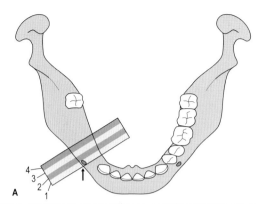

Fig. 16.11A   Diagram showing the relationship between the mandible and one typical set of four cross-sectional (transverse) tomographic images. B An example of four 4-mm wide Scanora® spiral tomographic slices corresponding to the sections illustrated in diagram A. The mental canal is demonstrated clearly on slice (1) (arrowed). The vertical opaque metal markers in the localization stent are evident on all four slices.

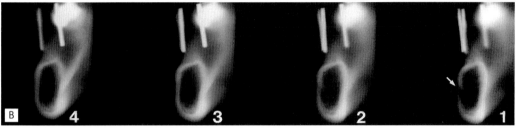

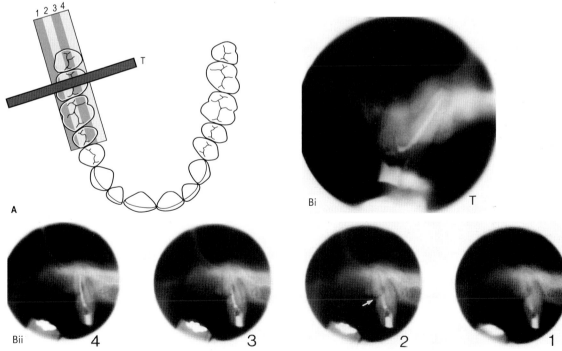

Fig. 16.12A   Diagram of the maxillary arch showing the relationship between the right maxillary molar teeth and one set of four tangential tomographic images and one cross-sectional (transverse) image (T). B An example of Scanora® spiral tomographic slices corresponding to the various sections illustrated in diagram A, through the 7⌋. (i) Cross-sectional or transverse slice (T) demonstrating the root filling in the palatal root canal. (ii) Four tangential slices. A fracture through the distobuccal root is demonstrated on slice (2) (arrowed).

Chapter 17

Panoramic radiography (dental panoramic tomography)

INTRODUCTION

Panoramic radiography or *dental panoramic tomography* has become a very popular technique in dentistry. The main reasons for this include:

- All the teeth and their supporting structures are shown on one image (see Fig. 17.1)
- The technique is relatively simple
- The radiation dose is relatively low, particularly with modern DC units and when using rare-earth intensifying screens or digital image receptors.

The major drawback to the technique is that the resultant film is a *sectional radiograph* produced by moving equipment, and like all other forms of *tomography* (see Ch. 16) only structures within the *section* will be evident and in focus on the final film. In panoramic tomography, the *section* or *focal trough* is designed to be approximately horseshoe-shaped, corresponding to the shape of the dental arches. Image quality is generally inferior to that obtained using intra-oral radiographic techniques – irrespective of the type of image receptor used – and interpretation is more complicated.

SELECTION CRITERIA

In the UK, the 2004 *Selection Criteria in Dental Radiography* booklet recommends panoramic radiography in general practice in the following circumstances:

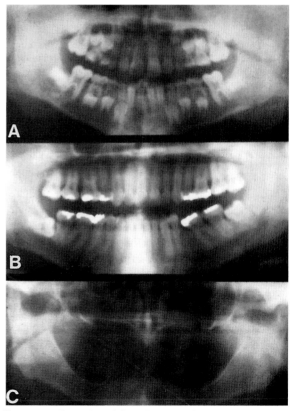

Fig. 17.1 Examples of dental panoramic radiographs. **A** A child in mixed dentition. **B** A dentate adult. **C** An edentulous adult.

- Where a bony lesion or unerupted tooth is of a size or position that precludes its complete demonstration on intra-oral radiographs
- In the case of a grossly neglected mouth
- As part of an assessment of periodontal bone support where there is pocketing greater than 6 mm
- For the assessment of wisdom teeth prior to planned surgical intervention. Routine radiography of unerupted third molars is not recommended
- As part of an orthodontic assessment where there is a clinical need to know the state of the dentition and the presence/absence of teeth. The use of clinical criteria to select patients rather than routine screening patients is essential.

In addition, in dental hospitals panoramic radiographs are also used to assess:

- Fractures of all parts of the mandible except the anterior region
- Antral disease — particularly to the floor, posterior and medial walls of the antra
- Destructive diseases of the articular surfaces of the TMJ
- Vertical alveolar bone height as part of pre-implant planning.

The 2004 *Selection Criteria* booklet specifically states that 'panoramic radiographs should only be taken in the presence of specific clinical signs and symptoms', and goes on to say that 'there is no justification for review panoramic radiography at arbitrary intervals' (see Ch. 8 on *justification*).

THEORY

The theory of dental panoramic tomography is complicated. Nevertheless, an understanding of how the resultant radiographic image is produced and which structures are in fact being imaged, is necessary for a critical evaluation, and for the interpretation of this type of radiograph.

The difficulty in panoramic tomography arises from the need to produce a final shape of *focal trough* which approximates to the shape of the dental arches.

An explanation of how this final horseshoe-shaped focal trough is achieved is given below.

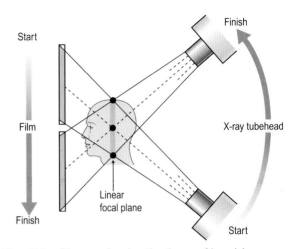

Fig. 17.2 Diagram showing the theory of broad-beam linear tomography to produce a vertical coronal section with the synchronized movement of the X-ray tubehead and the film in the vertical plane. Using a broad beam, there will be multiple centres of rotation (three are indicated: •), all of which will lie in the shaded zone. As all these centres of rotation will be in focus, this zone represents the focal plane or section that will appear in focus on the resultant tomograph. **Note** — the broad X-ray beam exposes the **entire** film throughout the exposure.

But first, other types of tomography — which form the basis of panoramic tomography — are described, showing how they result in different shapes of focal trough. These include:

- Linear tomography using a wide or broad X-ray beam
- Linear tomography using a narrow or slit X-ray beam
- Rotational tomography using a slit X-ray beam.

Broad–beam linear tomography

This was described in detail in Chapter 16 and is illustrated again in Figure 17.2. The synchronized movement of the tubehead and film, in the *vertical* plane, results in a straight linear focal trough. The broad X-ray beam exposes the entire film throughout the exposure.

Slit or narrow–beam linear tomography

A similar straight linear tomograph can also be produced by modifying the equipment and using a narrow or slit X-ray beam. The equipment is

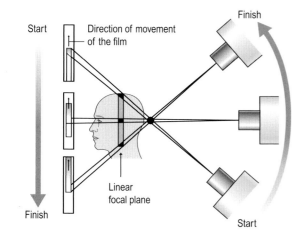

Fig. 17.3 Diagram showing the theory of narrow-beam linear tomography to produce a vertical coronal section. The tomographic movement is produced by the synchronized movement of the X-ray tubehead and the cassette carrier, in the vertical plane. The film, placed behind the metal protective front of the cassette carrier, also moves during the exposure, in the same direction as the X-ray tubehead. The narrow X-ray beam traverses the patient and film, exposing a **different** part of the film throughout the cycle.

designed so that the narrow beam traverses the film exposing different parts of the film during the tomographic movement. Only by the end of the tomographic movement has the entire film been exposed. The following equipment modifications are necessary:

- The X-ray beam has to be collimated from a broad beam to a narrow beam.
- The film cassette has to be placed behind a protective metal shield. A narrow opening in this shield is required to allow a small part of the film to be exposed to the X-ray beam at any one instant.
- A cassette carrier, incorporating the metal shield, has to be linked to the X-ray tubehead to ensure that they move in the **opposite** direction to one another during the exposure. This produces the synchronized tomographic movement in the *vertical* plane.
- Within this carrier, the film cassette itself has to be moved in the **same** direction as the tubehead. This ensures that a different part of the film is exposed to the X-ray beam throughout the exposure.

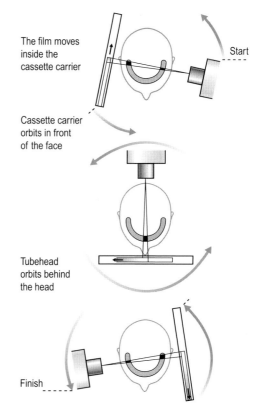

Fig. 17.4 Diagrams showing the theory of narrow beam rotational tomography. The tomographic movement is provided by the circular synchronized movement of the X-ray tubehead in one direction and the cassette carrier in the opposite direction, in the horizontal plane. The equipment has a single centre of rotation. The film also moves inside the cassette carrier so that a **different** part of the film is exposed to the narrow beam during the cycle, thus by the end the entire film has been exposed. The focal plane or trough (shaded) is curved and forms the arc of a circle.

The principle of narrow-beam linear tomography using this equipment is illustrated in Figure 17.3.

Narrow–beam rotational tomography

In this type of tomography, narrow-beam equipment is again used, but the synchronized movement of the X-ray tubehead and the cassette carrier are designed to rotate in the *horizontal* plane, in a *circular* path around the head, with a *single* centre of rotation. The resultant focal trough is curved and forms the arc of a circle, as shown in Figure 17.4.

Important points to note

- The X-ray tubehead orbits around the **back** of the head while the cassette carrier with the film orbits around the **front** of the face.
- The X-ray tubehead and the cassette carrier move in **opposite** directions to one another.
- The film moves in the **same** direction as the X-ray tubehead, behind the protective metal shield of the cassette carrier.
- A different part of the film is exposed to the X-ray beam at any one instant, as the equipment orbits the head.
- The simple circular rotational movement with a single centre of rotation produces a curved **circular** focal trough.
- As in conventional tomography, shadows of structures not within the focal trough will be out of focus and blurred owing to the tomographic movement.

DENTAL PANORAMIC TOMOGRAPHY

The dental arch, though curved, is not the shape of an arc of a circle. To produce the required elliptical, horseshoe-shaped focal trough, panoramic tomographic equipment employs the principle of narrow-beam rotational tomography, but uses two or more centres of rotation.

There are several dental panoramic units available; they all work on the same principle but differ in how the rotational movement is modified to image the elliptical dental arch. Four main methods (see Fig. 17.5) have been used including:

- Two stationary centres of rotation, using two separate circular arcs
- Three stationary centres of rotation, using three separate circular arcs
- A continually moving centre of rotation using multiple circular arcs combined to form a final elliptical shape
- A combination of three stationary centres of rotation and a moving centre of rotation.

However the focal troughs are produced, it should be remembered that they are three-dimensional. The focal trough is thus sometimes described as a *focal corridor*. All structures within the corridor, including the mandibular and maxillary teeth, will be in focus on the final radiograph. The

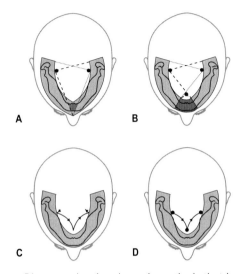

A   **B**

C   **D**

Fig. 17.5 Diagrams showing the main methods that have been used to produce a focal trough that approximates to the elliptical shape of the dental arch using different centres of rotation. **A** 2 stationary, **B** 3 stationary, **C** continually moving, **D** combination of 3 stationary and moving centre.

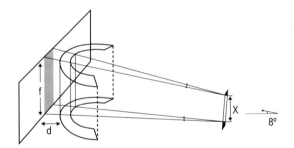

Fig. 17.6 Diagram showing how the height of the three-dimensional focal corridor is determined. The height (x) of the X-ray beam is collimated to just cover the height (f) of the film. The separation of the focal trough and the film (d), coupled with the 8° upward angulation of the X-ray beam results in the final image being slightly magnified.

vertical height of the corridor is determined by the shape and height of the X-ray beam and the size of the film as shown in Figure 17.6.

As in other forms of narrow-beam tomography, a different part of the focal trough is imaged throughout the exposure. The final radiograph is thus built up of sections (see Fig. 17.7), each created separately, as the equipment orbits around the patient's head.

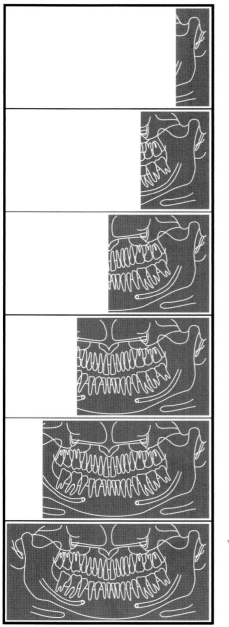

Fig. 17.7 Diagram showing the gradual build-up of a panoramic tomograph over an 18-second cycle, illustrating how a different part of the patient is imaged at different stages in the cycle.

Equipment

There are several different panoramic units available. Although varying in design and apperance all consist of four main components, namely:

- An *X-ray tubehead*, producing a narrow fan-shaped X-ray beam, angled upwards at approximately 8° to the horizontal (see Fig. 17.6)
- *Control panel* (see Fig. 17.9)
- *Patient-positioning apparatus* including chin and temporal supports and light beam markers
- *An image receptor* (film or digital) with or without an associated carriage assembly.

Traditional panoramic equipment was designed to use indirect-action radiographic film in an extra-oral cassette as the image receptor. With the advent of digital imaging several variations in image receptor now exist, including:

- Cassettes containing indirect-action film and rare-earth intensifying screens
- Cassettes containing a digital phosphor plate
- Flat cassette-sized solid-state sensors designed to fit into existing equipment
- Specially designed solid-state sensors—an integral part of new equipment (see Ch. 6).

Examples of two typical machines are shown in Figure 17.8. The regulations relating to the technical aspects of panoramic equipment are summarized in Chapter 8.

Control panel

The control panel design also varies from one machine to another but a typical panel is shown in Figure 17.9. The main features usually allow the operator to:

- Select the field size
- Select a limited range of arch shapes and sizes
- Select the mA and kV exposure factors
- Adjust the anteroposterior position of the bite-peg
- Select the size of the patient to be X-rayed
- Adjust the height of the equipment
- Select a range of field limitation options.

Equipment movement

A diagrammatic example of how a typical panoramic machine, using film or digital phosphor plate as the image receptor, functions is shown in Figure 17.10.

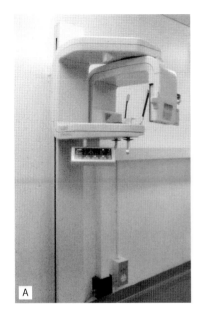

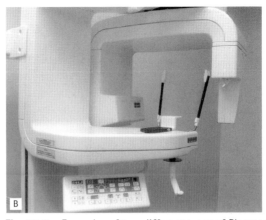

Fig. 17.8 Examples of two different types of Planmeca panoramic radiography machines. **A** Traditional unit incorporating a cassette suitable for film-based or digital phosphor plate imaging. **B** Dedicated digital unit with specifically designed built-in solid-state digital sensor. The basic components including the X-ray tubehead, the control panel and the patient positioning apparatus are common to both units.

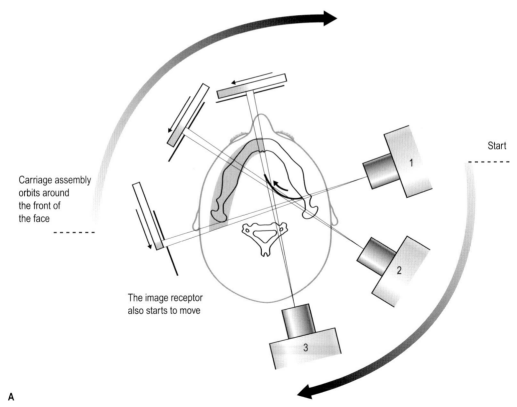

Fig. 17.10A Diagram from above, showing the relative movements of the X-ray tubehead, carriage assembly and image receptor (film or phosphor plate) during the first half of the panoramic cycle when the **left** side of the jaw is imaged. As the X-ray tubehead moves behind the patient's head to image the anterior teeth, the carriage assembly moves in front of the patient's face and the centre of rotation moves forward along the dark arc (arrowed) towards the midline. Note that the X-ray beam has to pass through the cervical spine.

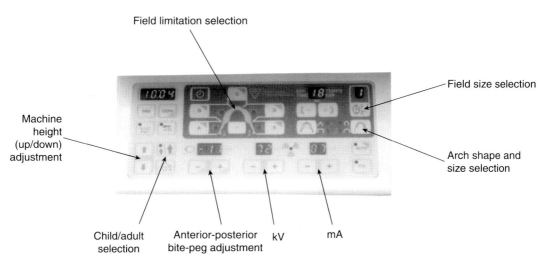

Field limitation selection

Field size selection

Machine
height
(up/down)
adjustment

Arch shape and
size selection

Child/adult
selection

Anterior-posterior
bite-peg adjustment

kV

mA

Fig. 17.9   An example of a typical panoramic control panel showing the main adjustment features.

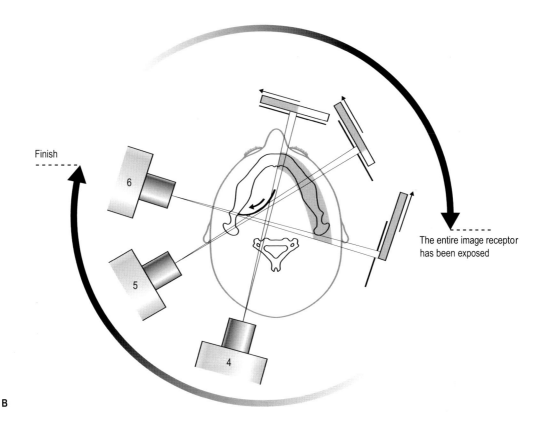

Finish

6

5

4

The entire image receptor
has been exposed

B

Fig. 17.10B   Diagram from above, showing the relative movements during the second half of the panoramic cycle when the **right** side of the jaw is imaged. The X-ray tubehead and carriage assembly continue to move around the patient's head to image the opposite side, and the centre of rotation moves backwards along the dark arc (arrowed) a way from the midline. Throughout the cycle the film or phosphor plate is also continuously moving as illustrated, so that a different part of the image receptor is exposed at any one time.

Technique and positioning

The exact positioning techniques vary from one machine to another. However, there are some general requirements that are common to all machines and these can be summarized as follows:

Patient preparation

- Patients should be asked to remove any earrings, jewellery, hair pins, spectacles, dentures or orthodontic appliances.
- The procedure and equipment movements should be explained, to reassure patients and if necessary use a test exposure to show them the machine's movements.

Equipment preparation

- The cassette containing the film or phosphor plate should be inserted into carriage assembly (if appropriate).
- The operator should put on suitable protective gloves (e.g. latex or nitrile) (see Ch. 9).
- The collimation should be set to the size of field required.
- The appropriate exposure factors should be selected according to the size of the patient— typically in range 70–100 kV and 4–12 mA.

Patient positioning

- The patient should be positioned in the unit so that their spine is straight and instructed to hold any stabilizing supports or handles provided (see Fig. 17.11).
- The patient should be instructed to bite their upper and lower incisors edge-to-edge on the bite-peg with their chin in good contact with the chin support.
- The head should be immobilized using the temple supports.
- The light beam markers should be used so that the mid-sagittal plane is vertical, the Frankfort plane is horizontal and the canine light lies between the upper lateral incisor and canine.
- The patient should be instructed to close their lips and press their tongue on the roof of their mouth so that it is in contact with their hard palate and not to move throughout the exposure cycle (approximately 15–18 seconds).

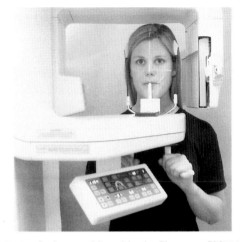

Fig. 17.11 Patient positioned in the Planmeca PM2002, Note the bite-peg, chin and temple supports and the three light-beam markers to facilitate accurate positioning.

Important points to note

- Panoramic radiography is generally considered to be unsuitable for children under six years old, because of the length of the exposure and the need for the patient to keep still.
- A protective lead apron should not be used. In the UK the 2001 *Guidance Notes* confirm that there is no justification for using a protective lead apron. If used, it can interfere with the final image (see Fig. 17.23F).

After exposure

- The temple supports should release automatically to enable the patient to leave the machine.
- The equipment should be wiped down with a surface disinfectant and the bite-peg sterilized (see Ch. 9).
- Gloves should be discarded as clinical waste.
- The film or phosphor plate should be processed.

The importance of accurate patient positioning

The positioning of the patient's head within this type of equipment is critical — it must be positioned accurately so that the teeth lie within the *focal trough*. The effects of placing the head too far forward, too far back or asymmetrically in relation to the focal trough, are shown in Figure 17.12. The parts of the jaws outside the focal trough will be out of focus. The fan-shaped X-ray beam causes patient malposition to be represented mainly as distortion in the horizontal plane, i.e. teeth appear too wide or too narrow rather than foreshortened or elongated. Thus, if the patient is rotated to the left (as shown in Fig. 17.12C), the left teeth are nearer the film and will be narrower, while the teeth on the right will be further away from the film and wider. These and other positioning errors are shown later (see Fig. 17.24).

However accurately the patient's head is positioned, the inclination of the incisor teeth, or the underlying skeletal base pattern, may make it impossible to position both the mandibular **and** maxillary teeth ideally within the focal corridor (see Fig. 17.13).

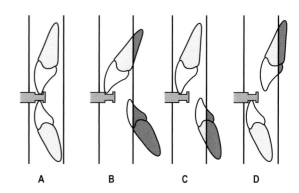

Fig. 17.13 Diagrams showing the vertical walls of the focal trough in the incisor region and the relative positions of the teeth with different underlying dental or skeletal abnormalities. **A** Class I. **B** Gross class II division 1 malocclusion with large overjet. **C** Angle's class II skeletal base. **D** Angle's class III skeletal base. The shaded areas outside the focal trough will be blurred and out of focus.

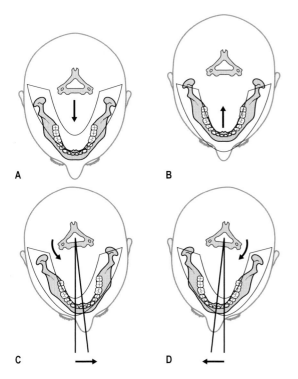

Fig. 17.12 Diagrams showing the position of the mandible in relation to the focal trough when the patient is not positioned correctly. **A** The patient is too close to the film and in front of the focal trough. **B** The patient is too far away from the film and behind the focal trough. **C** and **D** The patient is placed asymmetrically within the machine.

Technique variations

There are a number of technique variations possible with modern equipment, including:

- *Edentulous patient positioning* — the chin support is used instead of the bite-peg and the canine positioning light beam is centred on the corner of the mouth.
- *TMJ programmes* — (see Ch. 31).
- *Cross-sectional imaging* for implant assessment (see Ch. 24).
- *Collimation* — restricting the size of the beam so restricting the field of view e.g. the height of the beam is automatically reduced when selecting the settings for children.
- *Field limitation* techniques — only preselected parts of the patient are exposed and imaged on the final film as illustrated in Figure 17.14.

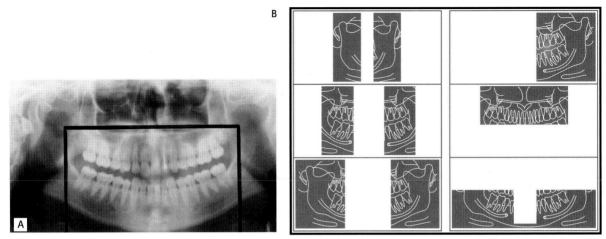

Fig. 17.14A The effect of selecting collimation to reduce the height of the beam **and** field limitation techniques to exclude the rami and parotid producing the so-called *dentition only* image. This has been reported to reduce the effective dose by approximately 50%. **B** Diagram showing a selection of images that can be obtained by using collimation and field limitation techniques.

Normal anatomy

The normal anatomical shadows that are evident on panoramic radiographs vary from one machine to another, but in general they can be subdivided into:

- *Real* or *actual shadows* of structures in, or close to, the focal trough
- *Ghost* or *artefactual shadows* created by the tomographic movement and cast by structures on the opposite side or a long way from the focal trough. The 8° upward angulation of the X-ray beam means that these ghost shadows appear at a higher level than the structures that have caused them.

These two types of shadows are clearly demonstrated in Figures 17.17 and 17.18.

Real or actual shadows

Important hard tissue shadows (see Fig. 17.15)
These include:

- Teeth
- Mandible
- Maxilla, including the floor, medial and posterior walls of the antra
- Hard palate

- Zygomatic arches
- Styloid processes
- Hyoid bone
- Nasal septum and conchae
- Orbital rim
- Base of skull.

Air shadows
- Mouth/oral opening
- Oropharynx.

Important soft tissue shadows (see Fig. 17.16)
These include:

- Ear lobes
- Nasal cartilages
- Soft palate
- Dorsum of tongue
- Lips and cheeks
- Nasolabial folds.

Ghost or artefactual shadows (see Fig. 17.19)

The more important ghost shadows include:
- Cervical vertebrae
- Body, angle and ramus of the contralateral side of the mandible
- Palate.

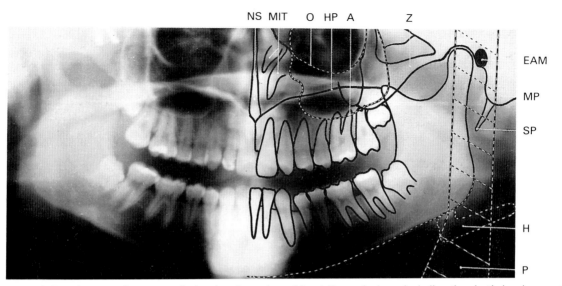

Fig. 17.15 A dental panoramic tomograph showing the main **real hard tissue** shadows, including the plastic head support, drawn in on one side of the radiograph, **NS** — nasal septum, **MIT** — middle and inferior turbinates, **O** — orbital margin, **HP** — hard palate, **A** — floor of antrum, **Z** — zygomatic arch, **EAM** — external auditory meatus, **MP** — mastoid process, **SP** — styloid process, **H** — hyoid, **P** — plastic head support.

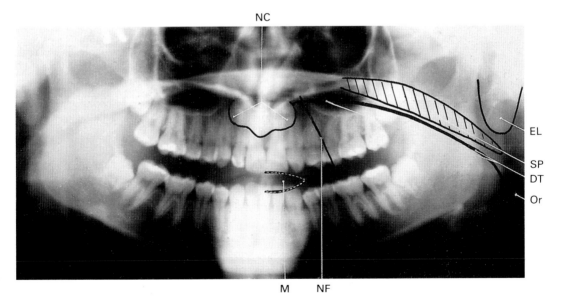

Fig. 17.16 A dental panoramic tomograph showing the main **real soft tissue** and **air** shadows drawn in on one side of the radiograph, **NC** — nasal cartilages, **EL** — ear lobe, **SP** — soft palate, **DT** — dorsum of tongue, **Or** — oropharynx, **NF** — naso-labial fold, **M** — mouth.

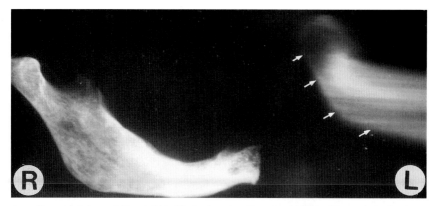

Fig. 17.17 Panoramic radiograph taken of the *right* half of a hemisectioned mandible. The **real** shadows are clearly shown on the *right*. The **ghost** shadow of the mandible is shown on the *left* (arrowed). Note these ghost shadows are at a higher level on the film than the real shadows because of the 8° rising X-ray beam that is used (kindly provided by Dr N. Drage).

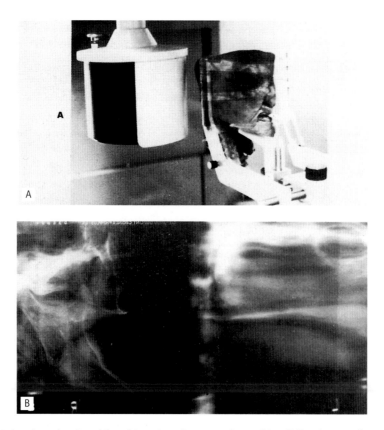

Fig. 17.18 Hemisected cadaver head positioned in a dental panoramic machine. **B** Resultant radiograph showing the real hard and soft tissue shadows on the right and the ghost shadows on the left. (Reproduced from *Oral Radiology*, by kind permission of Paul W. Goaz and Stuart C. White and The C.V. Mosby Company.)

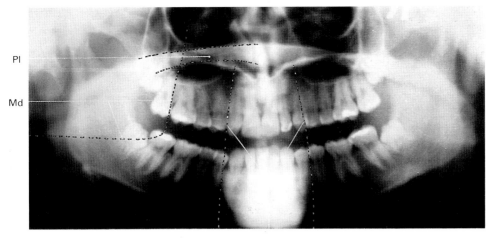

PI

Md

CV

Fig. 17.19 A dental panoramic tomograph showing the main anatomical **ghost** or **artefactual shadows** drawn in on one side of the radiograph, **PI** — palate, **Md** — mandible, **CV** — cervical vertebrae.

Advantages and disadvantages

Advantages

- A large area is imaged and all the tissues within the focal trough are displayed, including the anterior teeth, even when the patient is unable to open the mouth.
- The image is easy for patients to understand, and is therefore a useful teaching aid.
- Patient movement in the vertical plane distorts only that part of the image being produced at that instant.
- Positioning is relatively simple and minimal expertise is required.
- The overall view of the jaws allows rapid assessment of any underlying, possibly unsuspected, disease.
- The view of both sides of the mandible on one film is useful when assessing fracures and is comfortable for the injured patient.
- The overall view is useful for evaluation of periodontal status and in orthodontic assessments.
- The antral floor, medial and posterior walls are well shown.
- Both condylar heads are shown on one film, allowing easy comparison (see Ch. 31).
- The radiation dose (*effective dose*) is about one-fifth of the dose from a full-mouth survey of intra-oral films (see Ch. 3).

- Development of field limitation techniques which result in further dose reduction.

Disadvantages

- The tomographic image represents only a section of the patient. Structures or abnormalities not in the focal trough may not be evident (Fig. 17.20).
- Soft tissue and air shadows can overlie the required hard tissue structures (Fig. 17.21).
- Ghost or artefactual shadows can overlie the structures in the focal trough (Fig. 17.22).
- The tomographic movement together with the distance between the focal trough and film produce distortion and magnification of the final image (approx. x 1.3).
- The use of indirect-action film and intensifying screens results in some loss of image quality but image resolution can be improved by using digital image receptors.
- The technique is not suitable for children under six years or on some disabled patients because of the length of the exposure cycle.
- Some patients do not conform to the shape of the focal trough and some structures will be out of focus.
- Movement of the patient during the exposure can create difficulties in image interpretation (Fig. 17.23).

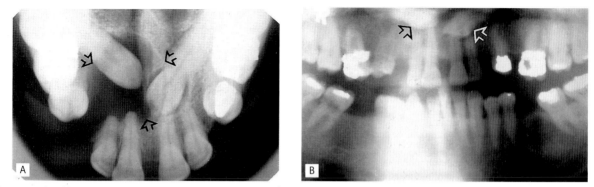

Fig. 17.20A Upper standard occlusal showing unerupted 3|3 and a large dentigerous cyst (arrowed) associated with 3|. **B** Dental panoramic radiograph showing the two unerupted canines out of focus (arrowed) and only a suggestion of the dentigerous cyst, because they are all outside the focal trough.

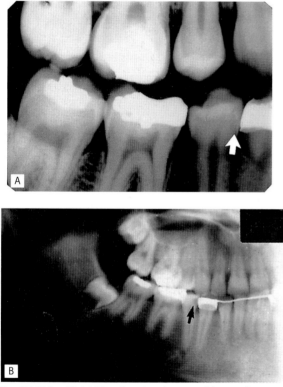

Fig. 17.21A Right bitewing showing no evidence of mesial caries in 5| (arrowed). **B** Dental panoramic radiograph showing an apparent lesion in this tooth (arrowed). This appearance is created by the overlying air shadow of the corner of the mouth.

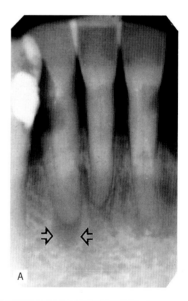

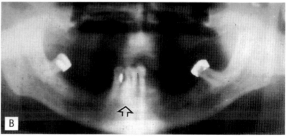

Fig. 17.22A Periapical of 21|12 region showing an area of radiolucency at the apex of 1| (arrowed). **B** Dental panoramic radiograph showing no evidence of the lesion (arrowed) owing to superimposition of the shadow of the cervical vertebrae.

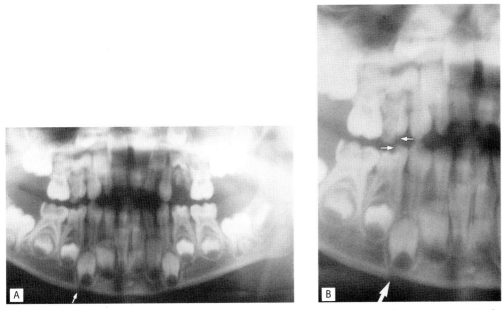

Fig. 17.23 **A** Panoramic radiograph of a young child, who had fallen over, showing a step deformity (arrowed) in the lower border suggesting a fracture. **B** Same radiograph enlarged showing the step deformity (large arrow), but also notice the step deformities in the crowns of the upper and lower first deciduous molars (small arrows). Sudden slight vertical movement of the patient makes interpretation difficult.

Assessment of image quality

As mentioned in previous chapters, in relation to all other radiographs, image quality assessment essentially involves three separate stages, namely:

- Comparison of the image against ideal quality criteria
- Subjective rating of image quality using published standards
- Detailed assessment of rejected films to determine the source of error.

Ideal quality criteria

Irrespective of the type of image receptor being used, typical quality criteria for a full field of view panoramic radiograph include:

- All the upper and lower teeth and their supporting alveolar bone should be clearly demonstrated
- The whole of the mandible should be included

- Magnification in the vertical and horizontal planes should be equal
- The right and left molar teeth should be equal in their mesiodistal dimension
- The density across the image should be uniform with no air shadow above the tongue creating a radiolucent (black) band over the roots of the upper teeth
- The image of the hard palate should appear above the apices of the upper teeth
- Only the slightest ghost shadows of the contralateral angle of the mandible and the cervical spine should be evident
- There should be no evidence of artefactual shadows due to dentures, earrings and other jewellery
- The patient identification label should not obscure any of the above features
- The image should be clearly labelled with the patient's name and date of the examination
- The image should be clearly marked with a **R**ight and/or **L**eft letter.

Subjective rating of image quality

The simple three-point subjective rating scale published in the 2001 *Guidance Notes* was introduced in Chapter 10 and is discussed in detail, together with the errors associated with exposure factors and chemical processing, in Chapter 18. The summary is shown again in Table 17.1. Panoramic patient preparation and positioning errors are described below.

Assessment of rejected films and determination of errors

Patient preparation errors (Fig. 17.24)

These can include:

- Failure to remove jewellery
  - Earrings
  - Necklaces
  - Piercings
- Failure to remove dentures
- Failure to remove orthodontic appliances
- Failure to remove spectacles
- Inappropriate use of the lead apron.

Patient positioning errors (Figs 17.25 and 17.26)

These can include:

- Failure to ensure that the spine is straight (ghosting shadow error)

- Failure to ensure the incisors are biting edge-to-edge on the bite-peg (anteroposterior error)
- Failure to use the light beam marker to ensure midsagittaal plane is vertical and the head is not rotated (horizontal error)
- Failure to use the light beam marker to ensure the Frankfort plane is horizontal (vertical error)
- Failure to instruct the patient to press the tongue against the roof of the mouth (air shadow error)
- Failure to instruct the patient to remain still throughout the exposure (movement error).

Equipment positioning errors (Fig. 17.27)

These can include:

- Failure to set height adjustment correctly
- Failure to select correct exposure settings (see Ch. 18)
- Failure to use the cassette correctly.

Footnote

Dental panoramic radiographs should not be considered an alternative to high-resolution intra-oral radiographs. However, they are commonly considered as an alternative to right and left *oblique lateral* radiographs or the bimolar projection (see Ch. 13) mainly because it is assumed that less operator expertise is required to produce panoramic images of adequate diagnostic quality. Unfortunately, the multiple and varied causes of error in panoramic radiography make the technique very operator-dependent, no matter how sophisticated the equipment and the image receptors become. The use of digital sensors (solid-state or phosphor plate) improves the resolution of panoramic images when compared to those captured using indirect-action film and intensifying screen combinations. In addition, digital images can be enhanced and manipulated using computer software (see Ch. 7).

The diagnostic value of all panoramic images is increased considerably if clinicians understand that the image created is a tomograph (whatever the image receptor) and are aware of the limitations that this imposes. A suggested systematic approach to interpretation of panoramic images is outlined in Chapter 20.

Table 17.1 Subjective quality rating criteria for film-captured images published in the 2001 *Guidance Notes for Dental Practitioners on the Safe Use of X-ray equipment*

Rating	Quality	Basis
1	Excellent	No errors of patient preparation, exposure, positioning, processing or film handling
2	Diagnostically acceptable	Some errors of patient preparation, exposure, positioning, processing or film handling, but which do not detract from the diagnostic utility of the radiograph
3	Unacceptabe	Errors of patient preparation, exposure, positioning, processing or film handling, which render the radiograph diagnostically unacceptable

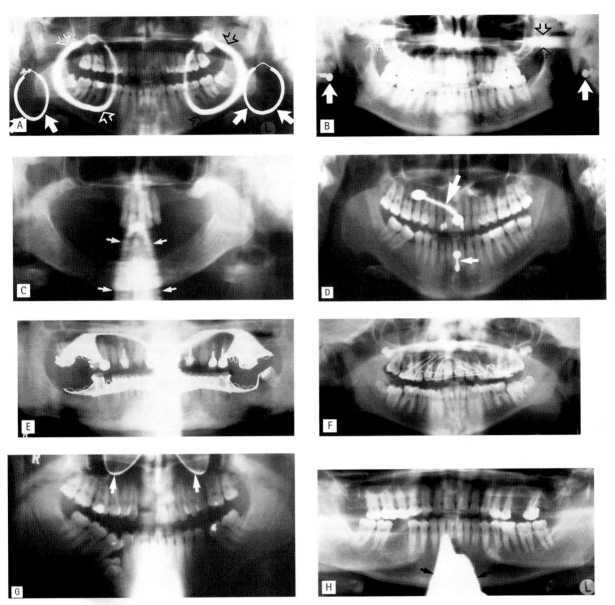

Fig. 17.24 Examples of common patient preparation errors.

A Failure to remove large ring-shaped earrings — note each earring casts two shadows, one real (in focus, solid arrows) and one ghost (blurred, open arrows). The ghost shadow of the LEFT earring is marked with white open arrows, that of the RIGHT earring with black open arrows.

B Failure to remove stud earring, real shadows (solid arrows) with ghost shadows (open arrows).

C Failure to remove a necklace — blurred ghost shadow (arrowed).

D Failure to remove piercing in the tongue (large arrow) and lower lip (small arrow).

E Failure to remove upper and lower metallic partial dentures.

F Failure to remove an upper orthodontic appliance.

G Failure to remove spectacles (arrowed).

H Inappropriate use of a protective lead apron — too high on the neck casting a dense radiopaque shadow (arrowed) over the anterior part of the mandible.

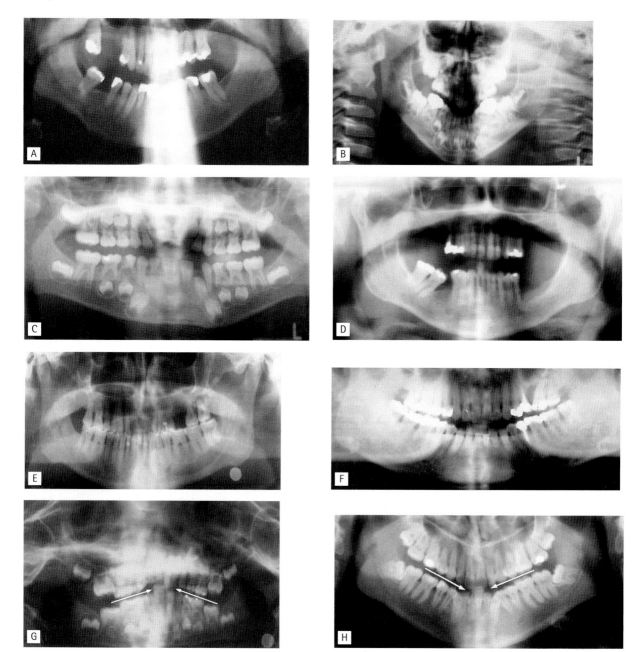

Fig. 17.25 Examples of common patient positioning errors. **A** Failure to position the neck correctly — extension of the neck causing excessive spinal ghosting shadows over the anterior teeth. **B** Anteroposterior error — patient positioned too far forwards (too close to the image receptor) and vertical error — Frankfort plane not horizontal (chin tipped down) creating narrow, out of focus anterior teeth, distorted occlusal plane (so-called *smiley face*) and excessive peripheral spinal shadowing. **C** Anteroposterior error — patient positioned too far back (too far away from the image receptor) creating widened, magnified and out of focus anterior teeth. **D** Anteroposterior error — patient positioned too far forwards (too close to the image receptor) creating narrowed incisors **and** failure to instruct patient to keep their tongue in contact with the palate creating the radiolucent band across the film. **E** Horizontal error — patient asymmetrical, rotated to the RIGHT. The RIGHT molars are closer to the image receptor and smaller, the LEFT molars are further away from the image receptor and larger. **F** Vertical error — Frankfort plane not horizontal (chin tipped down) creating out of focus lower incisors and excessive ghosting shadows of the contralateral angles of the mandible. **G** Vertical error — Frankfort plane not horizontal (chin tipped up) creating out-of-focus upper incisors and distorted occlusal plane (arrowed) (so-called *grumpy face*). **H** Vertical error — Frankfort plane not horizontal (chin tipped down) creating out of focus lower incisors and distorted occlusal plane (arrowed) (so-called *smiley face*).

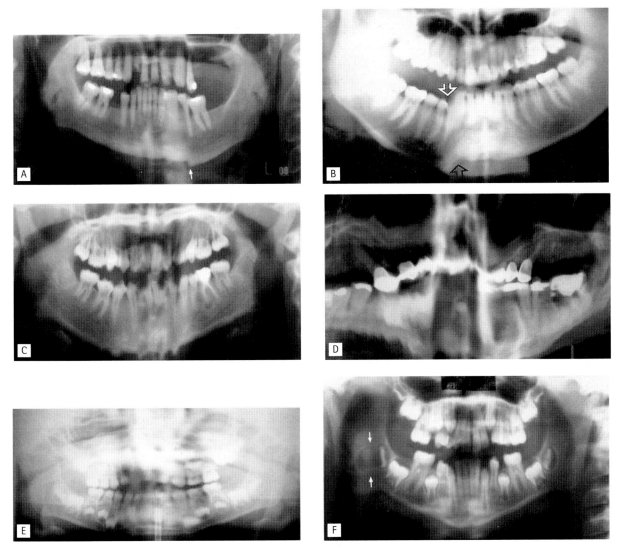

Fig. 17.26   Examples of failure to instruct the patient to keep still during the full panoramic cycle.
A Sudden movement in the vertical plane — distortion of the image 45 region creating a step-deformity in the lower border (see also Fig. 17.23).
B Movement in the vertical plane caused by the patient opening their mouth causing distortion in the $\overline{43}$ region (arrowed).
C Multiple vertical movements while the anterior teeth were being imaged.
D Continuous shaking movements throughout the cycle.
E Sudden side-to-side horizontal movement while the anterior teeth were being imaged causing them to be blurred.
F Horizontal movement towards the end of the cycle causing horizontal elongation and stretching of the shadow of the developing lower right third molar (arrowed).

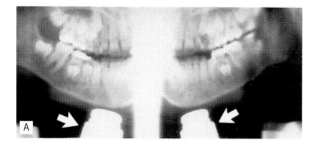

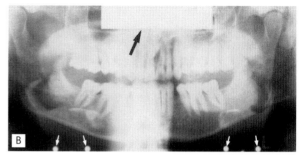

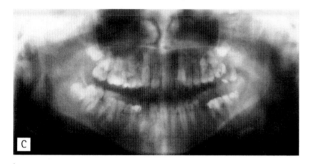

Fig 17.27 Examples of equipment positioning errors.
A The X-ray tubehead and image receptor carriage assembly positioned too low relative to the patient—the antra and condyles are not imaged but shadows of the chin rest are evident (arrowed).
B Cassette positioned back-to-front in the carriage assembly. Name plate and hinge screws are evident (arrowed).
C Cassette inadvertently used twice and double-exposed.

Chapter 18

The quality of radiographic images and quality assurance

INTRODUCTION

The factors that can affect the quality of radiographic images depends on:

- How the image was taken (radiographic technique)
- What image receptor was used (film or digital)
- How the visual image was created
  - Chemical processing (film)
  - Computer processing (digital).

The effects of poor radiographic technique are the same whatever type of image receptor is used. These technique errors have already been covered in detail in relation to the three main projections used in dentistry, namely: periapicals (Ch. 10), bitewings (Ch. 11) and panoramic radiographs (Ch. 17).

The creation of the visual *digital* image was described in Chapter 7, together with how computer software can be used to alter and manipulate the image with regards to contrast, brightness (degree of blackening), magnification, inversion, enhancement and pseudocolourization.

Creation of the black/white/grey image on *film* using chemical processing was also described in Chapter 7. This film-captured image can however be affected by many other factors. This chapter therefore is designed for revision, bringing together and summarizing from earlier chapters all these various factors. It also includes a quick reference section as an aid to fault-finding of film-captured images. Various film faults are illustrated together with their possible causes. This is followed by a section on quality assurance (QA) and suggested quality control measures.

IMAGE QUALITY

As mentioned in Chapter 1, image quality and the amount of detail shown on a radiographic film depends on several factors including:

- Contrast
- Image geometry
- Characteristics of the X-ray beam
- Image sharpness and resolution.

Contrast

Radiographic contrast, i.e. the final visual difference between the various black, white and grey shadows depends on:

- Subject contrast
- Film contrast
- Fog and scatter.

Subject contrast

This is the difference caused by different degrees of attenuation as the X-ray beam is transmitted through different parts of the patient's tissues. It depends upon:

- Differences in tissue thickness
- Differences in tissue density

- Differences in tissue atomic number (photo-electric absorption $\propto Z^3$ (see Ch. 2))
- Quality (voltage (kV)) or penetrating power of the radiation beam (kV↑, contrast↓ — *kV kills contrast*).

Film contrast

This is an inherent property of the film itself (see Ch. 6). It determines how the film will respond to the different exposures it receives after the X-ray beam has passed through the patient. Film contrast depends upon four factors:

- The characteristic curve of the film
- Optical density or degree of blackening of the film
- Type of film — direct or indirect action
- Processing.

Fog and scatter

Stray radiation reaching the film either as a result of background fog, or owing to scatter from within the patient, produces unwanted film density (blackening), and thus reduces radiographic contrast.

Image geometry

As mentioned and illustrated in Chapter 1, the geometric accuracy of any image depends upon the position of the X-ray beam, object and image receptor (film or digital) satisfying certain basic geometrical requirements:

- The object and the film should be in contact or as close together as possible
- The object and the film should be parallel to one another
- The X-ray tubehead should be positioned so that the beam meets the object and the film at right angles.

Characteristics of the X-ray beam

The ideal X-ray beam used for imaging should be:

- Sufficiently penetrating to pass through the patient, to a varying degree, and react with the film emulsion to produce good *contrast* between the various black, white and grey shadows (see earlier)

- Parallel, i.e. non-diverging, to prevent magnification of the image (see Ch. 5)
- Produced from a point source to reduce blurring of the image margins and the *penumbra effect* (see Ch. 5).

Image sharpness and resolution

Sharpness is defined as the ability of the X-ray film to define an edge. The main causes of loss of edge definition include:

- Geometric unsharpness including the *penumbra effect* (see above)
- Motion unsharpness, caused by the patient moving during the exposure
- Absorption unsharpness — caused by variation in object shape, e.g. cervical *burn-out* at the neck of a tooth (see Ch. 21)
- Screen unsharpness, caused by the diffusion and spread of the light emitted from intensifying screens (see Ch. 6)
- Poor resolution. Resolution, or resolving power of the film, is a measure of the film's ability to differentiate between different structures and record separate images of small objects placed very close together, and is determined mainly by characteristics of the film including:
  – type — direct or indirect action
  – speed
  – silver halide emulsion crystal size.
  Resolution is measured in line pairs per mm.

PRACTICAL FACTORS INFLUENCING IMAGE QUALITY

In practical terms, the various factors that can influence overall image quality can be divided into factors related to:

- The X-ray equipment
- The image receptor — film or film/screen combination
- Processing
- The patient
- The operator and radiographic technique.

As a result of all these variables, film faults and alterations in image quality are inevitable. However, since the diagnostic yield from radiography is related directly to the quality of the image, regular checks and monitoring of these variables are essential to achieve and maintain good quality radiographs. It is these checks which form the basis of *quality assurance (QA) programmes*.

Clinicians using film need to be able to recognize the cause of the various film faults so that appropriate corrective action can be taken.

TYPICAL FILM FAULTS

Examples of typical film faults are shown below and summarized later in Table 18.1.

Film too dark (Figs 18.1 and 18.2)

Possible causes

- Overexposure owing to:
  - Faulty X-ray equipment, e.g. timer
  - Incorrect exposure time selected
- Overdevelopment owing to:
  - Excessive time in the developer solution
  - Developer solution too hot
  - Developer solution too concentrated
- Fogging owing to:
  - Poor storage conditions:
    * Allowing exposure to stray radiation
    * Too warm
  - Old film stock used after expiry date
  - Faulty cassettes allowing ingress of light
  - Faulty darkroom/processing unit:
    * Allowing leakage of stray light
    * Faulty safe-light
- Thin patient tissues.

Film too pale (Fig. 18.3)

Possible causes

- Underexposure owing to:
  - Faulty X-ray equipment, e.g. timer
  - Incorrect exposure time setting by the operator
  - Failure to keep timer switch depressed throughout the exposure
- Underdevelopment owing to:
  - Inadequate time in the developer solution
  - Developer solution too cold
  - Developer solution too dilute
  - Developer solution exhausted
  - Developer contaminated by fixer
- Excessive thickness of patient's tissues
- Film packet back to front (film also marked).

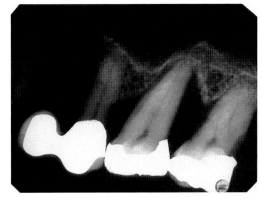

Fig. 18.1   Example of a periapical that is too dark with poor contrast.

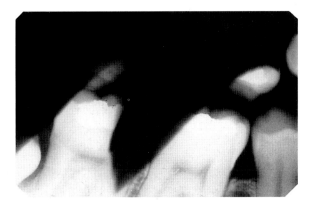

Fig. 18.2   Example of a fogged (blackened) film. Bitewing fogged in the darkroom by inadvertently exposing the upper part of the film to light. The lower part was protected by the operator's fingers.

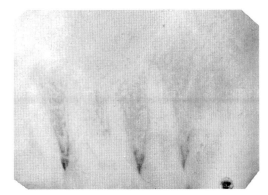

Fig. 18.3   Example of a periapical that is too pale with poor contrast.

Film with inadequate or low contrast (Figs 18.1, 18.2, 18.3)

Possible causes

- Processing error owing to:
  - Underdevelopment (film also pale)
  - Overdevelopment (film also dark)
  - Developer contaminated by fixer
  - Inadequate fixation time
  - Fixer solution exhausted
- Fogging owing to:
  - Poor storage conditions:
    * Allowing exposure to stray radiation
    * Too warm
  - Poor stock control and film used after expiry date
  - Faulty cassettes allowing the ingress of stray light
  - Faulty darkroom/processing unit.

Image unsharp and blurred (Fig. 18.4)

Possible causes

- Movement of the patient during the exposure (see also Chs 10, 11 and 17)
- Excessive bending of the film packet during the exposure (see also Ch. 10)
- Poor film/screen contact within a cassette
- Film type — image definition is poorer with indirect-action film than with direct-action film
- Speed of intensifying screens — fast screens result in loss of detail
- Overexposure — causing *burn-out* of the edges of a thin object
- Poor positioning in panoramic radiography (see Ch. 17).

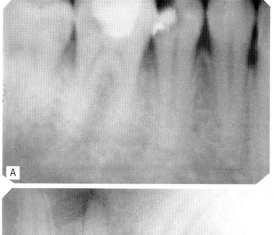
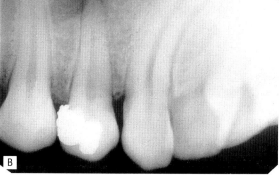

Fig. 18.4 Examples of unsharp and blurred films. **A** As a result of patient movement. **B** As a result of excessive bending of the film packet during the exposure.

Film marked (Fig. 18.5)

Possible causes

- Film packet bent by the operator
- Careless handling of the film in the darkroom resulting in marks caused by:
  - Finger prints
  - Finger nails
  - Bending
  - Static discharge
- Processing errors owing to:
  - Chemical spots
  - Under fixation — residual silver halide emulsion remaining
  - Roller marks
  - Protective black paper becoming stuck to the film
  - Insufficient chemicals to immerse films fully
- Patient biting too hard on the film packet
- Dirty intensifying screens in cassettes.

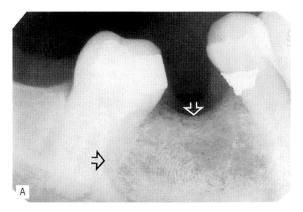

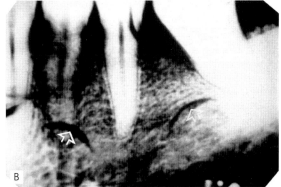

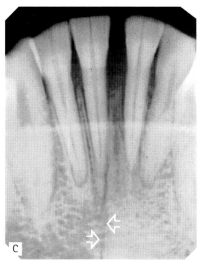

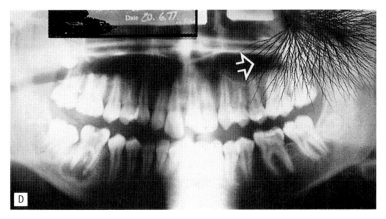

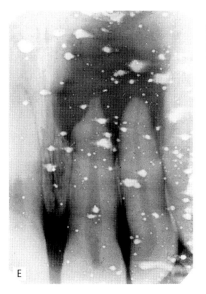

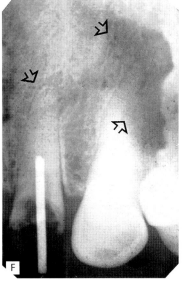

Fig. 18.5 Examples of marked films.
A Finger print impression in the emulsion (arrowed).
B Finger nail marks (arrowed).
C Sharply bent film (arrowed) damaging the emulsion.
D Discharge of static electricity (arrowed).
E Fixer splashes on the emulsion before the film was placed in the developer.
F Marks (arrowed) caused by residual emulsion remaining following inadequate fixation (these are usually brown).

Table 18.1 Summary of common film quality problems and their possible causes. (Reproduced, with modifications, from *Dental Update* with kind permission of Professor K. Horner and George Warman Publications)

Reason for rejection	Possible causes General	Particular	Remedy to each particular fault
Film too dark	Processing fault (overdevelopment)	Developer concentration too high	Dilute or change chemicals
		Development time too long	Adjust as necessary
		Developer temperature too high	Adjust as necessary
	Excessive X-ray exposure	Incorrect exposure setting	Adjust and repeat examination
		Faulty timer on X-ray set	Arrange service and repair of X-ray set
		Thin patient tissues	Decrease exposure and repeat
	Fogged film	Light leak in darkroom	Check and correct
		Faulty safelighting	Inspect safelights visually, coin test, and correct any fault detected
		Old film stock	Discard film
		Poor film storage	Discard film and re-assess storage facilities
		Light leak in cassette	Check hinges and catches and repair or replace if required
Film too pale	Processing fault (underdevelopment)	Overdiluted developer	Change chemicals
		Inadequate development time	Adjust as necessary
		Developer temperature too low	Adjust as necessary
		Exhausted developer	Change chemicals
		Developer contaminated by fixer	Change chemicals
	Inadequate X-ray exposure	Incorrect exposure setting	Adjust and repeat
		Faulty timer on X-ray set	Arrange service and repair of X-ray set
		Excessive thickness of patient's tissues	Increase exposure and repeat
	Technique error	Film back to front	Adjust and repeat
Inadequate or low contrast	Processing fault	Overdevelopment (plus dark films)	Check development and time/temperature relationship
		Underdevelopment (plus pale films)	As above
		Developer contaminated by fixer	Change chemicals
		Inadequate fixation time (films opaque; milky sheen)	Adjust as necessary
		Fixer exhausted (films opaque; milky sheen)	Change fixer solution
	Fogged film	See above	See above

Problem	Cause	Detail	Remedy
Unsharp image	Technique error	Patient movement	Assess and instruct patient carefully
		Excessive bending of the film packet during exposure	Adjust and repeat
		Poor patient positioning (in panoramic radiography)	Greater care in positioning and full use of positioning aids
	Cassette error	Poor film/screen contact	Check cassette and repair or replace if necessary
		Incorrect intensifying screen speed	Change screens
	Excessive X-ray exposure	Incorrect exposure setting for thin object causing *burn-out*	Decrease exposure setting and repeat
Film marked	Handling fault	Film packet bent	Careful handling
		Careless handling in darkroom	As above
	Processing fault	Chemical spots	Careful chemical handling
		Insufficient chemicals to allow full immersion of film	Check chemical tanks and adjust
		Automatic roller marks	Clean processor
		Patient biting too hard on the film	Instruct patient correctly and repeat
		Dirt on intensifying screens	Clean screens regularly
Poor positioning (Chs, 10, 11 and 17)	Film packet incorrectly positioned	Film back to front (plus pale film)	Use film holders for intraoral radiography when possible
		Not covering area of interest	As above
		Film used twice (plus dark film)	Greater care in film handling
	X-ray tubehead incorrectly positioned	Too steep an angle producing foreshortening	Use beam-aiming devices when possible
		Too shallow an angle producing elongation	As above
	Patient incorrectly positioned	Patient incorrectly placed (in panoramic unit)	Greater care in positioning and full use of positioning aids

PATIENT PREPARATION AND POSITIONING (RADIOGRAPHIC TECHNIQUE) ERRORS (Fig. 18.6)

These errors can happen whatever image receptor is being used and were described in detail and illustrated in Chapters 10, 11 and 17. They are summarized below and can be divided into intraoral and panoramic technique errors.

Intraoral technique errors

These can include:

- Failure to position the image receptor correctly to capture the area of interest
- Failure to position the image receptor correctly causing it to bend (if flexible) creating geometrical distortion
- Failure to orientate the image receptor correctly and using it back-to front
- Failure to align the X-ray tubehead correctly in the horizontal plane causing:
  - *coning off* or *cone cutting*
  - overlapping and geometrical distortion
  - superimposition
- Failure to align the X-ray tubehead correctly in the vertical plane causing:
  - *coning off* or *cone cutting*
  - foreshortening and geometrical distortion
  - elongation and geometrical distortion

- Failure to instruct the patient to remain still during the exposure with subsequent movement resulting in blurring
- Failure to set correct exposure settings (image too dark or too pale — see earlier)
- Careless inadvertent use of the image receptor twice.

Panoramic technique errors

These can include:

- Failure to remove jewellery
- Failure to remove dentures
- Failure to remove orthondontic appliances
- Failure to remove spectacles
- Inappropriate use of a protective lead apron
- Failure to ensure the spine is straight
- Failure to ensure the incisors are biting on the bite-peg (anteroposterior error)
- Failure to use the light beam markers to ensure mid-sagittal plane is vertical and Frankfort plane is horizontal (horizontal and vertical errors)
- Failure to instruct the patient to press the tongue against the roof of the mouth
- Failure to instruct the patient to remain still throughout the exposure cycle
- Failure to set machine height adjustment correctly
- Failure to set correct exposure settings (image too dark or too pale — see earlier)
- Failure to use the cassette/image receptor correctly.

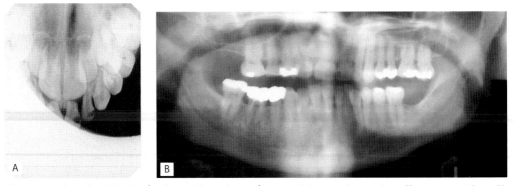

A　　　B

Fig. 18.6 Two examples of positioning (radiographic technique) errors. **A** Intraoral – *coning off* or *cone cutting* – X-ray tubehead incorrectly positioned, anterior part of image receptor not exposed. **B** Panoramic — patient too far away from the image receptor — incisor teeth magnified (anteroposterior error) **and** patient rotated to the LEFT, left molars narrowed, right molars widened (horizontal error).

QUALITY ASSURANCE IN DENTAL RADIOLOGY

The World Health Organization has defined radiographic quality assurance (QA) programmes as '... an organised effort by the staff operating a facility to ensure that the diagnostic images produced by the facility are of sufficiently high quality so that they consistently provide adequate diagnostic information at the lowest possible cost and with the least possible exposure of the patient to radiation'.

Quality control measures are therefore as essential in a general dental practice *facility*, as they are in a specialized radiography department. This importance of **quality** is acknowledged in the UK in the Ionising Radiations Regulations 1999 (see Ch. 8) which make quality assurance in dental radiography a mandatory requirement. A section in the 2001 *Guidance Notes for Dental Practitioners on the Safe Use of X-ray Equipment* is devoted to quality assurance and should be regarded as essential reading. This chapter is based broadly on the recommendations in the 2001 *Guidance Notes*.

Terminology

The main terms in quality procedures include:

- *Quality control* — the specific measures for ensuring and verifying the quality of the radiographs produced.
- *Quality assurance* — the arrangements to ensure that the quality control procedures are effective and that they lead to relevant change and improvement.
- *Quality audit* — the process of external reassurance and assessment that quality control and quality assurance mechanisms are satisfactory and that they work effectively.

Quality assurance programme

A basic principle of quality assurance is that, within the overall QA programme, all necessary procedures should be laid down in writing and in particular:

- Implementation should be the responsibility of a named person
- Frequency of operations should be defined
- The content of the essential supporting records should be defined and the frequency for the formal checking of such records.

As stated in the 2001 *Guidance Notes* and implied by the WHO definition, a well-designed QA programme should be comprehensive but inexpensive to operate and maintain. The standards should be well researched but once laid down would be expected to require only infrequent verification or modification. The procedures should amount to little more than 'written down common sense'. The aims of these programmes, whether using film-based or digital radiography, can be summarized as follows:

- To produce diagnostic radiographs of consistently high standard
- To reduce the number of repeat radiographs
- To determine all sources of error to allow their correction
- To increase efficiency
- To reduce costs
- To ensure that radiation doses to patients and staff are kept as low as reasonably practicable (ALARP).

Quality control procedures for film–based radiography

The essential quality control procedures relate to:

- Image quality and film reject analysis
- Patient dose and X-ray equipment
- Darkroom, image receptors and processing
- Working procedures
- Staff training and updating
- Audits.

Image quality and film reject analysis

Image quality assessment is an important test of the entire QA programme. Hence the need for clinicians to be aware of all the various factors, outlined earlier, that affect image quality and to monitor it on a regular basis. This assessment should include:

- A day-to-day comparison of the quality of every radiograph to a high standard reference film positioned permanently on the viewing screen and an investigation of any significant deterioration in quality.
- A formal analysis of film quality, either retrospective or prospective, approximately every six months. The 2001 *Guidance Notes* recommended the simple three-point subjective rating scale shown in Table 18.2, and shown previously in Chapters 10, 11 and 17, be used for film-based intra-oral and extra-oral radiography.
- Based on these quality ratings, performance targets can be set. Suitable targets recommended in the *Guidance Notes* are shown in Table 18.3 with the advice that practices should aim to achieve these targets within three years of implementing the QA programme. The 'interim targets' should be regarded as the minimum achievable standard in the shorter term.
- Analysis of all unacceptable films given a rating of 3 sometimes referred to as *film reject analysis* (see below).

Film reject analysis

This is a simple method of identifying all film faults and sources of error and amounts to a *register of reject radiographs*. To do this, it is necessary to collect all rejected (grade 3) radiographs and record

- Date
- Nature of the film fault/error, as shown earlier, e.g.:
  a. Film too dark
  b. Film too pale
  c. Low or poor contrast
  d. Unsharp image
  e. Poor positioning
- Known or suspected cause of the error or fault and corrective action taken (see Table 18.1)
- Number of repeat radiographs (if taken)
- Total number of radiographs taken during the same time period. This allows the percentage of faulty films to be calculated.

Regular review of film reject analysis records is an invaluable aid for identifying a range of problems, including a need for equipment maintenance,

additional staff training as well as processing faults that could otherwise cause unnecessary radiation exposure of patients and staff.

Patient dose and X-ray equipment

One of the aims of QA stated earlier is to ensure that radiation doses are kept as low as reasonably practicable. It is therefore necessary to measure patient doses on a regular basis and compare them against national diagnostic reference levels. To achieve this, X-ray equipment must comply with current recommendations, as described in Chapter 8. These include:

Table 18.2 Subjective quality rating criteria for film-captured images published in 2001 *Guidance Notes for Dental Practitioners on the Safe Use of X-ray Equipment*

Rating	Quality	Basis
1	Excellent	No errors of patient preparation, exposure, positioning, processing or film handling
2	Diagnostically acceptable	Some errors of patient preparation, exposure, positioning, processing or film handling, but which do not detract from the diagnostic utility of the radiograph
3	Unacceptable	Errors of patient preparation, exposure, positioning, processing or film handling, which render the radiograph diagnostically unacceptable

Table 18.3 Minimum and interim targets for radiographic quality from the 2001 *Guidance Notes*

	Percentage of radiographs taken	
Rating	Target	Interim target
1	Not less than 70%	Not less than 50%
2	Not greater than 20%	Not less than 40%
3	Not greater than 10%	Not greater than 10%

- The initial *critical examination and report* — carried out by the installer
- The *acceptance test* — carried out by the radiation protection adviser before equipment is brought into clinical use and includes measurement of patient dose
- A *re-examination report* following any relocation, repair or modification of equipment that may have radiation protection implications
- Day-to-day checks of important features that could affect radiation protection including:
  - correct functioning of warning lights and audible alarms
  - correct operation of safety devices
  - satisfactory performance of the counter-balance for maintaining the correct position of the tubehead
- Written records and an equipment log should be maintained and include:
  - all installer's formal written reports describing the checks made, the results obtained and action taken
  - results of all equipment checks in chronological order
  - details of all routine or special maintenance
- The Ionizing Radiation (Medical Exposure) Regulations 2000 require that an up-to-date inventory of each item of X-ray equipment is maintained, and available, at each practice and contains:
  - name of the manufacturer
  - model number
  - serial number or other unique identifier
  - year of manufacture
  - year of installation
- Compliance with the recommendations in Ch. 9 of *Recommended standards for the routine performance testing of diagnostic X-ray imaging systems*, Report 91 of the Institute of Physics and Engineering in Medicine (IPEM) published in 2005.

Darkroom, image receptors and processing

Darkroom
The QA programme should include instructions on all the regular checks that should be made, and how frequently, with all results recorded in a log. Important areas include:

- General cleanliness (daily), but particularly of work surfaces and film hangers (if used).
- Light-tightness (yearly), by standing in the darkroom in total darkness with the door closed and safelights switched off and visually inspecting for light leakage
- Safelights (yearly), to ensure that these do not cause fogging of films. Checks are required on:
  - Type of filter — this should be compatible with the colour sensitivity of film used, i.e. blue, green or ultraviolet (see Ch. 6)
  - Condition of filters — scratched filters should be replaced
  - Wattage of the bulb — ideally it should be no more than 25W
  - Their distance from the work surface — ideally they should be at least 1.2m (4ft) away
  - Overall safety (i.e. their fogging effect on film) — the simple quality control measure for doing this is known as the *coin test*:
  1. Expose a piece of screen film in a cassette to a very small even exposure of X-rays (so-called *flash* exposure) to make the emulsion ultra-sensitive to subsequent light exposure
  2. In the darkroom, remove the film from the cassette and place on the worksurface underneath the turned-off safelight
  3. Place a series of coins (e.g. seven) in a row on the film and cover them all with a piece of card
  4. Turn on the safelight and then slide the card to reveal the first coin and leave for approximately 30 seconds
  5. Slide the card along to reveal the second coin and leave again for approximately 30 seconds
  6. Repeat until all the coins have been revealed
  7. Process the film in the normal way.

A simulated result is shown in Figure 18.7. Fogging (blackening) of the film owing to the safelight will then be obvious when compared to the clear area protected by the coin. The part of the film adjacent to the first coin will have been exposed to the safelight for the longest time and will be the darkest. In practice, the normal film-handling time under the safelight can be measured and the effect of safelight fogging established.

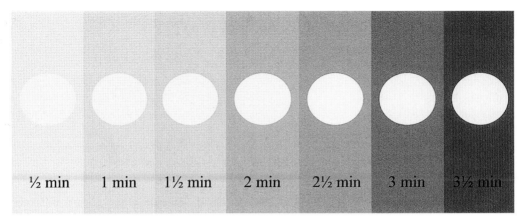

| ½ min | 1 min | 1½ min | 2 min | 2½ min | 3 min | 3½ min |

Fig. 18.7 A simulated coin test result. The film, with seven coins on it, has been gradually uncovered every 30 seconds. The coin-covered part of the film remains white while the surrounding film is blackened or fogged. The longer the film is exposed to the safelight the darker it becomes. (Kindly provided by Mr N. Drage.)

Note. The *coin test* can also be used to assess the amount of light transmission through the safety glass of automatic processors by performing the test within the processor under the safety glass under normal daylight loading conditions.

Image receptors

The QA programme requires written information, usually obtained from the suppliers, on film speed, expiry date and storage conditions as well as details regarding the maintenance and cleaning instructions of cassettes and/or digital image receptors. Typical requirements could include:

X-ray film

This requires:

- Ideal storage conditions — cool, dry and away from all sources of ionizing radiation — as recommended by the manufacturers
- Strict stock control with records to ensure usage before the expiry date
- Careful handling.

Cassettes

These require:

- Regular cleaning of intensifying screens with a proprietary cleaner
- Regular checks for light-tightness, as follows:
  1. Load a cassette with an unexposed film and place the cassette on a window sill in the daylight for a few minutes

  2. Process the film — any ingress of light will have fogged (darkened) the film (see Fig. 18.8(i))
- Regular checks for film/screen contact, as follows:
  1. Load a cassette with an unexposed film and a similar sized piece of graph paper
  2. Expose the cassette to X-rays using a very short exposure time
  3. Process the film — any areas of poor film/screen contact will be demonstrated by loss of definition of the image of the graph paper (see Fig. 18.8(ii))
- A simple method of identification of films taken in similar looking cassettes, e.g. a Letraset letter on one screen.

Processing

The QA programme should contain written instructions about each of the following:

Chemical solutions

These should be:

- Always made up to the manufacturers' instructions taking special precautions to avoid even trace amounts of contamination of the developer by the fixer, e.g. always fill the fixer tank first so that any splashes into the developer tank can be washed away **before** pouring in the developer
- Always at the correct temperature

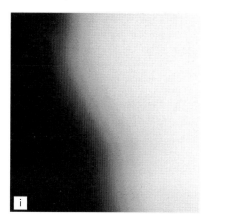

Fig. 18.8(i)   Radiograph from a faulty cassette being checked for light-tightness. The light that has got into the cassette has blackened one side of the film.

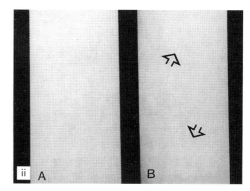

Fig. 18.8(ii)   Examples of the radiographs following the graph paper test for film/screen contact. **A** Good film/screen contact — the fine detail of the graph paper is evident over the whole film. **B** Poor film/screen contact — note the loss of detail in several areas.

- Changed or replenished regularly — ideally every 2 weeks — and records should be kept to control and validate these changes
- Monitored for deterioration. This can be done easily using radiographs of a *step-wedge phantom*:
  1. Make a simple step-wedge phantom using the lead foil from inside intra-oral film packets, as shown in Figure 18.9(i)
  2. Radiograph the step-wedge using known exposure factors
  3. Process the film in **fresh** solutions to produce a *standard reference film*
  4. Repeat, using the same exposure factors, every day as the solutions become exhausted
  5. Compare each day's film with the standard reference film to determine objectively any decrease in blackening of the processed film which would indicate deterioration of the developer (see Fig. 18.9(ii))
  6. Record the results.

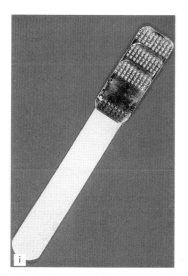

Fig. 18.9(i)   A simple step-wedge phantom constructed using pieces of lead foil taped to a tongue spatula.

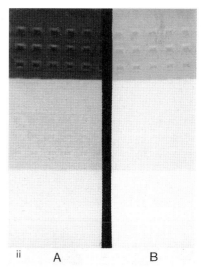

Fig. 18.9(ii)   **A** The *standard reference* film of the step-wedge phantom on DAY ONE processed using newly made-up chemical solutions. **B** Test film processed in chemical solutions 1 week old — note the reduced amount of blackening of the second film owing to the weakened action of the developer.

Processing equipment

- Manual processing requires the use of accurate timers, thermometers and immersion heaters. Instructions on their proper use should be provided.
- Automatic processors require regular replenishment of chemical solutions and regular cleaning, especially of the rollers. All cleaning procedures should be written down including how often they should be carried out.
- Record log confirming that all cleaning procedures have been carried out should be kept.

Working procedures

These include:

- *Local rules* — required in the UK under the Ionising Radiations Regulations 1999 (see Ch. 8). These rules should contain the procedural and operational elements that are essential to the safe use of X-ray equipment, including guidance on exposure times, and as such should contain much of what is relevant to the maintenance of good standards in QA.
- *Employers' written procedures* — required in the UK under the Ionising Radiation (Medical Exposure) Regulations 2000 (see Ch. 8).
- *Operational procedures or systems of work* — these include written procedures that provide for all actions that indirectly affect radiation safety and diagnostic quality, e.g. instructions for the correct preparation and subsequent use of processing chemicals (as explained earlier).
- *Procedures log* — the QA programme should include the maintenance of a procedures log to record the existence of appropriate *Local Rules* and *Employers' Written Procedures*, together with a record of each occasion on which they are reviewed or modified (ideally every 12 months).

Staff training and updating

As mentioned in Chapter 8, it is a legal requirement under the Ionising Radiation (Medical Exposure) Regulations 2000 that all *practitioners* and *operators* are adequately trained and that continuing professional development (CPD) is undertaken. The details of the training required in the UK are given in Chapter 8. The QA programme should incorporate a register of all staff involved with any aspect of radiography and should include the following information:

- Name
- Responsibility
- Date, nature and details of training received
- Recommended date for a review of training needs.

Audits

Each procedure within the QA programme will include a requirement for written records to be made by the responsible person at varying intervals. In addition, the person with overall responsibility for the QA programme should check the full programme at intervals not exceeding 12 months. This is an essential feature of demonstrating effective implementation of the programme. Clinical audits may include:

- The QA programme and associated records
- The justification and authorisation of radiographs
- The appropriateness of requests/investigations
- The clinical evaluation of radiographs.

QUALITY CONTROL PROCEDURES FOR DIGITAL RADIOGRAPHY

The overall quality control procedures for digital radiography are similar, and in some instances identical, to those required for film-based radiography. They relate to:

- Image quality assessment
- Patient dose and X-ray equipment
- Image processing and manipulation
- Working procedures
- Staff training and updating
- Audits.

Quality control procedures for digital *image quality assessment* and *image processing and manipulation* are currently not well defined or documented, although some of the recommendations in the 2005 IPEM Report 91, mentioned earlier, apply to dental digital imaging. Theoretically image quality overall should be improved as:

- Chemical processing errors are eliminated
- Most exposure errors can be compensated for by using computer software particularly when using phosphor plates with their wide latitude, although overexposure of solid-state sensors can cause *blooming* (see Ch. 7 and Fig. 7.14).

However, radiographic technique errors are just as important as in film-based radiography and need to be monitored. Clinicians using digital radiography are still required to have a quality assurance (QA) programme. The 2001 *Guidance Notes* make the additional recommendation that because of the ease with which digital radiographs can be retaken, it is essential to ensure that all retakes are properly justified, recorded and included in QA statistics.

Footnote

The requirement for quality assurance and quality control measures in general dental practice applies equally to specialized radiography departments. However, in view of the cost implications, the expensive, sophisticated equipment available for precise quality assurance measurements and accurate monitoring in X-ray departments are often inappropriate to general practice. The practical suggestions in this chapter for film-based radiography, based on the 2001 *Guidance Notes*, are designed to satisfy the WHO definition by bringing an element of objectivity to quality assurance in practice, but at the same time being simple, easily done and inexpensive.

Chapter 19

Alternative and specialized imaging modalities

INTRODUCTION

An array of medical imaging modalities has been developed in recent years and these continue to be developed at a phenomenal rate. Totally new imaging techniques have been introduced, while the resolution and image quality of existing systems are continually being refined and improved. Research and development have focused on manipulating and altering all three of the basic requirements for image production — the patient, the image-generating equipment (to find alternatives to ionizing radiation) and the image receptor. Digital image receptors (solid-state and photostimulable phosphor plates) are now used routinely (see Ch. 6). More and more sophisticated computer software is being developed to manipulate the image itself, once it has been captured. Many of these imaging modalities are playing an increasingly important role in dentistry. As a result, clinicians need to be aware of them and their application in the head and neck region. The main specialized imaging modalities include:

- Contrast studies
- Radioisotope imaging (nuclear medicine)
- Computed tomography (CT)
- Cone beam CT (CBCT)
- Ultrasound
- Magnetic resonance (MR).

This chapter provides a summary of these modalities and their main applications in the head and neck region.

CONTRAST STUDIES

These investigations use *contrast media*, radiopaque substances that have been developed to alter artificially the density of different parts of the patient, so altering *subject contrast* — the difference in the X-ray beam transmitted through different parts of the patient's tissues (see Ch. 18). Thus, by altering the patient, certain organs, structures and tissues, invisible using conventional means, can be seen (see Fig. 19.1). Contrast studies, and the tissues imaged, include:

- Sialography — salivary glands
- Arthrography — joints
- Angiography — blood vessels
- Lymphography — lymph nodes and vessels
- Urography — kidneys
- Barium swallow, meal and enema — GI tract
- Computed tomography — general enhancement (see later).

Types of contrast media

The main types include:

- Barium sulphate suspensions for investigating the gastrointestinal tract

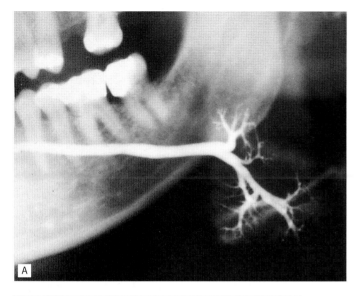

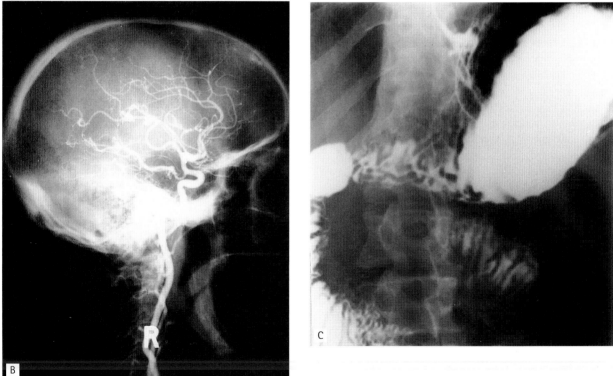

Fig. 19.1 Examples of different contrast studies. **A** A left submandibular gland sialograph. **B** A lateral skull angiograph showing contrast media in the branches of the right internal carotid artery (courtesy of Mrs J. E. Brown). **C** An abdominal radiograph following a barium meal showing contrast media in the stomach, duodenum and small bowel.

- Iodine-based aqueous solutions used for all other investigations and divided into:
  - *Ionic monomers*, including:
    * iothalmate (e.g. Conray®)
    * metrizoate (e.g. Isopaque®)
    * diatrizoate (e.g. Urografin®)
  - *Ionic dimers*, including:
    * ioxaglate (e.g. Hexabrix®)
  - *Non-ionic monomers*, including:
    * iopamidol (e.g. Niopam®)
    * iohexol (e.g. Omnipaque®)
    * iopromide (e.g. Ultravist®)
- Iodine-based oil solutions such as Lipiodol® (iodized poppy seed oil) used for lymphography and sialography
- MR contrast agents (e.g. gadolinium)

Harmful effects of contrast media

Ideally, contrast media should have no harmful effects at all. However, there is a small risk associated with their use, especially with the iodine-based aqueous solutions (the so-called *general contrast media*) when they are introduced into the blood stream. Considering a single dose of contrast medium contains more than 2000 times as much iodine as the body's total physiological content, adverse or residual effects are remarkably rare.

Important point to note
Several of the newer imaging modalities now being used more routinely in dentistry, as discussed later, rely heavily on the use of these contrast-enhancing agents and clinicians should therefore be aware of the risks involved.

Complications
The main complications associated with contrast media can be divided into:

- *Mild*, e.g. headache, nausea, warmth and/or pain, flushing, sneezing and constipation (GI investigations)
- *Moderate*, e.g. vomiting, bronchospasm, urticaria and hypotension
- *Severe*, e.g. cardiac arrhythmias, cardiac arrest, convulsions, anaphylactic shock and pulmonary oedema
- *Fatal*.

Patients particularly at risk
- The elderly and very young children
- Patients with a history of allergy to contrast media
- Diabetics
- Patients suffering from:
  - Cardiac failure
  - Renal failure
  - Severe pulmonary disorders, including asthma.

Causes of complications
Complications are due mainly to:

- Allergy
- Chemotoxicity
- Osmolality (osmotic pressure of the solution) — with ionic monomer contrast media, the *osmolality* is three times greater than that of other agents; the risk of complications arising when using these substances is therefore also greater
- Anxiety.

Prophylactic measures to minimize complications
- Use of low osmolality contrast agents
- Skin pre-testing (the value of this is in doubt)
- Prophylactic steroids
- Prophylactic antihistamines
- Reassurance to reduce levels of anxiety
- Ask specifically about previous history of iodine allergy.

Main contrast studies used in the head and neck

These include:

- Sialography — (see Ch. 33)
- Arthrography — (see Ch. 29)
- Computed tomography — to provide general enhancement (see later)
- Angiography — this involves the introduction of aqueous iodine-based contrast media into selected blood vessels. In the head and neck region, this involves usually the carotids (common, internal or external) or the vertebral arteries.

The procedure usually entails introducing a catheter into a femoral artery followed by selective catheterization of the carotid or vertebral arteries, as required, using fluoroscopic control. Once the catheter is sited correctly, the contrast medium is injected and radiographs of the appropriate area taken (see Fig. 19.1B).

Main indications for angiography in the head and neck
- To show the vascular anatomy and feeder vessels associated with haemangiomas.
- To show the vascular anatomy of arteriovenous malformations.
- Investigation of suspected subarachnoid haemorrhage resulting from an aneurysm in the Circle of Willis.
- Investigation of transient ischaemic attacks possibly caused by emboli from atheromatous plaques in the carotid arteries.

RADIOISOTOPE IMAGING

Radioisotope imaging relies upon altering the patient by making the tissues radioactive and the patient becoming the source of ionizing radiation. This is done by injecting certain radioactive compounds into the patient that have an affinity for particular tissues — so-called *target tissues*. The radioactive compounds become concentrated in the target tissue and their radiation emissions are then detected and imaged, usually using a stationary *gamma camera* (see Fig. 19.2). This investigation allows the function and/or the structure of the target tissue to be examined under both static and dynamic conditions.

Radioisotopes and radioactivity

Radioisotopes, as defined in Chapter 2, are *isotopes with unstable nuclei which undergo radioactive disintegration*. This disintegration is often accompanied by the emission of radioactive particles or radiation. The important emissions include:

- Alpha particles
- Beta− (electron) and beta+ (positron) particles
- Gamma radiation.

The main properties and characteristics of these emissions are summarized in Table 19.1.

Radioisotopes used in conventional nuclear medicine

Several radioisotopes are used in conventional nuclear medicine, depending on the organ or tissue under investigation. Typical examples together with their *target tissues* or *target diseases* include:
- Technetium (^{99m}Tc) — salivary glands, thyroid, bone, blood, liver, lung and heart
- Gallium (^{67}Ga) — tumours and inflammation
- Iodine (^{123}I) — thyroid
- Krypton (^{81}K) — lung.

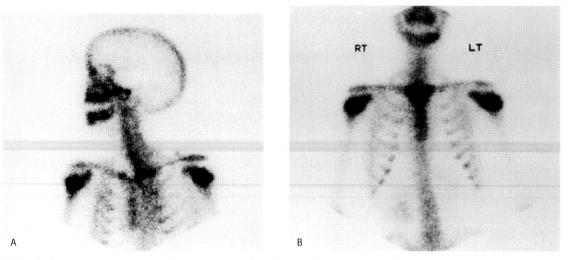

A   B

Fig. 19.2 Technetium bone scan. **A** Left lateral head and neck image. **B** Anterior chest image.

^{99m}Tc is the most commonly used radioisotope. Its main properties include:

- Single 141 keV gamma emissions which are ideal for imaging purposes
- A short half-life of $6\frac{1}{2}$ hours which ensures a minimal radiation dose
- It is readily attached to a variety of different substances that are concentrated in different organs, e.g.:
  - Tc + MPD (methylene diphosphonate) in bone
  - Tc + red blood cells in blood
  - Tc + sulphur colloid in the liver and spleen
- It can be used on its own in its ionic form (pertechnetate ^{99m}TcO^{4-}), since this is taken up selectively by the thyroid and salivary glands
- It is easily produced, as and when required, on site.

Main indications for conventional isotope imaging in the head and neck

- Tumour staging — the assessment of the sites and extent of bone metastases.
- Investigation of salivary gland function, particularly in Sjögren's syndrome (see Ch. 33)
- Evaluation of bone grafts.
- Assessment of continued growth in condylar hyperplasia.
- Investigation of the thyroid.
- Brain scans and assessment of a breakdown of the blood–brain barrier.

Advantages over conventional radiography

- Target tissue function is investigated.
- All similar target tissues can be examined during one investigation, e.g. the whole skeleton can be imaged during one bone scan.
- Computer analysis and enhancement of results are available.

Disadvantages

- Poor image resolution — often only minimal information is obtained on target tissue anatomy.
- The radiation dose to the whole body can be relatively high.
- Images are not usually disease-specific.
- Difficult to localize exact anatomical site of source of emission.
- Some investigations take several hours.
- Facilities are not widely available.

Further developments in radioisotope imaging techniques include:

- *Single photon emission computed tomography (SPECT)*, where the photons (gamma rays) are emitted from the patient and detected by a gamma camera rotating around the patient and the distribution of radioactivity is displayed as a cross-sectional image or SPECT scan enabling the exact anatomical site of the source of the emissions to be determined.
- *Positron emission tomography (PET)*. As shown in Table 19.1, some radioactive isotopes decay by

Table 19.1   Summary of the main properties and characteristics of radioactive emissions

Property	Alpha particles	Beta$^-$ particles	Gamma rays	Beta$^+$ particles
Nature	Particulate – two protons and two neutrons	Particulate – electrons	Electromagnetic radiation – identical to X-rays	Particulate – positron, interacts very rapidly with a negative electron to produce 2 gamma rays – *annihilation radiation* – properties as shown in adjacent column
Size	Large	Small	Nil	
Charge	Positive	Negative	Nil	
Speed	Slow	Fast	Very fast	
Range in tissue	1–2 mm	1–2 cm	As with X-rays	
Energy range carried	4–8 MeV	100 keV–6 MeV	1.24 keV–12.4 MeV	
Damage caused	Extensive ionization	Ionization	Ionization – similar damage to X-rays	
Use in nuclear medicine	Banned	Very limited	Main emission used	PET

the emission of a positively charged electron (positron) from the nucleus. This positron usually travels a very short distance (1–2 mm) before colliding with a free electron. In the ensuing reaction, the mass of the two particles is annihilated with the emission of two (photons) gamma rays of high energy (511 keV) at almost exactly 180° to each other. These emissions, known as *annihilation radiation*, can then be detected simultaneously (in coincidence) by opposite radiation detectors which are arranged in a ring around the patient. The exact site of origin of each signal is recorded and a cross-sectional slice is displayed as a PET scan. The major advantages of PET as a functional imaging technique are due to this unique detection method and the variety of new radioisotopes which can now be used clinically. These include:

– Carbon (^{11}C)
– Fluorine (^{18}F)
– Oxygen (^{15}O)
– Nitrogen (^{13}N).

As in conventional nuclear medicine, these radioisotopes can be used on their own or incorporated into diverse and biologically important compounds (e.g. glucose, amino acids, and ammonia) and then administered in trace amounts to study:

– Tissue perfusion
– Substrate metabolism, often using ^{18}F-fluorodeoxyglucose (^{18}FDG)
– Cell receptors
– Neurotransmitters
– Cell division
– Drug pharmacokinetics.

PET can therefore be used to investigate disease at a molecular level, even in the absence of anatomical abnormalities apparent on CT or MRI (see later). It is also possible to superimpose a PET scan on a CT scan, by a technique known as *co-localization*, to determine a lesion's exact anatomical position. Clinically it has been used in the management of patients with epilesy, cerebrovascular and cardiovascular disease, dementia and malignant tumours.

COMPUTED TOMOGRAPHY (CT)

CT scanners use X-rays to produce sectional or slice images, as in conventional tomography (see Ch. 16), but the radiographic film is replaced by very sensitive crystal or gas detectors. The detectors measure the intensity of the X-ray beam emerging from the patient and convert this into digital data which are stored and can be manipulated by a computer as described in Chapter 7. This numerical information is converted into a grey scale representing different tissue densities, thus allowing a visual image to be generated (see Fig. 19.3).

Equipment and theory

The CT scanner is essentially a large square piece of equipment (the gantry) with a central circular hole as shown in Figure 19.4A. The patient lies down with the part of the body to be examined within this circular hole. The gantry houses the X-ray tubehead and the detectors. The mechanical geometry of scanners varies. In so-called *third-generation scanners*, both the X-ray tubehead and the detector array revolve around the patient, as shown in Figure 19.4. In so-called

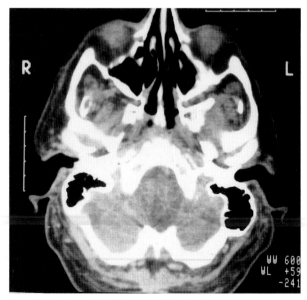

Fig. 19.3 An axial CT image of the head.

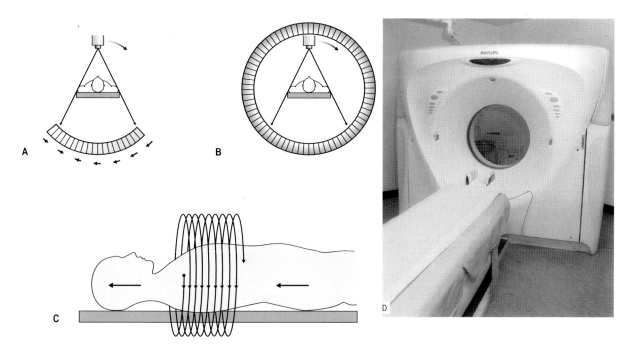

Fig. 19.4 Diagrams showing the principles of **A** a *third-generation* CT scanner — both the X-ray tubehead and the detector array rotate around the patient, **B** a *fourth-generation* CT scanner — the X-ray tubehead rotates within a stationary ring of detectors, and **C** *spiral CT* — the tubehead and detectors move in a continuous spiral motion around the patient as the patient moves continuously into the gantry in the direction of the solid arrows. **D** The Philips MX 8000 multislice spiral CT scanner.

fourth-generation scanners, there is a fixed circular array of detectors (as many as 1000) and only the X-ray tubehead rotates, as shown in Figure 19.4C. Whatever the mechanical geometry, each set of detectors produces an attenuation or penetration profile of the slice of the body being examined. The patient is then moved further into the gantry and the next sequential adjacent slice is imaged. The patient is then moved again, and so on until the part of the body under investigation has been completed. This stop–start movement means the investigation takes several minutes to complete and the radiation dose to the patient is high.

As a result, *spiral CT* has been developed in recent years. Acquiring spiral CT data requires a continuously rotating X-ray tubehead and detector system in the case of third-generation scanners or, for fourth-generation systems, a continuously rotating X-ray tubehead. This movement is achieved by slip-ring technology. The patient is now advanced continuously into

the gantry while the equipment rotates, in a spiral movement, around the patient, as shown in Figure 19.4D. The investigation time has been shortened to only a few seconds with a radiation dose reduction of up to 75%.

Whatever type of scanner is used, the level, plane and thicknesses (usually between 1.5 mm and 6 mm) of the slices to be imaged are selected and the X-ray tubehead rotates around the patient, scanning the desired part of the body and producing the required number of slices. These are usually in the axial plane, as was shown in Figure 19.3.

The sequence of events in image generation can be summarized as follows:

- As the tubehead rotates around the patient, the detectors produce the attenuation or penetration profile of the slice of the body being examined.
- The computer calculates the absorption at points on a grid or matrix formed by the

intersection of all the generation profiles for that slice.

- Each point on the matrix is called a *pixel* and typical matrix sizes comprise either 512 × 512 or 1024 × 1024 pixels. The smaller the individual pixel the greater the resolution of the final image (as described for digital imaging in Chs 6 and 7).
- The area being imaged by each pixel has a definite volume, depending on the thickness of the tomographic slice, and is referred to as a *voxel* (see Fig. 19.5).
- Each voxel is given a *CT number* or *Hounsfield unit* between, for example, +1000 and −1000, depending on the amount of absorption within that block of tissue (see Table 19.2).
- Each CT number is assigned a different degree of greyness, allowing a visual image to be constructed and displayed on the monitor.
- The patient moves through the gantry and sequential adjacent sections are imaged.
- The selected images are photographed subsequently to produce the hard copy pictures, with the rest of the images remaining on disc.

Image manipulation

The major benefits of computer-generated images are the facilities to manipulate or alter the image and to reconstruct new ones, without the patient having to be re-exposed to ionizing radiation (see also Ch. 7).

Window level and window width

These two variables enable the visual image to be altered by selecting the optimal range and level of densities to be displayed.

- **Window level** — this is the CT number selected for the centre of the range, depending on whether the lesion under investigation is in soft tissue or bone.
- **Window width** — the range selected to view on the screen for the various shades of grey, e.g. a narrow range allows subtle differences between very similar tissues to be detected.

Reconstructed images

The information obtained from the original axial scan can be manipulated by the computer to reconstruct tomographic sections in the coronal, sagittal or any other plane that is required, or to produce three-dimensional images, as shown in Figure 19.6. However, to minimize the *step effect* evident in these reconstructed images, the original axial scans need to be very thin and contiguous or overlapping with a resultant relatively high dose of radiation to the patient.

Main indications for CT in the head and neck

- Investigation of intracranial disease including tumours, haemorrhage and infarcts.
- Investigation of suspected intracranial and spinal cord damage following trauma to the head and neck.

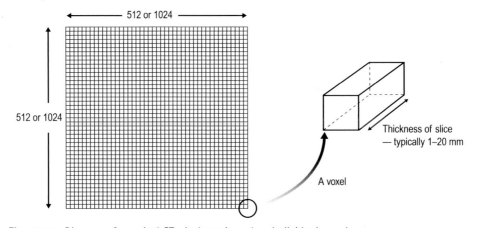

512 or 1024

512 or 1024

Thickness of slice — typically 1–20 mm

A voxel

Fig. 19.5 Diagram of a typical CT *pixel* matrix and an individual *voxel*.

Table 19.2	Typical CT numbers for different tissues	
Tissue	CT number	Colour
Air	−1000	Black
Fat	−100 to −60	
Water	0	
Soft tissue	+40 to +60	
Blood	+55 to +75	
Dense bone	+1000	White

- Assessment of fractures involving:
  - The orbits and naso-ethmoidal complex
  - The cranial base
  - The odontoid peg
  - The cervical spine.
- Assessment of the site, size and extent of cysts, giant cell and other bone lesions (see Fig. 19.7).
- Assessment of disease within the paranasal air sinuses (see Ch. 29).
- Tumour staging — assessment of the site, size and extent of tumours, both benign and malignant, affecting:
  - The maxillary antra
  - The base of the skull
  - The pterygoid region
  - The pharynx
  - The larynx.
- Investigation of tumours and tumour-like discrete swellings both intrinsic and extrinsic to the salivary glands.
- Investigation of osteomyelitis.
- Investigation of the TMJ.
- Preoperative assessment of maxillary and mandibular alveolar bone height and thickness before inserting implants (see Ch. 24).

Appropriate examples of CT scans are included in later chapters.

Advantages over conventional film–based tomography

- Very small amounts, and differences, in X-ray absorption can be detected. This in turn enables:
  - Detailed imaging of intracranial lesions
  - Imaging of **hard** and **soft** tissues
  - Excellent differentiation between different types of tissues, both normal and diseased.
- Images can be manipulated.

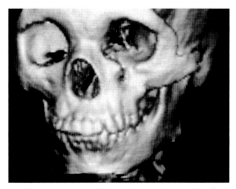

Fig. 19.6   A reconstructed three-dimensional CT image of the skull. (Kindly provided by Mr P. O'Driscoll.)

- Axial tomographic sections are obtainable.
- Reconstructed images can be obtained from information obtained in the axial plane.
- Images can be enhanced by the use of IV contrast media to delineate blood vessels.

Disadvantages

- The equipment is very expensive.
- Very thin contiguous or overlapping slices resulting in a generally high dose investigation (see Ch. 3).
- Metallic objects, such as fillings may produce marked streak or *star* artefacts across the CT image.
- Inherent risks associated with IV contrast agents (see earlier).

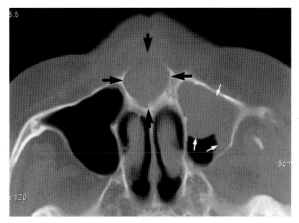

Fig. 19.7   Part of an axial CT scan showing an expansive cystic lesion in the anterior palate (black arrows). Mucosal thickening within the antrum is also evident (white arrows). (Kindly provided by Dr J. Kabala and Dr J. Luker).

CONE BEAM CT

Low dose cone beam CT technology has recently been developed specifically for use in the dental and maxillofacial regions and is rapidly establishing itself as the imaging modality of choice in many clinicaly situations. It is also referred to as *digital volume tomography.*

Equipment and theory

Several machines are currently available with new developments planned by most manufacturers of X-ray equipment. Designs vary from those resembling panoramic units to one resembling a medical CT unit, as shown in Figure 19.8.

The equipment employs a cone-shaped X-ray beam (rather than the flat fan-shaped beam used in conventional CT) and a special detector (e.g. an image intensifier or an amorphous silicon flat panel). The equipment orbits around the patient, taking approximately 20–40 seconds, and in **one** cycle or scan, images a cylindrical or spherical volume — described as the *field of view*. As all the information is obtained in the single scan, the patient must remain absolutely stationary throughout the exposure.

The size of the cylindrical or spherical *field of view* varies from one machine to another. Using a large field of view (typically 15 cm diameter) most of the maxillofacial skeleton fits within the cylindrical or spherical shape and is imaged in the one scan, as shown in Figure 19.9. Having obtained data from the one scan, the computer then collates the information into tiny cubes or voxels (typically 0.4 mm × 0.4 mm × 0.4 mm) — referred to as the *primary reconstruction.* Individual voxels are much smaller than in medical CT (see earlier Fig. 19.5). The voxel sizes in newer machines are even smaller (0.15 mm × 0.15 mm × 0.15 mm), so improving image resolution. Typically one scan contains over 100 million voxels. Computer software allows the operator to select whichever voxels are required in the sagittal, coronal or axial planes — referred to as *secondary (or multiplanar) reconstruction,* as shown in Figure 19.9.

Sagittal, coronal and axial images appear simultaneously on the computer monitor (see Fig. 19.10). Selecting and moving the cursor on one image, for example the sagittal image, automatically alters the other two reconstructed coronal and axial slices, so allowing images to be scrolled through in real time.

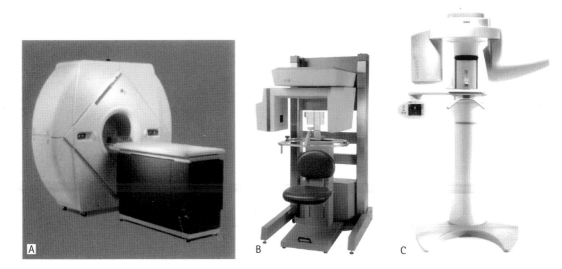

Fig. 19.8 Examples of three cone beam CT machines specially designed for imaging the maxillofacial skeleton **A** NewTom® 3G (NIM s.r.l. Italy). **B** I-CAT™ (Imaging Sciences International, Inc., USA). **C** Galileos (Sirona, Germany). (Figure **C** kindly provided by Mr Jochen Kusch and siCAT).

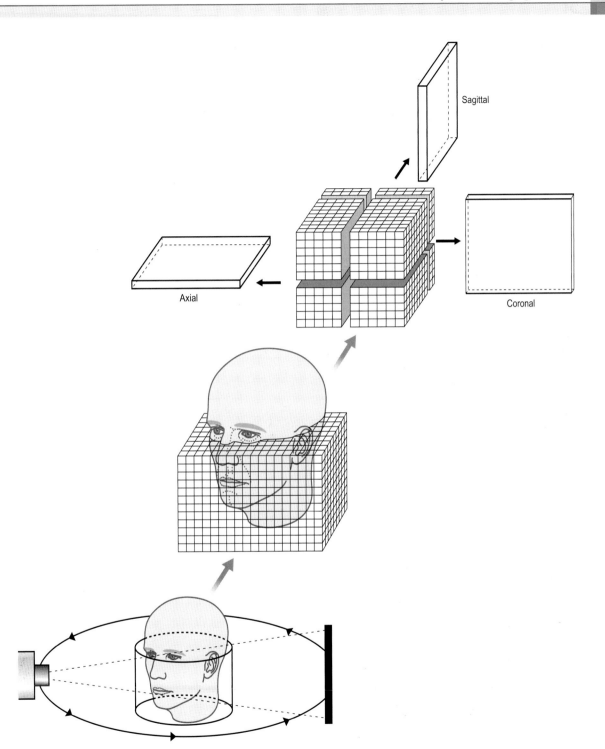

Fig. 19.9 Diagram showing the basic concept of cone beam CT. A cone-shaped X-ray beam is used which orbits once around the patient obtaining information in a cylindrical volume. The patient's maxillofacial skeleton is positioned within the cylinder and is divided up into tiny cubes or voxels. Computer manipulation (multiplanar reconstruction) of the data obtained allows separate images in the sagittal, coronal and axial planes to be created.

Multiplanar reconstruction also allows voxels in other planes to be selected. For example, it is possible to plot the curvature and shape of the dental arch to enable the computer to construct a panoramic image made up of the voxels that coincide with the plotted arch shape (see Fig. 19.11A and B). In addition, as with medical CT, it is also possible to reconstruct cross-sectional (also referred to as transaxial) images of any part of the jaw, and with appropriate software to produce three-dimensional images (see Fig. 19.12).

The equipment typically employs a high kV (90–110 kV) *pulsed* beam to minimize soft tissue absorption. For example, during a scan lasting 20 seconds, the patient is only exposed to ionizing radiation for about 3.5 seconds. The overall effective dose has been estimated to be in the order of 0.035–0.10 mSv, (using the proposed 2005 ICRP tissue weighting factors (see Ch. 3)), depending on the length of the scan, the size of the *field of view* and the type of equipment being used. This is equivalent to approximately 2–8

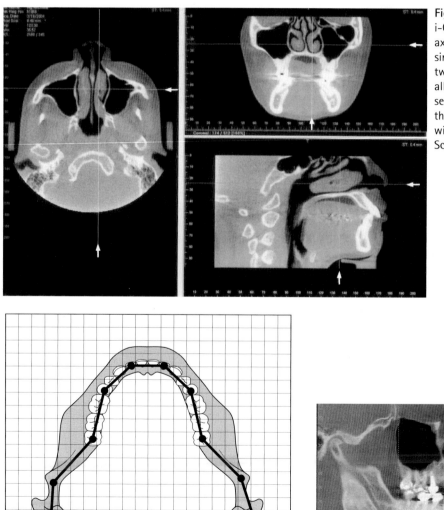

Fig. 19.10 An example of the i-CAT monitor screen showing axial, sagittal and coronal images simultaneously. Each image has two cursor lines (arrowed) allowing the images in the selected plane to be scrolled through in real time. (Reproduced with kind permision of Imaging Sciences International, Inc.)

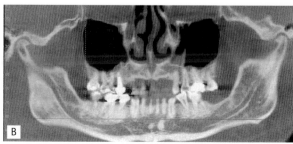

Fig. 19.11A Diagram showing how plotting the shape of the arch, identifies the cubes/voxels that are required for the computer to generate a panoramic image. **B** An example of a computer-generated cone beam CT panoramic image. (Image B reproduced with kind permission of Imaging Sciences International, Inc.)

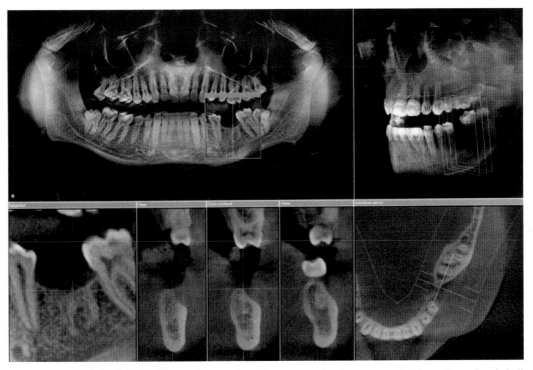

Fig. 19.12   An example of the Galileos (Sirona, Germany) monitor screen showing panoramic, three dimensional skull as well as sagittal, transaxial and axial images. (Kindly provided by Mr Jochen Kusch and siCAT).

conventional panoramic radiographs. It is considerably lower than a medical CT scan of the mandible and maxilla which is the equivalent of 200–300 conventional panoramic radiographs. The hard tissues — teeth and bones — are imaged well using cone beam CT, but very little detail is provided on the soft tissues.

One machine, the 3D Accuitomo shown in Figure 19.13, has been developed which only images a very small cylinder of information (4 cm in diameter and 3 cm tall). This enables high resolution images of specific teeth to be obtained, as shown in Figure 19.14, rather than the whole maxillofacial skeleton. The voxel size is a tiny 0.125 mm × 0.125 mm × 0.125 mm. The dose from this unit is very low and has been estimated to be in the order of 3–4 periapical radiographs.

Main indications in the head and neck

Cone beam CT has the potential to revolutionize imaging in all aspects of dental and maxillofacial

radiology. It has already been shown to be particularly valuable in:

- Investigation of all conditions affecting the mandible or maxilla including cysts, tumours, giant cell lesions and osseous dysplasias
- Investigation of the maxillary antra (see Ch. 29)

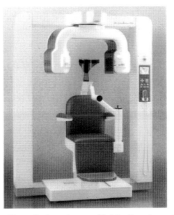

Fig. 19.13   The 3D Accuitomo (J. Morita, Japan) small volume cone beam CT machine.

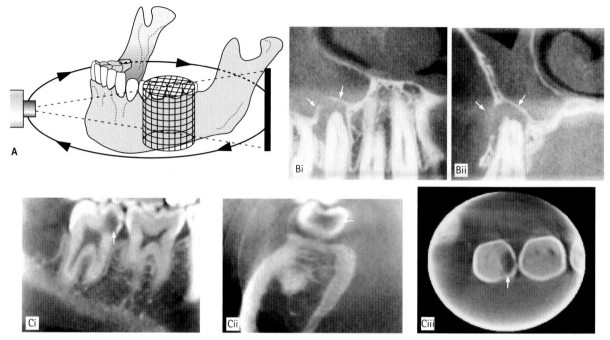

Fig. 19.14A   Diagram showing the basic concept of the low dose 3D Accuitomo (J. Morita, Japan) that images a small cylindrical volume (4 cm in diameter x 3 cm in height) to produce high resolution multiplanar images of the teeth. **B** (i) Sagittal and (ii) coronal high resolution images showing the apical radiolucency associated with 5| (arrowed). Mucosal thickening with the antrum is also evident. **C** Examples of high resolution (i) sagittal, (ii) coronal and (iii) axial images showing the mesial carious cavity in 7| (arrowed). (Figures **B** and **C** kindly provided by Professor D. Benn.)

- Investigation of the TMJ (see Ch. 31)
- Implant assessment (see Ch. 24)
- Orthodontic assessment
- Localization of unerupted teeth or odontomes (see Ch. 25)
- Assessment of lower third molars and identification of the relationship with the ID canal (see Ch. 25)
- Investigation of fractures of the mandible or middle third of the facial skeleton
- Multiplanar imaging of the teeth, periapical and periodontal tissues with the high resolution scanner. Examples of various cone beam CT images are included in later chapters.

Advantages

- Multi-plane imaging and manipulation allowing anatomy/pathological conditions to be viewed in different planes.

- Low radiation dose.
- Very fast scanning time.
- Relatively inexpensive and affordable compared to medical CT.
- Compatible with implant and cephalometric planning software.

Disadvantages

- Patient has to remain absolutely stationary.
- Soft tissues not imaged in detail.
- Computer constructed panoramic images are not directly comparable with conventional panoramic radiographs — particular care is needed in their interpretation.
- Metallic objects, such as fillings, may produce streak or star artefacts as with medical CT.
- Facilities not yet widely available.

ULTRASOUND

Diagnostic ultrasound is now established as the first choice imaging modality for soft tissue investigations of the face and neck, particularly of the salivary glands (see Ch. 33). It is a non-invasive investigation that uses a very high frequency (7.5–20 MHz) pulsed ultrasound beam, rather than ionizing radiation, to produce high resolution images of more superficial structures. The use of colour power Doppler allows blood flow to be detected.

Equipment and theory

Several machines are available — an example is shown in Figure 19.15. The high frequency ultrasound beam is directed into the body from a transducer placed in contact with the skin. Jelly is placed between the transducer and the skin to avoid an air interface, as shown in Figure 19.15A. As the ultrasound travels through the body, some of it is reflected back by tissue interfaces to produce *echoes*, which are picked up by the same transducer and converted into an electrical signal and then into a real-time black, white and grey visual *echo picture*, which is displaced on a computer screen. Examples are shown in Figure 19.16.

The ultrasound image is also a sectional image or *tomograph*, but it represents a topographical map of the depth of tissue interfaces, just like a sonar picture of the seabed. The thickness of the section is determined by the width of the ultrasound beam. Areas of different density in the black/white echo picture are described as *hypoechoic* (dark) or *hyperechoic* (light).

Utilization of the Doppler effect — a change in the frequency of sound reflected from a moving source — allows the detection of arterial and/or venous blood flow as shown in Figure 19.15. As can be seen, the computer adds the appropriate colour, red or blue, to the vascular structures in the visual echo picture image, making differentiation between structures straighforward.

The ultrasound wave must be able to travel through the tissue to return to the transducer. If it is absorbed by the tissue, no image will result.

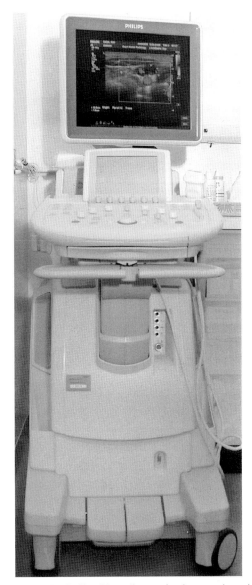

Fig. 19.15 The Philips iU 22 diagnostic ultrasound machine.

Since air, bone and other calcified materials absorb nearly all the low frequency ultrasound beam its diagnostic use is limited. However, the newer high frequency machines enable penetration of more superficial structures to provide high resolution images.

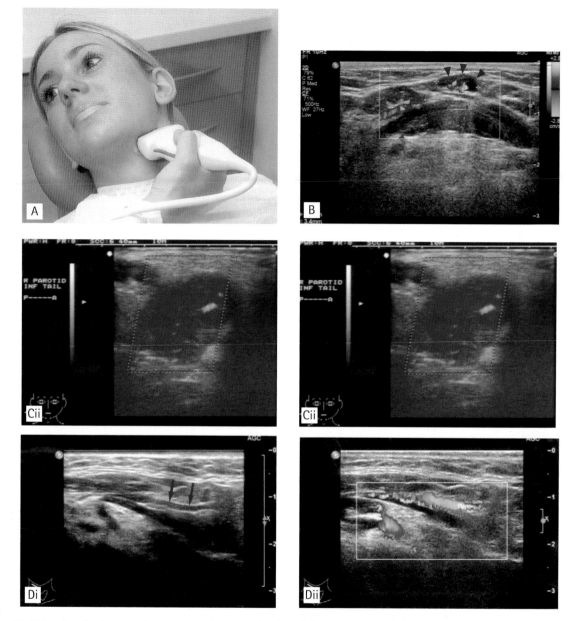

Fig. 19.16A A patient undergoing an ultrasound investigation of the left submandibular salivary gland. The transducer is placed against the skin overlying the gland. Note the jelly between the transducer and the skin. **B** Ultrasound image of the submental region showing the use of Doppler colour flow imaging to detect blood flow in the hilar vessels of a small submental lymph node (arrow heads). **C (i)** Ultrasound image of a pleomorphic adenoma in the parotid gland showing a hypoechoic (dark) mass with a well-defined, lobulated outline; **(ii)** Ultrasound image of the same patient with colour power Doppler showing blood flow in the fine vessels within the benign tumour. **D** Ultrasound image of the submental region demonstrating the value of colour Doppler imaging in differentiating vessels from other structures; **(i)** shows a submental vessel (arrowed) while **(ii)** illustrates blood flow within the vessel. (Figures **B**, **C** and **D** kindly provided by Mrs J.E. Brown.)

Main indications for ultrasound in the head and neck

- Evaluation of swellings of the neck, particularly those involving the thyroid, cervical lymph nodes or the major salivary glands — ultrasound is now regarded as the investigation of choice for detecting solid and cystic soft tissue masses.
- Detection of salivary gland and duct calculi (see Ch. 33).
- Determination of the relationship of vascular structures and vascularity of masses with the addition of colour flow Doppler imaging.
- Assessment of blood flow in the carotids and carotid body tumours.
- Assessment of the ventricular system in babies by imaging through the open fontanelles.
- Therapeutically, in conjunction with the newly developed sialolithotripter, to break up salivary calculi into approximately 2-mm fragments which can then pass out of the ductal system so avoiding major surgery.
- Ultrasound-guided fine-needle aspiration (FNA) biopsy.

Advantages over conventional X-ray imaging

- Sound waves are NOT ionizing radiation.
- There are no known harmful effects on any tissues at the energies and doses currently used in diagnostic ultrasound.
- Images show good differentiation between different **soft** tissues and are very sensitive for detecting focal disease in the salivary glands.
- Technique is widely available and relatively inexpensive.

Disadvantages

- Ultrasound has limited use in the head and neck region because sound waves are absorbed by bone. Its use is therefore restricted to the superficial structures.
- Technique is operator dependent.
- Images can be difficult to interpret for inexperienced operators.
- Real-time imaging means that the radiologist must be present during the investigation.

MAGNETIC RESONANCE (MR)

Magnetic resonance is another specialized imaging modality that does not involve the use of ionizing radiation. It is now widely available and is becoming increasingly sophisticated and important in imaging intracranial and soft tissue lesions.

Essentially it involves the behaviour of protons (positively charged nuclear particles (see Chap. 2)) in a magnetic field. The simplest atom is hydrogen, consisting of one proton in the nucleus and one orbiting electron, and it is the hydrogen protons that are used to create the MR image. The image itself is another example of a *tomograph* or sectional image that at first glance resembles a CT image.

Equipment and theory

An example of an MR machine is shown in Figure 19.17. The basic principles on how it works can be summarized as follows:

- The patient is placed within a very strong magnetic field (usually between 0.5–1.5 Tesla). The patient's hydrogen protons, which normally spin on an axis, behave like small

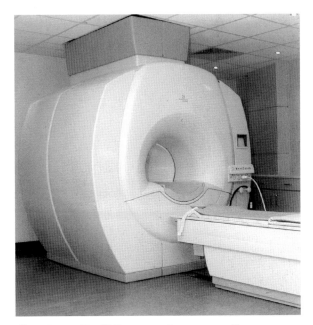

Fig. 19.17 The Philips magnetic resonance Gyroscan

magnets to produce the *net magnetization vector* (NMV) which aligns itself readily with the long axis of the magnetic field. This contributes to the longitudinal magnetic force or magnetic moment which runs along the long axis of the patient.

- Radiowaves are pulsed into the patient by the body coil transmitter at 90° to the magnetic field. These radiowaves are chosen to have the same frequency as the spinning hydrogen protons. This energy input is thus readily absorbed by the protons inducing them to resonate.

- The excited hydrogen protons then do two things:
  (i) First, they begin to precess like many small gyroscopes and their long axes move away from the long axis of the main magnetic field. This causes the *longitudinal magnetic moment* to diminish and the *transverse magnetic moment* to grow.
  (ii) Second, their spins synchronize so that they behave like many small bar magnets spinning like tops in phase with each other. Together their total magnetic moment can be detected as a magnetic force precessing within the patient.

- This magnetic moment now lies *transversely* across the patient and since it is moving around the patient, it is in effect a fluctuating magnetic force and is therefore capable of inducing an electrical current in a neighbouring conductor or receiver.

- Surface coils act as receiver coils and detect the small electrical current induced by the signal for a long time and appear white on so-called *T2-weighted images*. Fat on the other hand has a short T2, produces a weak signal and appears dark on a T2-weighted image.

- As the hydrogen atoms relax, they drop back into the long axis of the main magnetic field and the *longitudinal moment* begins to increase. The rate at which it returns to normal is described by the *time constant T1*. Fluids have a long T1 (i.e. they take a long time to re-establish their longitudinal magnetic moment), produce a weak signal and appear dark on so-called *T1-weighted images* (see Fig. 19.18). Again fat behaves in the opposite manner and has a short T1, produces a strong signal and appears white on a T1-weighted image.

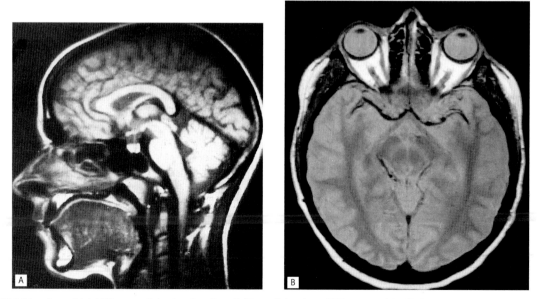

Fig. 19.18A   A sagittal MRI scan of the head and neck (T1-weighted, so CSF appears black). Bone does not give a signal and therefore appears dark, while bone marrow gives a strong signal and appears white. **B** An axial MRI scan, at the level of the orbits and ethmoidal air sinuses.

- The computer correlates this information and images may be produced that are either *T1-* or *T2-weighted* to show up differences in the T1 or T2 characteristics of the various tissues. Essentially T1-weighted images with a strong longitudinal signal show normal anatomy well, whereases T2-weighted images with a strong transverse signal show disease well.
- Alternatively, since the signal emanates principally from excited hydrogen protons, an image can be produced which indicates the distribution of protons in the tissues — the so-called *proton density image* where neither T1 or T2 effects predominate.
- By varying the frequency and timing of the radiofrequency input, the hydrogen protons can be excited to differing degrees allowing different tissue characteristics to be highlighted on a variety of imaging sequences. In addition, tissue characteristics can be changed by using gadolinium as a contrast agent, which shortens the T1 relaxation time of tissues giving a high signal on a T1-weighted image.
- Many different echo sequences are available including:
  - Static spin-echo, gradient echo and fat suppression sequences
  - Cineloop or pseudodynamic (used mainly for TMJ imaging)
  - Echoplanar or dynamic (used mainly as a research tool at present)
  - Time lapse subtraction (for vascular imaging — MR angiography).

Main indications for MR in the head and neck

- Assessment of intracranial lesions involving particularly the posterior cranial fossa, the pituitary and the spinal cord.
- Investigation of the salivary glands (see Ch. 33).
- Tumour staging — evaluation of the site, size and extent of soft and hard tissue tumours including nodal involvement, involving all areas in particular:
  - The salivary glands
  - The tongue and floor of mouth
  - The pharynx
  - The larynx
  - The sinuses (see Ch. 29)
  - The orbits
  - The jaws, to assess bone marrow involvement.
- Investigation of the TMJ to show both the bony and soft tissue components of the joint including the disc position (see Ch. 31). MR may be indicated:
  - When diagnosis of internal derangement is in doubt
  - As a preoperative assessment before disc surgery.
- Implant assessment (see Ch. 24).

Advantages

- Ionizing radiation is not used.
- No adverse effects have yet been demonstrated.
- Image manipulation available.
- High-resolution images can be reconstructed in all planes (using 3D volume techniques).
- Excellent differentiation between different soft tissues is possible and between normal and abnormal tissues enabling useful differentiation between benign and malignant disease and between recurrence and postoperative effects.
- Useful in determining intramedullary spread malignancy.

Disadvantages

- Bone does not give an MR signal, a signal is only obtainable from bone marrow, although this is of less importance now that radiologists are used to looking at MR images.
- Scanning time can be long and is thus demanding on the patient.
- It is contraindicated in patients with certain types of surgical clips, cardiac pacemakers, cochlear implants and in the first trimester of pregnancy.
- Equipment tends to be claustrophobic and noisy.
- Metallic objects, e.g. endotracheal tubes need to be replaced by non-ferromagnetic alternatives.
- Equipment is very expensive.
- The very powerful magnets can pose problems with siting of equipment although magnet shielding is now becoming more sophisticated.
- Bone, teeth, air and metallic objects all appear black, making differentiation difficult.

PART 5

Radiology

PART CONTENTS

20. Introduction to radiological interpretation   245

21. Dental caries and the assessment of restorations   251

22. The periapical tissues   265

23. The periodontal tissues and periodontal disease   277

24. Implant assessment   289

25. Development abnormalities   299

26. Radiological differential diagnosis – describing a lesion   323

27. Differential diagnosis of radiolucent lesions of the jaws   329

28. Differential diagnosis of lesions of variable radiopacity in the jaws   355

29. The maxillary antra   373

30. Trauma to the teeth and facial skeleton   387

31. The temporomandibular joint   411

32. Bone diseases of radiological importance   431

33. The salivary glands   445

Chapter 20

Introduction to radiological interpretation

Interpretation of radiographs can be regarded as an unravelling process — uncovering all the information contained within the black, white and grey radiographic images. The main objectives are:

- To identify the presence or absence of disease
- To provide information on the nature and extent of the disease
- To enable the formation of a differential diagnosis.

To achieve these objectives and maximize the diagnostic yield, interpretation should be carried out under specified conditions, following ordered, systematic guidelines.

Unfortunately, interpretation is often limited to a cursory glance under totally inappropriate conditions. Clinicians often fall victim to the problems and pitfalls produced by *spot diagnosis* and *tunnel vision*. This is in spite of knowing that in most cases radiographs are their main diagnostic aid.

This chapter provides an introductory approach to how radiographs should be interpreted, specifying the viewing conditions required and suggesting systematic guidelines.

ESSENTIAL REQUIREMENTS FOR INTERPRETATION

The essential requirements for interpreting dental radiographs can be summarized as follows:

- Optimum viewing conditions
- Understanding the nature and limitations of the black, white and grey radiographic image

- Knowledge of what the radiographs used in dentistry should look like, so a critical assessment of individual image quality can be made
- Detailed knowledge of the range of radiographic appearances of normal anatomical structures
- Detailed knowledge of the radiographic appearances of the pathological conditions affecting the head and neck
- A systematic approach to viewing the entire radiograph and to viewing and describing specific lesions
- Access to previous images for comparison.

Optimum viewing conditions

For film-captured images these include:

- An even, uniform, bright light viewing screen (preferably of variable intensity to allow viewing of films of different densities) (see Fig. 20.1)
- A quiet, darkened viewing room
- The area around the radiograph should be masked by a dark surround so that light passes only through the film
- Use of a magnifying glass to allow fine detail to be seen more clearly on intra-oral films
- The radiographs should be dry.

These ideal viewing conditions give the observer the best chance of perceiving all the detail contained within the radiographic image. With many simultaneous external stimuli, such as extraneous light and inadequate viewing

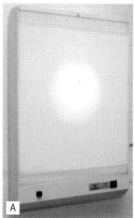
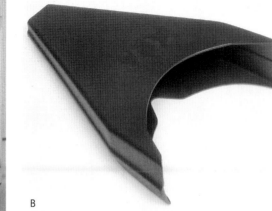

Fig. 20.1A Wardray viewing box incorporating an additional central bright-light source for viewing over-exposed dark films. **B** The SDI X-ray reader — an extraneous light excluding intraoral film viewer with built-in magnification.

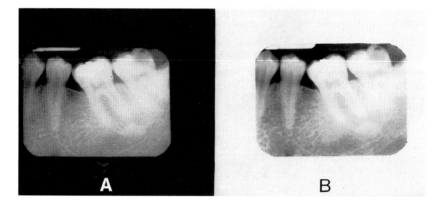

Fig. 20.2 The effect of different viewing conditions on the same periapical film. **A** With a black surround. **B** With a white surround. Note the increased detail visible in A, particularly around the molar teeth.

conditions, the amount of information obtained from the radiograph is reduced (see Fig. 20.2). Film-captured radiographs should be viewed once they have dried as films still wet from processing may show some distortion of the image.

Digital images should be viewed on bright, high-resolution monitors in subdued lighting.

The nature and limitations of different radiographic images

The importance of understanding the nature of different types of radiographic images — film-captured or digital (depending on the type of image receptor used) and their specific limitations was explained in Chapter 1. How the visual images are created by processing — chemical or computer was explained in Chapter 7. Revision of both of these chapters is recommended. To reiterate, the final image whether captured on film or digitally is 'a two-dimensional picture of three-dimensional structures superimposed on one another and represented as a variety of black, white and grey shadows' — a *shadowgraph*.

Critical assessment of image quality

To be able to assess and interpret any radiographic image correctly, clinicians have to know what that image should look like, how it was captured, and which structures should be shown. It is for this reason that the chapters on radiography included:

1. WHY each projection was taken
2. HOW the projections were taken using different image receptors
3. WHAT the resultant radiographic image should look like
4. WHICH anatomical structures they showed.

With this practical knowledge of radiography, clinicians are in a position to make an overall critical assessment of individual film-captured and digital images.

Film–captured images

The practical factors that can influence film quality were discussed in Chapter 18, and included:

- The X-ray equipment
- The image receptor-film or film/screen combination
- Processing
- The patient
- The operator and radiographic technique.

A critical assessment of radiographs can be made by combining these factors and by asking a series of questions about the final image. These questions relate to:

- Radiographic technique
- Exposure factors and film density
- Processing.

Here are some typical examples.

Technique (see Fig. 20.3)

- Which technique has been used?
- How were the patient, film and X-ray tubehead positioned?
- Is this a good example of this particular radiographic projection?
- How much distortion is present?

- Is the image foreshortened or elongated?
- Is there any rotation or asymmetry?
- How good are the image resolution and sharpness?
- Has the film been fogged?
- Which artefactual shadows are present?
- How do these technique variables alter the final radiographic image?

Exposure factors (see Fig. 20.4)

- Is the radiograph correctly exposed for the specific reason it was requested?
- Is it too dark and so possibly overexposed?
- Is it too light/pale and so possibly underexposed?
- How good is the contrast?
- What effect will exposure factor variation have on the zone under investigation?

Processing

- Is the radiograph correctly processed?
- Is it too dark and so possibly overdeveloped?
- Is it too pale and so possibly underdeveloped?
- Is it dirty with emulsion still present and so underfixed?
- Is the film wet or dry?

Digitally–captured images

The practical factors that can effect digitally-captured images, how the images are created and how they can be altered using computer soft-ware were discussed in Chapter 7 and included:

- The image receptor — solid-state or photostimulable phosphor plate

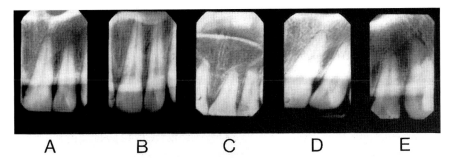

A   B   C   D   E

Fig. 20.3   Examples of how variations in radiographic technique can alter the images—film or digital—produced of the same object. **A** Correct projection. **B** Incorrect vertical angulation producing an elongated image. **C** Incorrect vertical angulation producing a foreshortened image. **D** and **E** Incorrect horizontal angulations producing distorted images.

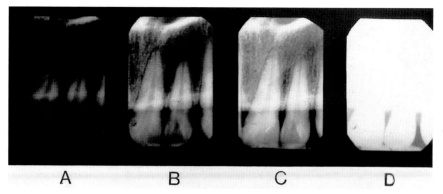

Fig. 20.4 The effect on the degree of blackening by altering *exposure* (mAs—current or exposure time) for film-captured images OR, by altering the *brightness* control for digital images.

- Computer image processing and enhancement
- The patient
- The operator and radiographic technique.

As with film-captured images a critical assessment of digital images can be made by combining these factors and by asking a series of questions about the final image. These questions relate to:

- Radiographic technique
- Image processing.

Technique

- Which technique has been used?
- How were the patient, digital receptor and X-ray tubehead positioned?
- Is this a good example of this particular radiographic projection?
- How much distortion is present?
- Has the whole area of interest been included?
- Is the image foreshortened or elongated?
- Is there any rotation or asymmetry?
- How good are the image resolution and sharpness?
- Which artefactual shadows are present?
- How do these technique variables alter the final radiographic image?

Note: These technique questions are almost identical to those relating to film-captured images. Image quality is totally dependent on high quality practical radiography whatever image receptor is chosen.

Image processing

- Is the contrast optimal?
- Is the brightness optimal?
- Is the image enhancement optimal?
- Is the magnification optimal?

With experience, this critical assessment of image quality is not a lengthy procedure but it is never one that should be overlooked. A poor radiographic image is a poor diagnostic aid and sometimes may be of no diagnostic value at all. Clinicians used to using film-captured images who decide to 'go digital' should take time to understand the nature of the digital image and the effect on the image of using powerful computer software manipulation.

Detailed knowledge of normal anatomy

A detailed knowledge of the radiographic appearances of **normal** anatomical structures is necessary if clinicians are to be able to recognize the **abnormal** appearances of the many diseases that affect the jaws.

Not only is a comprehensive knowledge of hard and soft tissue anatomy required but also a knowledge of:

- The type of radiograph being interpreted (e.g. conventional radiograph or tomograph)
- The position of the patient, image receptor and X-ray tubehead.

Only with **all** this information can clinicians appreciate how the various normal anatomical structures, through which the X-ray beam has passed, will appear on any particular radiograph.

Detailed knowledge of pathological conditions

Radiological interpretation depends on recognition of the typical patterns and appearances of different diseases. The more important appearances are described in Chapters 21–33.

Systematic approach

A systematic approach to viewing radiographs is necessary to ensure that no relevant information is missed. This systematic approach should apply to:

- The entire radiograph
- Specific lesions.

The entire radiograph

Any systematic approach will suffice as long as it is logical, ordered and thorough. Several suggested sequences are described in later chapters. By way of an example, a suggested systematic approach to the overall interpretation of dental panoramic radiographs (see Ch. 17) is shown in Figure 20.5.

This type of ordered sequential viewing of radiographs requires discipline on the part of the observer. It is easy to be sidetracked by noticing something unusual or abnormal, thus forgetting the remainder of the radiograph.

Specific lesions

A systematic description of a lesion should include its:

- Site or anatomical position
- Size
- Shape
- Outline/edge or periphery
- Relative radiodensity and internal structure
- Effect on adjacent surrounding structures
- Time present, if known.

Making a radiological differential diagnosis depends on this systematic approach. It is described in detail and expanded on later (see Ch. 26).

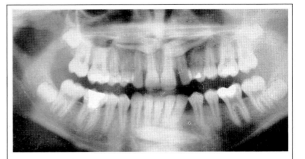

General overview of the entire film
1 Note the chronological and development age of the patient.
2 Trace the outline of all normal anatomical shadows and compare their shape and radiodensity.

The teeth
3 Note particularly:
   a The number of teeth present
   b Stage of development
   c Position
   d Condition of the crowns
     (i) Caries
     (ii) Restorations
   e Condition of the roots
     (i) Length
     (ii) Fillings
     (iii) Resorption
     (iv) Crown/root ratio.

The apical tissues
4 Note particularly:
   a The integrity of lamina dura
   b Any radiolucencies or opacities associated with the apices.

The peridontal tissues
5 Note particularly:
   a The width of the periodontal ligament
   b The level and quality of crestal bone
   c Any vertical or horizontal bone loss
   d Any furcation involvements
   e Any calculus deposits.

The body and ramus of the mandible
6 Note:
   a Shape
   b Outline
   c Thickness of the lower border
   d Trabeculae pattern
   e Any radiolucent or radiopaque areas
   f Shape of the condylar heads.

Other structures
7 These include:
   a The antra, note:
     (i) The outline of the floor, and anterior and posterior walls
     (ii) Radiodensity
   b Nasal cavity
   c Styloid processes.

Fig. 20.5 An example of a dental panoramic radiograph and a suggested systematic sequence for viewing this type of film.

Comparison with previous films

The availability of previous films for comparative purposes is an invaluable aid to radiographic interpretation. The presence, extent and features of lesions can be compared to ascertain the speed of development and growth, or the degree of healing.

Note: Care must be taken that views used for comparison have been taken with a comparable technique **and** are of comparable density.

Conclusion

Successful interpretation of radiographs, no matter what the quality, relies ultimately on clinicians understanding the radiographic image, being able to recognize the range of normal appearances as well as knowing the salient features of relevant pathological conditions.

The following chapters are designed to emphasize these requirements and to reinforce the basic approach to interpretation outlined earlier.

Chapter 21

Dental caries and the assessment of restorations

INTRODUCTION

The word *caries* is used to describe both the invisible *caries process* and the potentially visible *caries lesion*. Understanding this difference is important if the role and value of radiography is to be understood.

The *caries process* is the interaction of the biofilm of plaque with the dental hard tissues. The *biofilm* consists of a community of metabolically active micro-organisms capable of fermenting sugars (e.g. sucrose or glucose) to produce acid, which can lower the pH to 5 in 1–3 minutes and produce *demineralization* of the dental hard tissues. The acid can be neutralized by saliva and mineral regained resulting in *remineralization*. Together these processes produce the *caries lesion*, which may or may not be visible clinically and/or radiographically. Being able to see the lesion depends on the extent and balance between demineralization and remineralization.

The first half of this chapter concentrates on the detection of caries in posterior teeth from bitewing radiographs. The second half summarizes the important features to observe when assessing restorations and outlines a systematic approach to interpreting bitewing radiographs.

CLASSIFICATION OF CARIES

Lesions of caries are usually classified and/or described by the anatomical site of the tooth affected. Terminology used includes:

- Pit or fissure caries
- Smooth surface caries
- Enamel caries
- Root caries
- Primary caries — caries developing on unrestored surfaces
- Secondary or recurrent caries — caries developing adjacent to restorations
- Residual caries — demineralized tissue left behind before filling the tooth.

Lesions of caries are also classified and/or described by the activity of the *caries process*. Terminology used includes:

- Active caries
  - Rampant caries — multiple active lesions in the same patient, often on surfaces that are usually caries-free. In very small children this is sometimes referred to as *bottle caries* or *nursing caries*
  - Early childhood caries
- Arrested or inactive caries.

Levels of Disease

Caries is also described by the extent or size of the lesion. Typically 4 *levels of disease* are used:

- D1 — Clinically detectable enamel lesions with intact surfaces
- D2 — Clinically detectable cavities limited to enamel
- D3 — Clinically detectable lesions in dentine
- D4 — Lesions into the pulp.

These distinctions are important with regard to management. Lesions at levels D1 and D2 are generally managed using preventative measures, whereas lesions at the D3 or D4 level are likely to require restorative treatment. Detection of lesions of caries and being able to assess the level of disease are therefore crucial in determining clinical treatment.

DIAGNOSIS AND DETECTION OF CARIES

Diagnosis has been defined as identifying a disease from its signs and symptoms. In caries diagnosis that would involve both detecting the lesion and determining the activity of the process. Dental radiography is one method used to detect the lesion but it gives no information on the activity of the process. Various detection methods are available for different sites.

Occlusal caries

- Clinical examination using direct vision of clean, dry teeth
- Bitewing radiography
- Laser fluorescence (DIAGNOdent (KaVo, Germany)
- Electrical conductance measurements (ECM).

Approximal caries

- Clinical examination using direct vision of clean, dry teeth
- Gentle probing
- Bitewing radiography in adults and children (posterior teeth)
- Paralleling technique periapical radiography (anterior teeth)
- Fibreoptic transillumination (FOTI)
- Light fluorescence (QLF)
- Elective temporary tooth separation
- Ultrasound.

Secondary or recurrent caries (caries developing adjacent to a restoration)

- Clinical examination using direct vision of clean, dry teeth
- Gently probing
- Bitewing radiography.

Radiographic detection of lesions of caries

Bitewing radiographic techniques, using both film packets and digital sensors (solid-state and phosphor plates) as the image receptor, were described in Chapter 11. For caries detection, film packets and phosphor plates are preferred as the imaging area of the equivalent sized solid-state sensors is smaller. It has been reported that on average three fewer interproximal tooth surfaces are shown per image.

Approximal lesions of caries are detectable radiographically only when there has been 30%–40% demineralization, so allowing the lesion to be differentiated from normal enamel and dentine. The importance of optimum viewing conditions for both film and digital images, as described in Chapter 20, cannot be overemphasized when looking for these early subtle changes. Magnification is of particular importance, as shown in Figure 21.1.

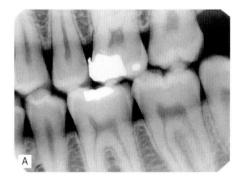

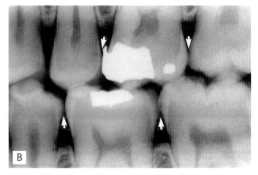

Fig. 21.1 The effect of magnification. **A** Bitewing radiograph showing almost invisible very early approximal lesions in the molar and premolar teeth. **B** Magnified central portion of the same bitewing showing the approximal lesions (arrowed) more clearly.

Radiographic assessment of caries activity

A single bitewing radiograph may illustrate one or more caries lesions but it gives no information on caries activity. As caries is a slowly progressing disease, this progression and therefore caries activity, can be assessed over time by periodic radiographic investigations.

In the UK, the 2004 Faculty of General Dental Practice (UK)'s booklet *Selection Criteria in Dental Radiography* recommends that the frequency of these follow-up radiographs be linked to the *caries risk* of the patient (see Ch. 8 and Table 8.1). The booklet contains a very helpful summary table entitled *Selection criteria for radiographs according to caries risk status for children and adults*, which is reproduced with kind permission of the Faculty as Table 21.1. As can be seen, for high-caries-risk children and adult and patients 6-monthly intervals are recommended, for medium-caries-risk patients 12-monthly intervals and for low-caries-risk patients 2-yearly intervals for adults and 12–18 monthly intervals for children in the primary dentition.

Radiographs used to monitor the progression of caries lesions need to be geometrically identical — hence the need for image receptor holders and beam-aiming devices (see Ch. 11). They should also be similarly exposed to give comparable contrast and density.

Geometrically reproducible digital images can be superimposed and the information in one image subtracted from the other to create the *subtraction image* which shows the changes that have taken place between the two investigations (see Ch. 7).

Radiographic appearance of caries lesions

As lesions of caries progress and enlarge, they appear as differently shaped areas of radiolucency in the crowns or necks of the teeth. These shapes are fairly characteristic and vary according to the *site* and *size* of the lesion. They are illustrated diagrammatically in Figure 21.2 and examples are shown in Figure 21.3.

Fig. 21.2 Diagrams illustrating the radiographic appearances and shapes of various lesions of caries.

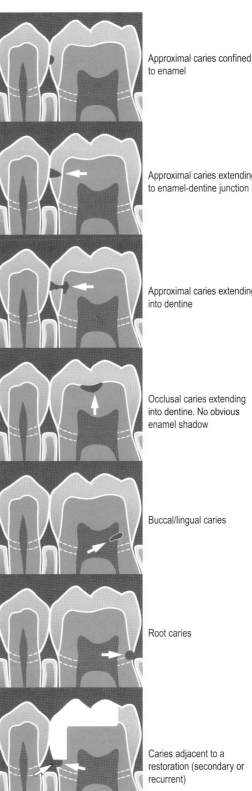

Approximal caries confined to enamel

Approximal caries extending to enamel-dentine junction (EDJ)

Approximal caries extending into dentine

Occlusal caries extending into dentine. No obvious enamel shadow

Buccal/lingual caries

Root caries

Caries adjacent to a restoration (secondary or recurrent)

Fig. 21.1 Summary of *Selection criteria for radiographs according to caries risk status for children and adults* reproduced with minor modifications from the 2004 *Selection Criteria in Dental Radiography* (with kind permission from the Faculty of General Dental Practice (UK) of the Royal College of Surgeons of England)

Selection criteria for radiographs according to caries risk status for children and adults

Risk category	Radiographic guidelines	CARIES RISK FACTORS						
		Social history	Medical history	Dietary habits	Use of fluoride	Plaque control	Saliva	Clinical evidence
HIGH CARIES RISK	Posterior bitewing radiographs at six-month intervals* until no new or active lesions are apparent and the individual has entered another risk category *Bitewings should not be taken more frequently and it is imperative to reassess caries risk in order to justify using this interval again.	• Socially deprived • High caries in siblings • Low knowledge of dental disease • Irregular attender • Ready availability of snacks • Low dental aspirations	• Medically compromised • Handicapped • Xerostomia • Long-term cariogenic medicine	• Frequent sugar intake	• Drinking-water not fluoridated • No fluoride supplements • No fluoride toothpaste	• Infrequent, ineffective cleaning • Poor manual control	• Low flow rate • Low buffering capacity • High *S Mutans* and *Lactobacillus* counts	• New lesions, premature extractions, anterior caries or restorations, multiple restorations • No fissure sealants • Fixed appliance orthodontics • Partial dentures
MODERATE CARIES RISK	Annual posterior bitewings unless risk status alters	INDIVIDUALS WHO DO NOT CLEARLY FIT INTO HIGH OR LOW CARIES RISK CATEGORIES ARE CONSIDERED TO BE AT MODERATE CARIES RISK						
LOW CARIES RISK	Posterior bitewing radiographs at approximately: 12–18 month intervals in primary dentition Two-year intervals in permanent dentition More extended radiographic recall intervals may be employed if there is explicit evidence of continuing low caries risk	• Socially advantaged • Low caries siblings • Dentally aware • Regular attender • Work does not allow regular snacks • High dental aspirations	• No medical problem • No physical problem • Normal salivary flow • No long-term medication	• Infrequent sugar intake	• Drinking-water fluoridated • Fluoride supplements used • Fluoride toothpaste used	• Frequent, effective cleaning • Good manual control	• Normal flow rate • High buffering capacity • Low *S Mutans* and *Lactobacillus* counts	• No new lesions • Nil extractions for caries • Sound anterior teeth • No or few restorations • Restorations inserted years ago • Fissure-sealed • No appliance

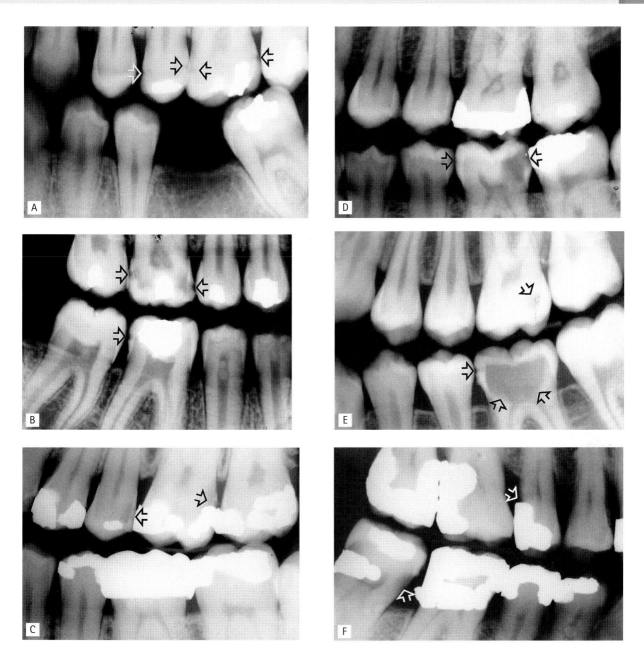

Fig. 21.3 Bitewing radiographs showing examples of typical caries lesions (arrowed). **A** Small approximal lesions |56. **B** Large approximal lesions with extensive dentine involvement 6| and a small lesion 6|. **C** Approximal lesion extending into dentine |5 and recurrent caries |6. **D** Small and extensive approximal lesions ⌐6. **E** Small occlusal lesion |6 and extensive occlusal lesion ⌐6, apart from the small approximal enamel lesion, the enamel cap appears intact. **F** Root caries 7| and recurrent caries 5|.

OTHER IMPORTANT RADIOGRAPHIC APPEARANCES

Radiographic detection of caries lesions is not always straightforward. It can be complicated by:

- Residual caries
- Radiodensity of adhesive restorations
- Cervical *burn-out* or cervical *translucency*
- Dentinal changes beneath amalgam restorations.

Residual caries

The rationale for removal of caries has changed in recent years. The primary aim nowadays when excavating dentine caries is to remove only the highly infected, irreversibly demineralized dentine in order to allow effective restoration of the cavity and surface anatomy of the tooth and to prevent disease progression. In other words, demineralized tissue (*residual caries)* is left behind in the base of the cavity and the tooth restored. Radiographically, this *inactive caries* may show a zone of radiolucency beneath the restoration. This appearance is identical to that of an *active caries lesion* under a restoration (see Fig. 21.4).

Radiodensity of adhesive restorations

The development of successful adhesive restorative materials in recent years, including dentine bonding agents and glass ionomer cements, has resulted in many teeth being restored with non-metallic fillings. These various adhesive materials vary considerably in their radiodensity and do not appear as white on radiographic images as traditional amalgam, as shown in Figure 21.5. Identifying subtle radiolucent lesions of caries adjacent to these materials can be very difficult, if not impossible.

Cervical burn–out or cervical translucency

This radiolucent shadow is often evident at the neck of the teeth, as illustrated in Figure 21.6. It is an artefactual phenomenon created by the anatomy of the teeth and the variable penetration of the X-ray beam.

Cervical *burn-out* can be explained by considering **all** the different parts of the tooth and supporting bone tissues that the same X-ray beam has to penetrate:

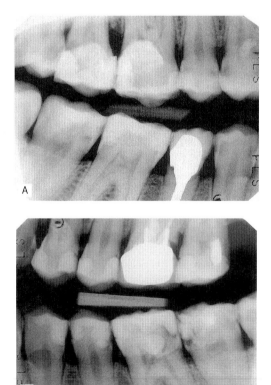

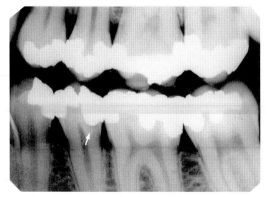

Fig. 21.4 Bitewing showing the radiolucency of residual caries beneath the restoration in ⌐5 (arrowed). It is impossible to assess whether the lesion is *active* or *inactive*.

Fig. 21.5A Right and **B** left bitewings showing numerous posterior teeth that have been filled with adhesive restorations. Note: the fillings look less radiopaque than amalgam, and as a result the reduced contrast difference between dentine and restoration makes identification of adjacent radiolucent caries difficult (kindly provided by Dr A. Banerjee).

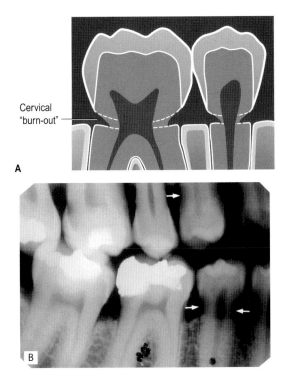

Cervical "burn-out"

A

B

Fig. 21.6A Diagram illustrating the radiographic appearance of cervical *burn-out*. **B** Bitewing radiograph showing extensive cervical *burn-out* of the premolars (arrowed). Compare this with the appearance of cervical caries on distal aspect 6̲|.

- In the crown — the dense enamel cap and dentine
- In the neck — only dentine
- In the root — dentine and the buccal and lingual plates of alveolar bone (see Fig. 21.7).

Thus, at the edges of the teeth in the cervical region, there is **less** tissue for the X-ray beam to pass through. Less attenuation therefore takes place and virtually no opaque shadow is cast of this area on the radiograph. It therefore appears radiolucent, as if some cervical tooth tissue does not exist or that it has been apparently *burnt-out*.

Cervical *burn-out* is of diagnostic importance because of its similarity to the radiolucent shadows of cervical and recurrent caries. However, *burn-out* can usually be distinguished by the following characteristic features:

- It is located at the neck of the teeth, demarcated above by the enamel cap or restoration and below by the alveolar bone level
- It is triangular in shape, gradually becoming less apparent towards the centre of the tooth
- Usually all the teeth on the radiograph are affected, especially the smaller premolars.

In contrast, *root* and *recurrent caries lesions*, although they also often affect the cervical region, have no apparent upper and lower demarcating borders. These lesions are saucer-shaped and tend to be localized, as shown in Figure 21.2. If in doubt, the diagnosis should be confirmed clinically by

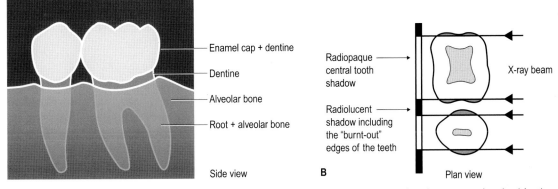

Enamel cap + dentine

Dentine

Alveolar bone

Root + alveolar bone

A   Side view

Radiopaque central tooth shadow

Radiolucent shadow including the "burnt-out" edges of the teeth

B   Plan view

X-ray beam

Fig. 21.7A   Diagrammatic representation of |5̄6̄ from the side showing the three-dimensional structures involved in the formation of the radiographic image. Note that in the cervical region there is less tissue present. **B** Plan view at the level of the necks of the teeth. Through the centre of the teeth there is a large mass of dentine to absorb the X-ray beam, while at the edges there is only a small amount. The edges of the necks of the teeth are therefore not dense enough to stop the X-ray beam, so their normally opaque shadows do not appear on the final radiograph.

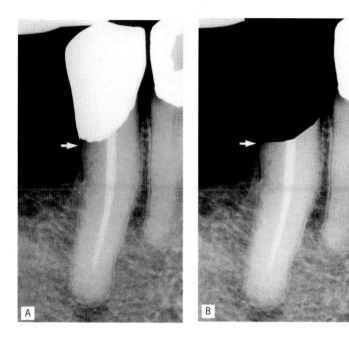

Fig. 21.8 The visual perceptual problem of contrast. **A** The zone at the distal cervical margin (arrowed), directly beneath the white metallic restoration shadow, appears radiolucent in the 5̄. **B** The same image but with the white restoration blacked out. The zone beneath the restoration (arrowed) now appears less radiolucent.

direct vision and gentle probing having cleaned and dried the area.

Important points to note

- *Burn-out* is more obvious when the exposure factors are increased, as required ideally for detecting approximal caries.
- It is also more apparent, by the perceptual problem of *contrast*, if the tooth contains a metallic restoration, which may make the zone above the cervical shadow completely radiopaque (see Fig. 21.8 and Ch. 1, Fig. 1.16). As this area is also the main site for recurrent caries, diagnosis is further complicated.

Dentinal changes beneath amalgam restorations

Following attack by caries, posterior teeth are still most commonly restored using dental amalgam. An *amalgam* is defined as an alloy of mercury with another metal or metals. In dental amalgam, mercury is mixed with an alloy powder. The alloy powders available principally contain silver, tin and copper with small amounts of zinc. It has been shown that, with time, tin and zinc ions are released into the underlying demineralized (but not necessarily infected) dentine producing a

radiopaque zone within the dentine which follows the S-shape curve of the underlying tubules (see Fig. 21.9). The radiopacity of this zone may make the normal dentine on either side appear more radiolucent by contrast. This somewhat more radiolucent normal dentine may simulate the radiolucent shadows of caries and lead to difficulties in diagnosis.

In addition, the pulp may also respond to both the carious attack and subsequent restorative treatment by laying down *reparative secondary dentine* which reduces the size of the pulp chamber.

LIMITATIONS OF RADIOGRAPHIC DETECTION OF CARIES

In addition to the problems of detection caused by the radiolucent and radiopaque shadows mentioned earlier, further limitations are imposed by the conventional two-dimensional radiographic image. The main problems include:

- Lesions of caries are usually larger clinically than they appear radiographically and very early lesions are not evident at all.
- Technique variations in image-receptor and X-ray beam positions can affect considerably the image of the caries lesion — varying the horizontal tubehead angulation can make a

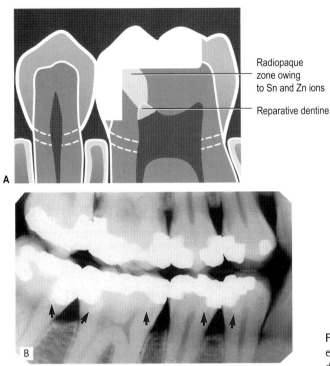

A

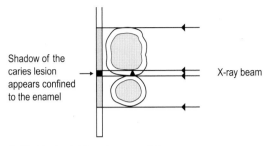

A Ideal horizontal X-ray beam angulation

Radiopaque zone owing to Sn and Zn ions

Reparative dentine

Shadow of the caries lesion appears confined to the enamel

X-ray beam

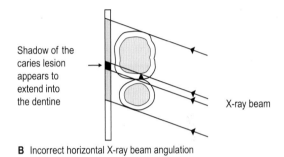

Shadow of the caries lesion appears to extend into the dentine

X-ray beam

B Incorrect horizontal X-ray beam angulation

Fig. 21.10 Diagrams showing how the appearance and extent of a caries lesion confined to enamel alters with different horizontal X-ray beam angulations.

B

Fig. 21.9A Diagram illustrating the S-shaped radiopaque zone caused by tin and zinc ions released into the underlying demineralized dentine beneath an amalgam restoration and the appearance of reparative dentine. **B** Bitewing radiograph showing the S-shaped radiopaque shadows (arrowed) in the heavily restored lower teeth.

lesion confined to enamel appear to have progressed into dentine (see Fig. 21.10) — hence the need for accurate, reproducible techniques as described in Chapter 11.

- Exposure factors can have a marked effect on the overall radiographic contrast (see Fig. 21.11) on film-captured images and thus affect the appearance or size of caries lesions on the film.
- Superimposition and a two-dimensional image (digital or film) mean that the following features cannot always be determined:
  - The exact site of a caries lesion, e.g. buccal or lingual
  - The buccolingual extent of a lesion
  - The distance between the caries lesion and the pulp horns. These two shadows can appear to be close together or even in contact but they may not be in the same plane

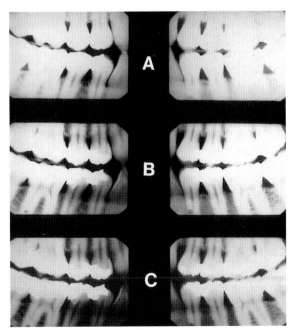

Fig. 21.11 Three pairs of film-captured bitewings taken with different exposure factors. **A** Considerably reduced exposure. **B** Slightly reduced exposure. **C** Slightly increased exposure. Note the varying contrast between enamel, dentine and the pulp.

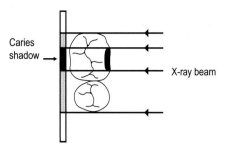

A(i) Buccal lesion

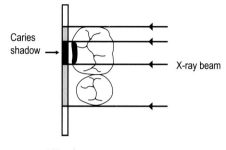

A(ii) Lingual lesion

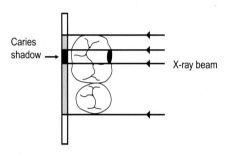

B(i) Shallow buccal lesion

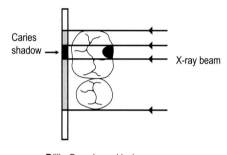

B(ii) Deep buccal lesion

C(i) Large lesion not
      involving the pulp

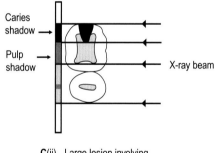

C(ii) Large lesion involving
       the pulp

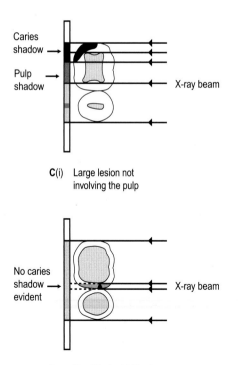

D Small lesion hidden by
   dense overlaying enamel

Fig. 21.12A Diagrams showing differently positioned caries lesions (i) buccal and (ii) lingual, producing similar radiographic shadows. **B** Diagrams showing different sized buccal lesions (i) shallow and (ii) deep, producing similar radiographic shadows. **C** Diagrams showing (i) a large approximal lesion superimposed over, but not involving the pulp and (ii) a large approximal lesion involving the pulp, both producing similar radiographic shadows. **D** Diagram showing how a small lesion may not be evident radiographically if dense radiopaque enamel shadows are superimposed.

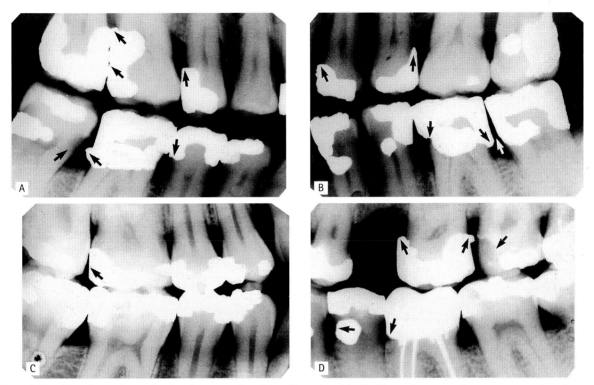

Fig. 21.13   Bitewing radiographs showing examples of heavily restored teeth. The major areas of concern — overhanging ledges, poor contour, defective contact points and caries adjacent to restorations — are arrowed.

– The presence of an enamel lesion — the density of the overlying enamel may obscure the zone of decalcification
– The presence of caries adjacent to restorations may be completely obscured by the restoration (see Fig. 21.12).

RADIOGRAPHIC ASSESSMENT OF RESTORATIONS

Critical assessment of the restoration

The important features to note include:

- The type and radiodensity of the restorative material, e.g.
  - amalgam
  - cast metal
  - adhesive materials such as composite or glass ionomer (see earlier and Fig. 21.5)
- Overcontouring
- Overhanging ledges
- Undercontouring

- Negative or reverse ledges
- Presence of contact points
- Adaptation of the restorative material to the base of the cavity
- Marginal fit of cast restorations
- Presence or absence of a lining material
- Radiodensity of the lining material.

Assessment of the underlying tooth

The important features to note include:

- Caries adjacent to restorations
- Residual caries (see earlier and Fig. 21.4)
- Radiopaque shadow of released tin and zinc ions (see earlier and Fig. 21.9)
- Size of the pulp chamber
- Internal resorption
- Presence of root-filling material in the pulp chamber
- Presence and position of pins or posts.

Examples showing several of these features are shown in Figure 21.13.

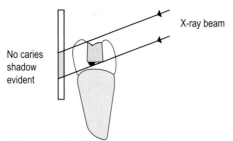

A Incorrect vertical X-ray beam angulation

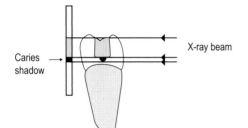

B Ideal vertical X-ray beam angulation

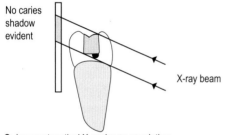

C Incorrect vertical X-ray beam angulation

Fig. 21.14 Diagrams illustrating the effect of incorrect vertical X-ray beam angulation in diagnosing recurrent lesions adjacent to the base of a restoration box.

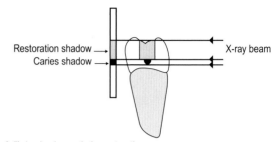

A (i) Lesion beneath the restoration

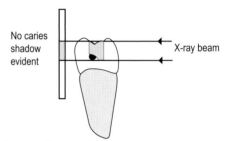

A (ii) Lesion hidden by the restoration

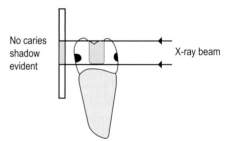

B Buccal and lingual lesions hidden by the restoration

Fig. 21.15A Diagrams illustrating the difficulty of assessing caries lesions beneath a restoration. **B** Diagram showing the difficulty of assessing buccal and lingual lesions in restored teeth.

LIMITATIONS OF THE RADIOGRAPHIC IMAGE

Once again, the radiographic image provides only limited information when assessing restorations. The main problems include:

- Technique variations in X-ray tubehead position may cause recurrent caries lesions to be obscured (see Fig. 21.14)
- Cervical *burn-out* shadows tend to be more obvious when their upper borders are demarcated by dense white restorations because of the increased contrast differences (see Fig. 21.8)
- Superimposition and a two-dimensional image mean that:
  - Only part of a restoration can be assessed radiographically
  - A dense radiopaque restoration may totally obscure a caries lesion in another part of the tooth
  - Recurrent caries adjacent to the base of an interproximal box may not be detected (see Fig. 21.15).

SUGGESTED GUIDELINES FOR INTERPRETING BITEWING IMAGES

Overall critical assessment

A typical series of questions that should be asked about the quality of a bitewing image based on the *ideal quality criteria* described in Chapter 11, include:

Technique (film OR digitally-captured images)

- Are all the required teeth shown?
- Are the crowns of upper and lower teeth shown?
- Is the occlusal plane horizontal?
- Are the contact areas overlapped?
- Has there been any *coning off* or *cone cutting*?
- Are the buccal and lingual cusps overlapped?
- Is it geometrically comparable to previous films?

Exposure factors (film-captured images)

- Is the image too dark — and so possibly over-exposed?
- Is the image too light — and so possibly under-exposed?
- Is the exposure sufficient to allow the enamel–dentine junction to be seen?
- What effect do the exposure factors have on the structures shown?
- How noticeable is the cervical *burn-out*?

Processing (film-captured images)

- Is the radiograph correctly processed?

- Is it overdeveloped?
- Is it underdeveloped?
- Is it correctly fixed?
- Has it been adequately washed?

Image processing (digitally-captured images)

- Is the contrast optimal?
- Is the brightness optimal?
- Is image enhancement optimal?
- Is magnification optimal?

Systematic viewing

Suggested systematic approaches to viewing bitewing radiographs are shown in Figures 21.16 and 21.17

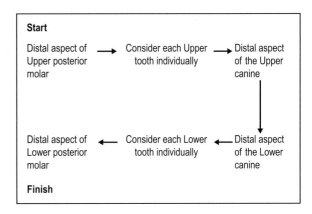

Fig. 21.16 Suggested sequence for examining a right bitewing radiograph.

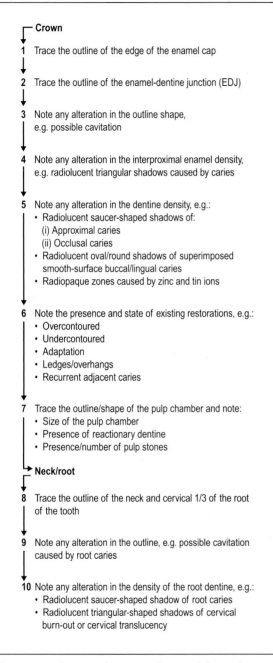

Crown

1 Trace the outline of the edge of the enamel cap

2 Trace the outline of the enamel-dentine junction (EDJ)

3 Note any alteration in the outline shape,
   e.g. possible cavitation

4 Note any alteration in the interproximal enamel density,
   e.g. radiolucent triangular shadows caused by caries

5 Note any alteration in the dentine density, e.g.:
   • Radiolucent saucer-shaped shadows of:
     (i) Approximal caries
     (ii) Occlusal caries
   • Radiolucent oval/round shadows of superimposed
     smooth-surface buccal/lingual caries
   • Radiopaque zones caused by zinc and tin ions

6 Note the presence and state of existing restorations, e.g.:
   • Overcontoured
   • Undercontoured
   • Adaptation
   • Ledges/overhangs
   • Recurrent adjacent caries

7 Trace the outline/shape of the pulp chamber and note:
   • Size of the pulp chamber
   • Presence of reactionary dentine
   • Presence/number of pulp stones

Neck/root

8 Trace the outline of the neck and cervical 1/3 of the root
   of the tooth

9 Note any alteration in the outline, e.g. possible cavitation
   caused by root caries

10 Note any alteration in the density of the root dentine, e.g.:
   • Radiolucent saucer-shaped shadow of root caries
   • Radiolucent triangular-shaped shadows of cervical
     burn-out or cervical translucency

Fig. 21.17 Suggested sequence for examining each
individual tooth.

Chapter 22

The periapical tissues

INTRODUCTION

This chapter explains how to interpret the radiographic appearances of the periapical tissues by illustrating the various normal appearances, and describing in detail the typical changes associated with apical infection and inflammation following pulpal necrosis. To help explain the different radiographic appearances, they are correlated with the various underlying pathological processes. In addition, there is a summary of the other, sometimes sinister, lesions that can affect the periapical tissues and may simulate simple inflammatory changes.

NORMAL RADIOGRAPHIC APPEARANCES

A reminder of the complex three-dimensional anatomy of the hard tissues surrounding the teeth in the maxilla and mandible, which contribute to the two-dimensional periapical radiographic image, is given in Figure 22.1.

The appearances of normal, healthy, periapical tissues vary from one patient to another, from one area of the mouth to another and at different stages in the development of the dentition. These different normal appearances are described below.

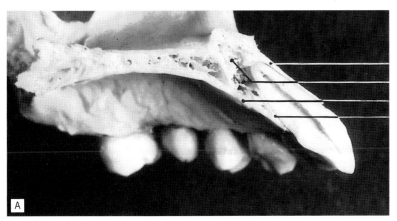

Buccal cortical plate of compact bone

Trabecular or cancellous bone
Palatal cortical plate of compact bone
Cortical bone of the socket

Fig. 22.1A Sagittal section through the maxilla and central incisor showing the hard tissue anatomy.

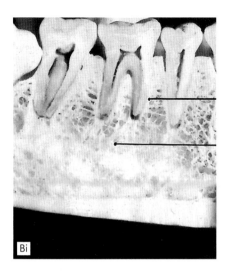

Cortical bone of the socket

Trabecular or cancellous bone

Fig. 22.1B (i) Sagittal and (ii) coronal sections through the mandible in the molar region showing the hard tissue anatomy.

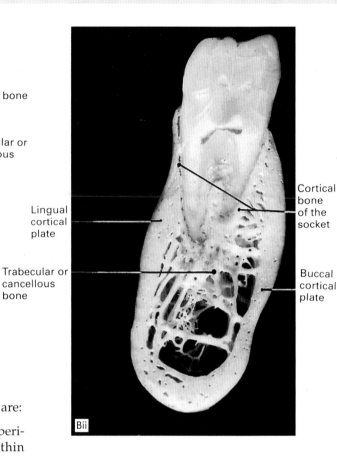

Cortical bone of the socket

Lingual cortical plate

Buccal cortical plate

Trabecular or cancellous bone

The periapical tissues of permanent teeth (Fig. 22.2)

The three most important features to observe are:

- The radiolucent line that represents the periodontal ligament space and forms a thin continuous black line around the root outline
- The radiopaque line that represents the lamina dura of the bony socket and forms a thin, continuous, white line adjacent to the black line
- The trabecular pattern and density of the surrounding bone:
  - In the mandible, the trabeculae tend to be relatively thick and close together, and are often aligned horizontally
  - In the maxilla, the trabeculae tend to be finer, and more widely spaced. There is no predominant alignment pattern.

These features hold the key to the interpretation of periapical radiographs, since changes in their thickness, continuity and radiodensity reflect the presence of any underlying disease, as described later.

Important points to note

- There is considerable variation in the definition and pattern of these features from one patient to another and from one area of the jaws to another, owing to variation in the density, shape and thickness of the surrounding bone.
- The limitations imposed by contrast, resolution and superimposition can make radiographic identification of these features particularly difficult, hence the need for ideal viewing conditions and digital image enhancement software.

The periapical tissues of deciduous teeth (Fig. 22.3)

The important features of normality (thin lamina dura and periodontal ligament shadows) are the same as for permanent teeth, but can be complicated by:

- The presence of an underlying permanent tooth and its crypt, the shadows of which may overlie the deciduous tooth apex
- Resorption of the deciduous tooth root during the normal exfoliation process.

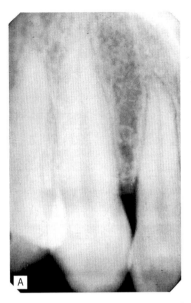
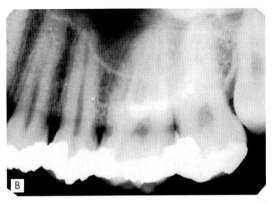
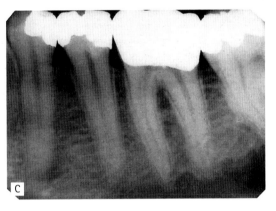

Fig. 22.2 Periapical radiographs of A 32|, B |4567, C |456 showing the normal radiographic anatomy of the periapical tissues in different parts of the jaws. Note the continuous radiolucent line of the periodontal ligament shadow and the radiopaque line of the lamina dura outlining the roots.

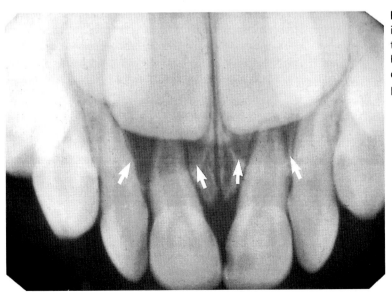

Fig. 22.3 Periapical radiograph of BA/AB in a 4-year-old, showing normal periapical tissues. Note the confusing shadows created by the radiopaque crowns and radiolucent crypts (arrowed) of the developing permanent incisors.

The periapical tissues of developing teeth (Fig. 22.4)

The important features of normal apical tissues, where the root is partially formed and the radicular papilla still exists, include:

- A circumscribed area of radiolucency at the apex
- The radiopaque line of the lamina dura is intact around the papilla
- The developing root is funnel-shaped
- Only after root development is complete does the thin continuous radiolucent line become evident.

The effects of normal superimposed shadows

Normal anatomical shadows superimposed on the apical tissues can be either *radiolucent* or *radiopaque*, depending on the structure involved.

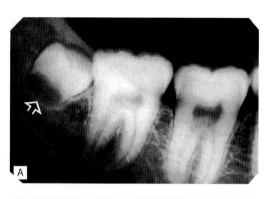

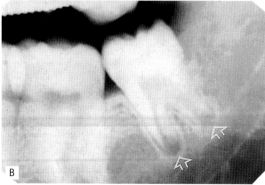

Fig. 22.4 Periapical radiographs showing the normal periapical tissues of developing teeth. A 8⌋, B 7⌋. Note the circumscribed areas of radiolucency of the radicular papillae (arrowed) and the funnel-shaped roots.

Radiolucent shadows

Examples include:

- The maxillary antra
- The nasopalatine foramen
- The mental foramina.

Such cavities in the alveolar bone decrease the total amount of bone that would normally contribute to the final radiographic image, with the following effects:

- The radiolucent line of the periodontal ligament may appear MORE radiolucent or widened, but will still be continuous and well demarcated
- The radiopaque line of the lamina dura may appear LESS obvious and may not be visible
- There will be an area of radiolucency in the alveolar bone at the tooth apex (see Figs 22.5 and 22.6).

Important points to note
- The fact that the radiopaque lamina dura shadow may not be visible does not mean that the bony socket margin is not present clinically. It only means that there is now not enough total bone in the path of the X-ray beam to produce a visible opaque shadow. Since the bony socket is in fact intact, it still defines the periodontal ligament space. Thus, the radiolucent line representing this space still appears continuous and well demarcated.
- Although confusing, this effect of normal anatomical radiolucent shadows on the apical tissues is very important to appreciate, so as not to mistake a normal area of radiolucency at the apex for a pathological lesion.

Radiopaque shadows

Examples include:

- The mylohyoid ridge
- The body of the zygoma
- Areas of sclerotic bone (so-called *dense bone islands*).

Such radiopacities complicate periapical interpretation by obscuring or obliterating the detailed shadows of the apical tissues, as shown in Figure 22.7.

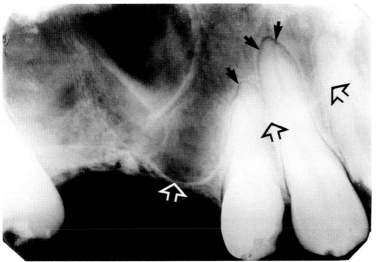

Fig. 22.5 Periapical of Q| showing normal healthy apical tissues but with the radiolucent shadow of the antrum superimposed (the antral floor is indicated by the open arrows). As a result the radiolucent line of the periodontal ligament appears widened and more obvious around the apices of the canine and premolar, but it is still well demarcated, while the radiopaque line of the lamina dura is almost invisible (solid arrows).

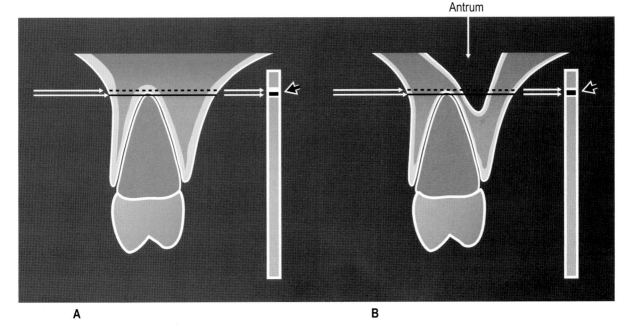

Fig. 22.6 Diagrams of 5| showing the anatomical tissues that the X-ray beam passes through to reach the film. **A** Without a normal anatomical cavity superimposed. **B** With the antral cavity in the path of the X-ray beam. The different resultant radiopaque (white) and radiolucent (black) lines of the apical lamina dura and periodontal ligament are shown on the film (arrowed).

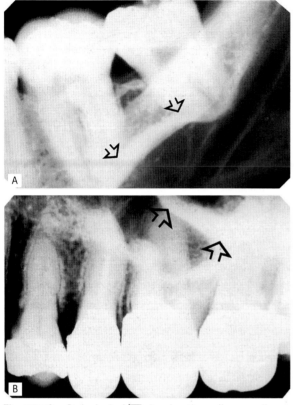

Fig. 22.7A   Periapical of |78 showing the radiopaque line of the mylohyoid ridge (arrowed) superimposed over the apices. **B** Periapical of |4567 showing the radiopaque shadow of the zygomatic buttress (arrowed) overlying and obscuring the apical tissues of the molars.

RADIOGRAPHIC APPEARANCES OF PERIAPICAL INFLAMMATORY CHANGES

Types of inflammatory changes

Following pulpal necrosis, either an acute or chronic inflammatory response is initiated in the apical tissues. The inflammatory response is identical to that set up elsewhere in the body from other toxic stimuli, and exhibits the same signs and symptoms.

Cardinal signs of acute inflammation
These include:

- Swelling — *tumor*
- Redness — *rubor*
- Heat — *calor*
- Pain — *dolor*
- Loss of function — *functio laesa*.

In the apical tissues, inflammatory exudate accumulates in the apical periodontal ligament space (*swelling*), setting up an **acute apical periodontitis**. The affected tooth becomes periostitic or tender to pressure (*pain*), and the patient avoids biting on the tooth (*loss of function*). *Heat* and *redness* are clinically undetectable. These signs are accompanied by destruction and resorption, often of the tooth root, and of the surrounding bone, as a **periapical abscess** develops, and radiographically a periapical radiolucent area becomes evident.

Hallmarks of chronic inflammation
These include the processes of *destruction* and *healing* which are going on simultaneously, as the body's defence systems respond to, and try to confine, the spread of the infection. In the apical tissues, a **periapical granuloma** forms at the apex and dense bone is laid down around the area of resorption. Radiographically, the apical radiolucent area becomes circumscribed and surrounded by dense sclerotic bone. Occasionally, under these conditions of chronic inflammation, the epithelial cell rests of Malassez are stimulated to proliferate and form an inflammatory **periapical radicular cyst** (see Ch. 27) or there is an acute exacerbation producing another abscess (the so-called *phoenix abscess*).

The type and progress of the inflammatory response at the apex and the subsequent spread of apical infection is dependent on several factors relating to:

- The infecting organism including its virulence
- The body's defence systems.

The result is a wide spectrum of events ranging from a very rapidly spreading acute periapical abscess to a very slowly progressing chronic periapical granuloma or cyst. This variation in the underlying disease processes is mirrored radiographically, although it is often not possible to differentiate between an abscess, granuloma or cyst.

A summary of the different inflammatory effects and the resultant radiographic appearances is shown in Table 22.1. The effects are shown diagrammatically in Figure 22.8. Various examples are shown in Figures 22.9–22.12.

Table 22.1 Summary of the effects of different inflammatory processes on the periapical tissues and the resultant radiographic appearances

State of inflammation	Underlying inflammatory changes	Radiographic appearances
Initial acute inflammation	Inflammatory exudate accumulates in the apical periodontal ligament space – *acute apical periodontitis*	Widening of the radiolucent line of the periodontal ligament space OR No apparent changes evident
Initial spread of inflammation	Resorption and destruction of the apical bony socket – *periapical abscess*	Loss of the radiopaque line of the lamina dura at the apex
Further spread of inflammation	Further resorption and destruction of the apical alveolar bone	Area of bone loss at the tooth apex
Initial low-grade chronic inflammation	Minimal destruction of the apical bone. The body's defence systems lay down dense bone in the apical region	No apparent bone destruction but dense sclerotic bone evident around the tooth apex (*sclerosing osteitis*)
Latter stages of chronic inflammation	Apical bone is resorbed and destroyed and dense bone is laid down around the area of resorption – *periapical granuloma* or *radicular cyst*	Circumscribed, well-defined radiolucent area of bone loss at the apex, surrounded by dense sclerotic bone

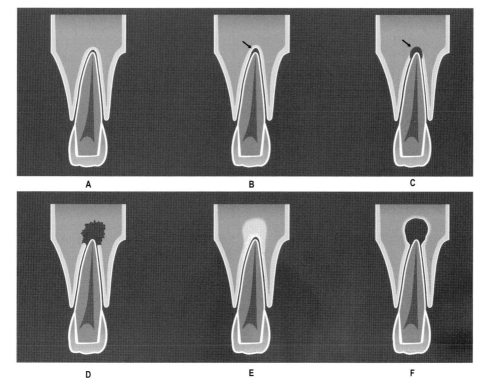

Fig. 22.8 Diagrams showing the various radiographic appearances of infection and inflammation in the apical tissues. **A** Normal. **B** Early apical change – widening of the radiolucent periodontal ligament space (*acute apical periodontitis*) (arrowed). **C** Early apical change – loss of the radiopaque lamina dura (*early periapical abscess*) (arrowed). **D** Extensive destructive acute inflammation – diffuse, ill-defined area of radiolucency at the apex (*periapical abscess*). **E** Low grade chronic inflammation – diffuse radiopaque area at the apex (*sclerosing osteitis*). **F** Longstanding chronic inflammation – well-defined area of radiolucency surrounded by dense sclerotic bone (*periapical granuloma or radicular cyst*).

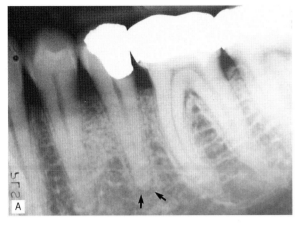

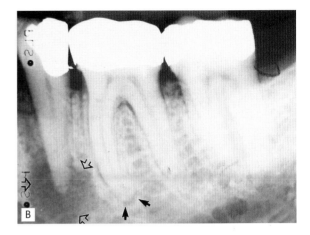

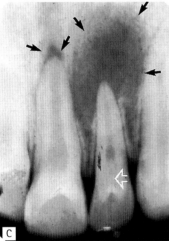

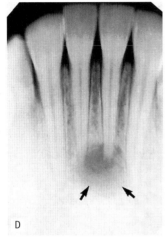

Fig. 22.9　Periapicals showing examples of inflammatory changes in the periapical tissues. **A** Early apical change on $\lfloor 5$ showing widening of the periodontal ligament space and thinning of the lamina dura (*acute apical periodontitis*) (arrowed). **B** Same patient 6 months later — the area of bone destruction at the apex $\lfloor 5$ has increased considerably (open arrows) and there is now early apical change associated with the mesial root $\lfloor 6$ (solid arrows). **C** Large, diffuse area of bone destruction associated with $\lfloor 2$ and a smaller area associated with $\lfloor 1$ (black arrows) (*periapical abscess*). $\lfloor 2$ shows evidence of a dens-in-dente (invaginated odontome) (open white arrow). **D** Reasonably well-defined area of bone destruction (arrowed) associated with $\overline{1\rfloor}$ (*periapical abscess, granuloma or cyst*).

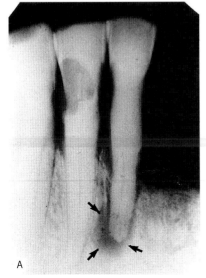

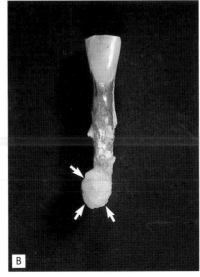

Fig. 22.10A　Periapical showing a well-defined area of radiolucency at the apex of $\overline{1\rfloor}$ (arrowed). The surrounding bone is relatively dense and opaque suggesting a chronic periapical granuloma or radicular cyst. **B** The extracted $\overline{1\rfloor}$, showing the granuloma attached to the root apex (arrowed).

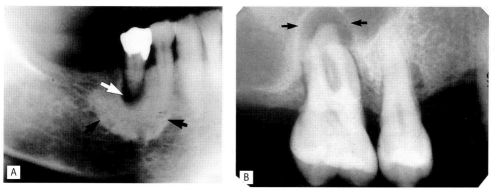

Fig. 22.11   Radiographic examples of other chronic inflammatory changes in the periapical tissues. **A** Long-standing low grade chronic infection associated with 5| resulting in a radiolucent periapical granuloma or radicular cyst (white arrow), surrounded by florid opaque sclerosing osteitis (black arrow). **B** Well-defined area of bone destruction associated with 6| which has resulted in remodelling of the antral floor, producing the so-called *antral halo* appearance (black arrow) (see also Fig. 29.6C).

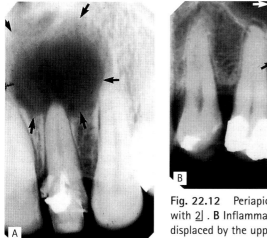

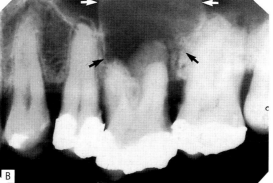

Fig. 22.12   Periapicals showing **A** Inflammatory radicular cyst (arrowed) associated with 2| . **B** Inflammatory radicular cyst (arrowed) associated with |6. The antrum has been displaced by the upper margin of the cyst which is not evident on this radiograph.

Treatment and radiographic follow-up

Most inflammatory periapical lesions are treated by conventional endodontic treatment. The Faculty of General Dental Practice (UK)'s 2004 booklet *Selection Criteria in Dental Radiography*, 2nd edn, recommends:

- A good quality pre-operative radiograph
- At least one good quality radiograph to determine working length
- A mid-fill radiograph if there is any doubt about the apical constriction
- A postoperative radiograph to assess success of the obturation and to act as a baseline for assessment of apical disease or healing

- A further follow-up radiograph after one year following completion of treatment (see Fig. 22.13), even for asymptomatic teeth and large periapical radiolucencies should be monitored more frequently.

If endodontic therapy is clinically unsuccessful, subsequent treatment involves either:

- Repeat conventional endodontics
- Surgical exploraton, curettage of the infected area and/or enucleation of the cyst, apicectomy and retrograde root filling
- Extraction of the tooth.

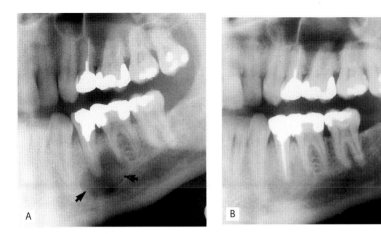

Fig. 22.13A Part of a panoramic radiograph showing a round, well-defined area of radiolucency — a likely radicular cyst (arrowed), associated with the poorly root-filled ⌐5. **B** Same patient 12 months later following successful root filling at ⌐5. Note the bony fill-in in the apical area.

OTHER IMPORTANT CAUSES OF PERIAPICAL RADIOLUCENCY

Many of the conditions described in Chapters 27 and 28 can present occasionally in the apical region of the alveolar bone. Some can simulate the simple inflammatory changes described above including:

- Benign and malignant bone tumours including secondary metastatic deposits (see Fig. 22.14)
- Lymphoreticular tumours of bone
- Langerhans cell disease
- Osseous dysplasia (early stages).

Although it is uncommon, clinicians should still be alert to the possibility that malignant lesions can present as apparently simple localized areas of infection. The signs of concern include:

- A vital tooth with minimal caries
- Spiking root resorption and an irregular radiolucent apical area with a ragged, poorly defined outline
- Tooth mobility in the absence of generalized periodontal disease
- Regional nerve anaesthesia
- Failure to respond to good endodontic therapy.

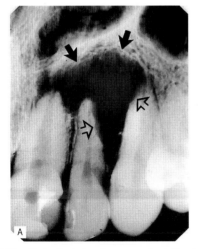

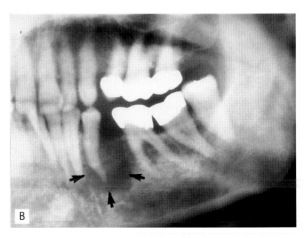

Fig. 22.14A Periapical showing a poorly defined area of radiolucency in the apical region of ⌊123. Features of concern are the ragged bone margin (solid arrows) and the extensive resorption of ⌊2 and ⌊3 (open arrows). Initial treatment involved unsuccessful root treatment of ⌊1. Biopsy revealed an osteosarcoma. **B** Part of a panoramic radiograph showing a large poorly defined area of radiolucency in 45 region (arrowed). Both premolars were caries-free and unrestored, but mobile. ⌐5 was extracted and histopathology revealed a secondary metastatic malignant tumour from a breast primary.

SUGGESTED GUIDELINES FOR INTERPRETING PERIAPICAL IMAGES

Although somewhat repetitive, this methodical approach to radiographic interpretation is so important, and so often ignored, that it is described again.

Overall critical assessment

A typical series of questions that should be asked about the quality of a periapical radiographic image based on the *ideal quality criteria* described in Chapter 10 include:

Technique (film OR digitally-captured images)

- Is the required tooth shown?
- Is the apical alveolar bone shown?
- Has the image been taken using the bisected angle or paralleling technique?
- How much distortion is present?
- Is the image foreshortened or elongated?
- Are the crowns overlapped?
- Has there been any *coning off* or *cone cutting?*

Exposure factors (film-captured images)

- Is the image too dark and so possibly over-exposed?
- Is the image too light and so possibly under-exposed?
- What effect do the exposure factors have on the appearance of the apical tissues?

Processing (film-captured images)

- Is the radiograph correctly processed?
- Is it overdeveloped?
- Is it underdeveloped?
- Is it correctly fixed?
- Has it been adequately washed?

Image processing (digitally-captured images)

- Is the contrast optimal?
- Is the brightness optimal?
- Is image enhancement optimal?
- Is magnification optimal?

Systematic viewing

A systematic approach to viewing periapical radiographs is shown in Figure 22.15. This approach ensures that **all** areas of the film are observed and that the important features of the tooth apex are examined.

General overview of entire radiograph
1 Note the chronological and development age of the patient
2 Note the position, outline and density of all the normal superimposed anatomical shadows including any developing teeth

Examine each tooth on the radiograph and assess

3 **The crown**
   Note particularly:
   - The presence of caries
   - The state of existing restorations

4 **The root(s)**
   Note particularly:
   - The length of the root
   - The number(s)
   - The morphology
   - The size and shape of canals
   - The presence of:
     a Pulp stones
     b Root fillings
     c Internal resorption
     d External resorption
     e Root fractures

5 **The apical tissues**
   Note particularly:
   - The integrity, continuity and thickness of:
     a The radiolucent line of the periodontal ligament space
     b The radiopaque line of the lamina dura
   - Any associated radiolucent areas
   - Any associated radiopaque areas
   - The pattern of the trabecular bone

5 **The peridontal tissues**
   Note particularly:
   - The width of the periodontal ligament
   - The level and quality of the crestal bone
   - Any vertical or horizontal bone loss
   - Any calculus deposits
   - Any furcation involvements

Fig. 22.15   A systematic sequence for viewing periapical images.

Chapter 23

The periodontal tissues and periodontal disease

INTRODUCTION

An overall assessment of the periodontal tissues is based on both the clinical examination and radiographic findings — the two investigations complement one another. Unfortunately, like many other indicators of periodontal disease, radiographs only provide retrospective evidence of the disease process. However, they can be used to assess the morphology of the affected teeth and the pattern and degree of alveolar bone loss that has taken place. *Bone loss* can be defined as *the difference between the present septal bone height and the assumed normal bone height for any particular patient*, taking age into account. In fact radiographs actually show the amount of alveolar bone *remaining* in relation to the length of the root. But this information is still important in the overall assessment of the severity of the disease, the prognosis of the teeth and for treatment planning.

Radiographs are therefore used to:

- Assess the extent of bone loss and furcation involvement
- Determine the presence of any secondary local causative factors
- Assess root length and morphology
- Assist in treatment planning
- Evaluate treatment measures particularly following *guided tissue regeneration* (GTR).

SELECTION CRITERIA

Several radiographic projections can be used to show the periodontal tissues. Those recommended by the Faculty of General Dental Practice (UK) in 2004 in their booklet *Selection Criteria in Dental Radiography* are summarized in Table 23.1.

In addition, digital radiography and image manipulation including subtraction and densitometric image analysis (see Ch. 7), may assist in showing and measuring subtle changes in fine

Table 23.1 Summary of radiographs recommended for periodontal assessment based on the Faculty of General Practice (UK)'s *Selection Criteria in Dental Radiography* in 2004

Clinical indication	Radiographs
Uniform pocketing < 6 mm	Horizontal bitewings
Uniform pocketing > 6 mm	Vertical bitewings + selected paralleling technique periapicals
Irregular pocketing	Bitewings — horizontal or vertical + selected paralleling technique periapicals
Widespread pocketing and other dental problems	Panoramic radiograph + selected paralleling technique periapicals
Periodontal/endodontic lesions	Paralleling technique periapicals

alveolar and crestal bone pattern. However, these techniques require the inclusion of a reference object of known density and a highly reproducible positioning technique to be helpful.

Important points to note

- In the interpretation of the periodontal tissues, images of excellent quality are essential — perhaps more so than in other dental specialties — because of the fine detail that is required.
- Exposure factors should be reduced when using film-based techniques to avoid *burn-out* of the interdental crestal bone.

RADIOGRAPHIC FEATURES OF HEALTHY PERIODONTIUM

A *healthy* periodontium can be regarded as *periodontal tissue exhibiting no evidence of disease*. Unfortunately, *health* cannot be ascertained from radiographs alone, clinical information is also required.

However, to be able to interpret radiographs successfully clinicians need to know the usual radiographic features of healthy tissues where there has been no bone loss. The only reliable radiographic feature is the relationship between the crestal bone margin and the cemento–enamel junction (CEJ). If this distance is within normal limits (2–3 mm) and there are no clinical signs of loss of attachment, then it can be said that there has been no periodontitis.

The usual radiographic features of *healthy* alveolar bone are shown in Figures 23.1 and 23.2 and include:

- Thin, smooth, evenly corticated margins to the interdental crestal bone in the posterior regions.
- Thin, even, pointed margins to the interdental crestal bone in the anterior regions.
- Cortication at the top of the crest is not always evident, owing mainly to the small amount of bone between the teeth anteriorly.
- The interdental crestal bone is continuous with the lamina dura of the adjacent teeth. The junction of the two forms a sharp angle.
- Thin even width to the mesial and distal periodontal ligament spaces.

Important points to note

- Although these are the usual features of a healthy periodontium, they are not always evident.
- Their absence from radiographs does not necessarily mean that periodontal disease is present.
- Failure to see these features may be due to:
  - Technique error
  - Overexposure
  - Normal anatomical variation in alveolar bone shape and density.
- Following successful treatment, the periodontal tissues may appear healthy clinically, but radiographs may show evidence of earlier bone loss when the disease was active. Bone loss observed on radiographs is therefore not an indicator of the presence of inflammation.

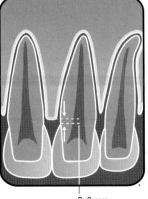

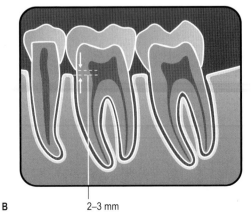

A   2–3 mm   B   2–3 mm

Fig. 23.1 Diagrams illustrating the radiographic appearances of a healthy periodontium. **A** The upper incisor region. **B** The lower molar region. The normal distance of 2–3 mm from the crestal margin to the cemento–enamel junction is indicated.

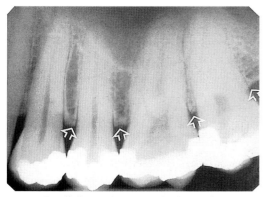

Fig. 23.2 Paralleling technique periapical radiograph of ⌊4567 (slightly reduced exposure) showing the radiographic features of a healthy periodontium (arrowed).

CLASSIFICATION OF PERIODONTAL DISEASE

Various classifications of periodontal disease have been put forward over the years. The most comprehensive, although not universally agreed, was produced by the International Workshop of the American Academy of Periodontology and the European Federation of Periodontology in 1999. A simplified version is shown in Table 23.2.

Table 23.2 Simplified classification of periodontal diseases and conditions based broadly on that produced by the International Workshop of the American Academy of Periodontology and the European Federation of Periodontology in 1999

I	Gingival diseases	A. Plaque induced gingival diseases
		1. Gingivitis associated with dental plaque only
		(a) Without local factors
		(b) With local factors
		2. Gingival diseases modified by systemic factors,
		e.g. Smoking
		Pregnancy
		Uncontrolled diabetes
		3. Gingival diseases modified by medications,
		e.g. Phenytoin, Nifedipine
		4. Gingival diseases modified by malnutrition,
		e.g. Vitamin C deficiency
		B. Non-plaque induced gingival lesions
II	Chronic periodontitis	A. Localized
		B. Generalized
III	Aggressive periodontitis	A. Localized
		B. Generalized

IV	Periodontitis as a manifestation of systemic disease	A. Associated with haematological disorders,
		     e.g. Leukaemia
		        Acquired neutropenia

		B. Associated with genetic disorders,
		     e.g. Down's syndrome
		        Papillon–Lefevre syndrome
		        Langerhans cell disease
		        (histiocytosis X)

		C. Not otherwise specified, *e.g. HIV*
V	Necrotizing periodontal diseases	A. Necrotizing ulcerative gingivitis (NUG)
		B. Necrotizing ulcerative periodontitis (NUP)
VI	Abscesses of the periodontium	A. Gingival abscess
		B. Periodontal abscess
		C. Pericoronal abscess
VII	Periodontitis in association with endodontic lesions	
VIII	Developmental or acquired deformities and conditions	

RADIOGRAPHIC FEATURES OF PERIODONTAL DISEASE AND THE ASSESSMENT OF BONE LOSS AND FURCATION INVOLVEMENT

It is beyond the scope of this book to describe the features of all the periodontal diseases and conditions shown in the classification in Table 23.2. Discussion will be restricted to:

- Gingival diseases
- Periodontitis
  - Chronic
  - Aggressive
- Abscesses of the periodontium.
.

Gingival diseases

Radiographs provide no direct evidence of the soft tissue involvement in gingival diseases. However, in severe cases of necrotizing ulcerative gingivitis (NUG) or acute ulcerative gingivitis (AUG) where there has been extensive cratering of the interdental papilla, inflammatory destruction of the underlying crestal bone may be observed.

Periodontitis

Periodontitis is the name given to periodontal disease when *the superficial inflammation in the gingival tissues extends into the underlying alveolar bone and there has been loss of attachment.* The destruction of the bone can be either *localized*, affecting a few areas of the mouth, or *generalized* affecting all areas. In *chronic periodontitis* the rate of this progression and subsequent bone destruction is usually slow and continues intermittently over many years, whereas in *aggressive periodontitis* it is usually rapid. The radiographic features of the different forms of periodontitis are similar; it is the distribution and the rate of bone destruction that varies.

Terminology
The terms used to describe the various appearances of bone destruction include:

- Horizontal bone loss
- Vertical bone loss
- Furcation involvements.

The terms *horizontal* and *vertical* have been used traditionally to describe the direction or pattern of bone loss using the line joining two adjacent teeth at their cemento-enamel junctions as a line of reference. The amount of bone loss is then assessed as mild, moderate or severe as shown diagrammatically in Figure 23.3.

Severe vertical bone loss, extending from the alveolar crest and involving the tooth apex, in

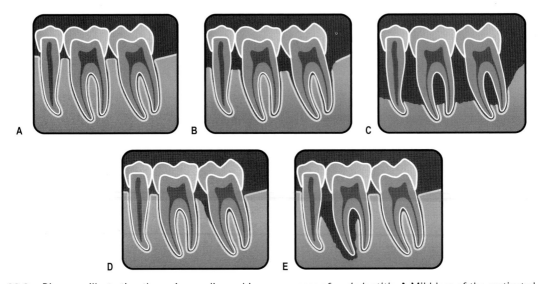

Fig. 23.3 Diagrams illustrating the various radiographic appearances of *periodontitis*. **A** Mild loss of the corticated crestal bone, widening of the periodontal ligament and loss of the normally sharp angle between the crestal bone and the lamina dura. **B** Moderate horizontal bone loss. **C** Severe generalized horizontal bone loss with furcation involvement. **D** Localized vertical bone loss affecting ⎯7|. **E** Extensive localized bone loss involving the apex of ⎯6| — the so-called *perio-endo* lesion.

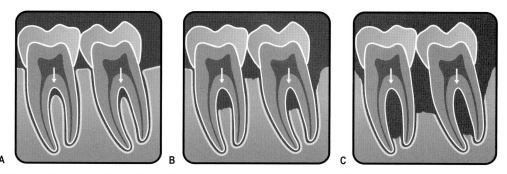

Fig. 23.4 Diagrams illustrating the radiographic appearances of varying degrees of furcation involvement in lower molars (arrowed). **A** Very early involvement showing widening of the furcation periodontal ligament shadow. **B** Moderate involvement. **C** Severe involvement.

which necrosis of pulp tissue is also believed to be a contributory factor, is classified as *periodontitis associated with an endodontic lesion*, often abbreviated to a *perio-endo lesion* (see Figs 23.3E and 23.14).

The term *furcation involvement* describes the radiographic appearance of bone loss in the furcation area of the roots which is evidence of advanced disease in this zone, as shown diagrammatically in Figure 23.4. Although central furcation involvements are seen more readily in mandibular molars, they can also be seen in maxillary molars despite the superimposed shadow of the overlying palatal root. In addition, early maxillary molar furcation involvement between the mesiobuccal or distobuccal roots and the palatal root produces a characteristic triangular-shaped radiolucency at the edge of the tooth (see Figs 23.8C and 23.10A).

Chronic periodontitis (Figs 23.5—23.11)

This is the most common and important form of periodontal disease, affecting the majority of the dentate and partially dentate population. It is the main cause of loss of teeth in later adult life. The main pathological features of this disease are:

- Inflammation (usually a progression from chronic gingivitis)
- Destruction of periodontal ligament fibers
- Resorption of the alveolar bone
- Loss of epithelial attachment
- Formation of pockets around the teeth
- Gingival recession.

It is the resorption of the alveolar bone that provides the main radiographic features of chronic periodontitis. These include:

- Loss of the corticated interdental crestal margin, the bone edge becomes irregular or blunted
- Widening of the periodontal ligament space at the crestal margin
- Loss of the normally sharp angle between the crestal bone and the lamina dura — the bone angle becomes rounded and irregular
- Localized or generalized loss of the alveolar supporting bone
- Patterns of bone loss — *horizontal* and/or *vertical* — resulting in an even loss of bone or the formation of complex intra-bony defects
- Loss of bone in the furcation areas of multirooted teeth — this can vary from widening of the furcation periodontal ligament to large zones of bone destruction
- Widening of the interdental periodontal ligament spaces

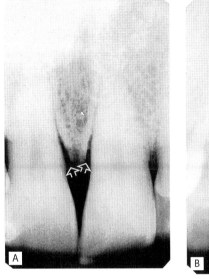
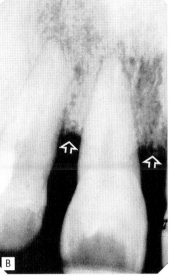

Fig. 23.5 Periapical radiographs showing the typical radiographic features of horizontal bone loss (arrowed) in periodontitis affecting maxillary incisors. **A** Moderate bone loss. **B** Severe bone loss.

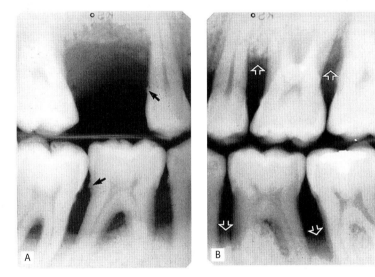

Fig. 23.6A Right and **B** Left vertical bitewings showing severe bone loss (open arrows) typical of chronic periodontitis. The black arrows indicate calculus deposits.

- Associated complicating *secondary local factors* — although the primary cause of periodontal disease is bacterial plaque, many complicating secondary local factors may also be involved. Some of these factors can be detected on radiographs (see Fig. 23.11) and include:
  - Calculus deposits
  - Carious cavities
  - Root resorption
  - Overhanging filling ledges
  - Poor restoration margins
  - Lack of contact points
  - Poor restoration contour, including pontic design
  - Perforations by pins or posts
  - Endodontic status in relation to perio-endo lesions
  - Overerupted opposing teeth
  - Tilted teeth
  - Root approximation
  - Gingivally fitting partial dentures,
  - Developmental grooves
  - Dens-in-dente.

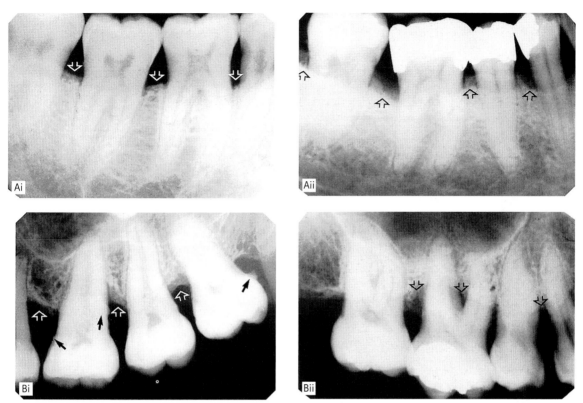

Fig. 23.7   Periapical radiographs showing the typical radiographic features of horizontal bone loss in chronic periodontitis affecting poster teeth. **A** (i) Early or mild and (ii) moderate bone loss (arrowed) affecting mandibular molars. **B** (i) Moderate and (ii) severe bone loss (open arrows) affecting maxillary molars. The black arrows indicate calculus deposits.

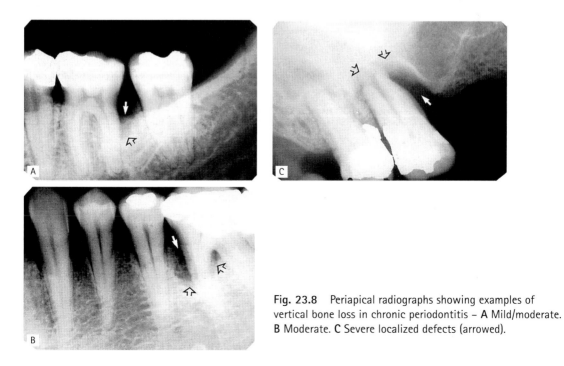

Fig. 23.8   Periapical radiographs showing examples of vertical bone loss in chronic periodontitis – **A** Mild/moderate. **B** Moderate. **C** Severe localized defects (arrowed).

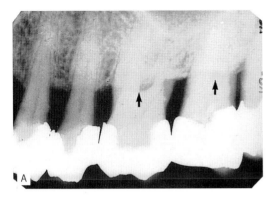

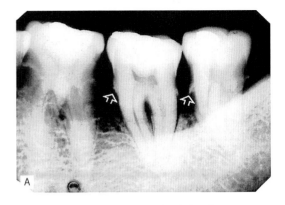

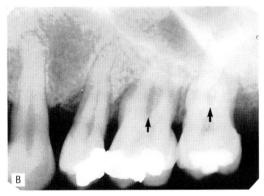

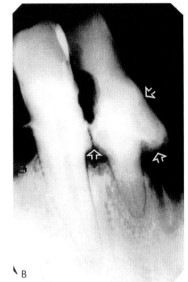

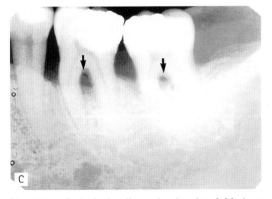

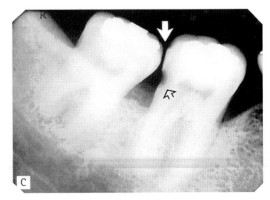

Fig. 23.9 Periapical radiographs showing **A** Moderate furcation involvement (black arrows) in maxillary molars. Note the characteristic mesial and distal cervical triangular radiolucent shadows indicating furcation involvement between the mesiobuccal and palatal roots and the distobuccal and palatal roots. **B** Severe degrees of furcation bone loss (arrowed) in maxillary molars. **C** Moderate and severe degrees of furcation bone loss (arrowed) in mandibular molars.

Fig. 23.10 Radiographic examples of some secondary local causative factors (arrowed) associated with periodontal disease. **A** Small calculus deposits. **B** Gross calculus deposits. **C** Defective contact point and root caries.

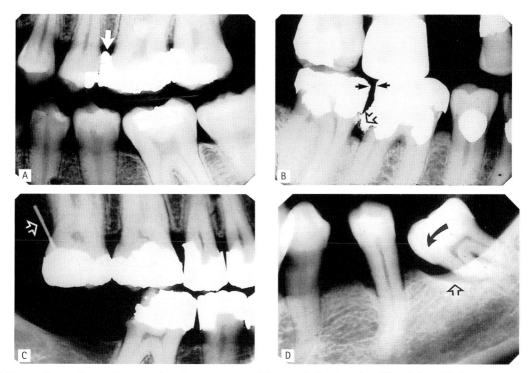

Fig. 23.11 Further radiographic examples of secondary local factors. **A** Overhanging filling ledge. **B** Defective contact point and overhanging filling ledge. **C** Pin perforated into the periodontal tissues. **D** Tilted tooth,

Aggressive periodontitis (Figs 23.12–23.13)

As mentioned earlier, in aggressive periodontitis the progression of the disease and subsequent bone destruction is rapid and can be either generalized or localized. One example is *early onset periodontitis* which includes *localized juvenile periodontitis* and *prepubertal periodontitis*. Radiographic features include:

- Severe vertical bone defects affecting the first molars and/or incisors
- Arch or saucer-shaped defects
- Sometimes the bone loss is more generalized
- Migration of the incisors with diastema formation
- Rapid rate of bone loss.

Abscesses of the periodontium

As was shown in the classification in Table 23.1, abscesses of the periodontium are divided into three groups. These included:

- Gingival abscess
- Periodontal abscess
  - Lateral periodontal abscess
  - Perio-endo lesion
- Pericoronal abscess.

Typically the patient presents with a localized acute exacerbation of underlying periodontal disease, usually originating in deep soft tissue pocket which may have become occluded. The diagnosis of an abscess is made clinically where the signs of acute inflammation and infection are evident. Vitality testing helps to differentiate between the lateral periodontal abscess and the perio-endo lesion. The underlying radiographic bone changes may be indistinguishable from other forms of periodontal bone destruction, as shown in Figure 23.14.

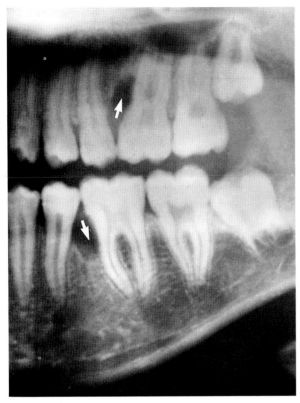

Fig. 23.12 Part of a panoramic radiograph showing the typical localized bone defects affecting the first molars (arrowed) of aggressive localized juvenile periodontitis.

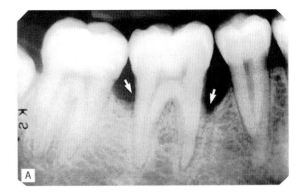

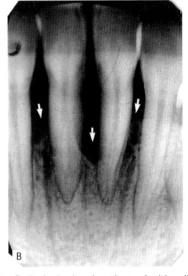

Fig. 23.13 Periapicals showing the typical localized bone defects (arrowed) of aggressive localized juvenile periodontitis affecting **A** the mandibular molars and **B** the mandibular incisors in an 18-year-old.

Fig. 23.14 Periapical radiograph showing an extensive area of bone loss (arrowed) associated with 4| — a so-called *perio-endo* lesion. The patient had presented clinically with a periodontal abscess.

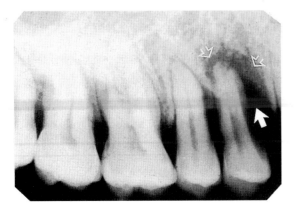

EVALUATION OF TREATMENT MEASURES

Traditional treatment of periodontal disease involves improving oral hygiene, scaling, polishing and root planing of affected teeth surfaces and the removal of any other secondary local factors in an attempt to slow down or arrest the disease process. In recent years, there has been an attempt to achieve the ultimate treatment aim of regeneration of lost tissue by the development of the procedure called *guided tissue regeneration*. This favours regeneration of the attachment complex to denuded root surfaces by allowing selective regrowth of periodontal ligament cells while excluding the gingival tissues from reaching contact with the root during wound healing. This is achieved by surgically interposing a barrier membrane between the gingiva and the root surface.

The success or otherwise of these treatment measures can be assessed by a combination of clinical examination, including probing and attachment loss measurements, and periodic radiographic investigation, as shown in Figures 23.15 and 23.16. **Note**: To provide useful information sequential radiographs ideally should be comparable in both technique and exposure factors.

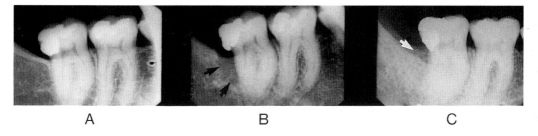

Fig. 23.15 Periapicals showing evaluation of treatment. **A** Initial film. **B** 9 years later showing overhanging filling margin and distal bony defect on 7⌐ (arrowed). **C** Follow-up film 3 years later following guided tissue regeneration showing the reduced defect (arrowed) and the bone in-fill. (Kindly supplied by Dr A. Sidi.)

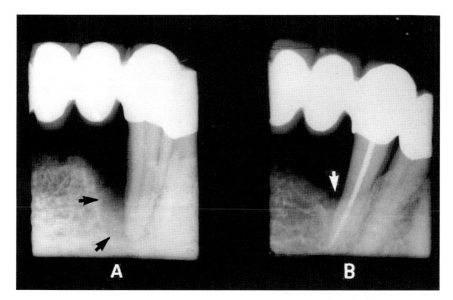

Fig. 23.16 Periapicals showing evaluation of treatment. **A** Preoperative film showing a perio-endo lesion affecting ⌐3 with severe bony defect on the mesial aspect of the root (arrowed). **B** Follow-up film 2 years later following successful endodontic therapy and guided tissue regeneration. Note the reduced bony defect (arrowed). (Kindly supplied by Dr A. Sidi.)

LIMITATIONS OF RADIOGRAPHIC DIAGNOSIS

Radiographic evaluation of the periodontal tissues is somewhat limited. The main limitations include:

- Superimposition and a two-dimensional image bringing about the following problems:
  - It is difficult to differentiate between the buccal and lingual crestal bone levels
  - Only part of a complex bony defect is shown
  - One wall of a bone defect may obscure the rest of the defect
  - Dense tooth or restoration shadows may obscure buccal or lingual bone defects, and buccal or lingual calculus deposits
  - Bone resorption in the furcation area may be obscured by an overlying root or bone shadow.
- Information is provided only on the hard tissues of the periodontium, since the soft tissue gingival defects are not normally detectable.
- Bone loss is detectable only when sufficient calcified tissue has been resorbed to alter the attenuation of the X-ray beam. As a result, the histological front of the disease process cannot be determined by the radiographic appearance.
- Technique variations in image receptor and X-ray beam positions can affect considerably the appearance of the periodontal tissues; hence the need for accurate, reproducible techniques as described in Chapter 11.
- Exposure factors can have a marked effect on the apparent crestal bone height — over-exposure causing *burn-out* when using film-based imaging.
- Complete reliance cannot be placed on the inherently inferior images of dental panoramic radiographs although they do provide a reasonable overview of the periodontal status (see Fig. 23.17 and Ch. 17).
- Some of the limitations of two-dimensional conventional radiography, in visualizing three-dimensional periodontal bone defects, can be overcome by high resolution cone beam CT (see Ch. 19).

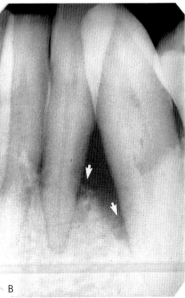

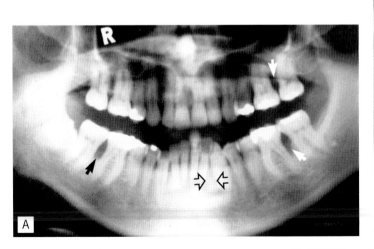

Fig. 23.17A Panoramic radiograph showing bony defects in the molar regions (arrowed) but no evidence of a similar defect in the $\overline{23}$ region (open arrows) owing to superimposition of the radiopaque artefactual shadow of the cervical vertebrae. **B** Periapical of $\overline{23}$ region taken at the same time showing the severe bony defect (arrowed) that was actually present.

Chapter 24

Implant assessment

INTRODUCTION

The restoration of edentulous and partially dentate jaws using a variety of implant-retained prostheses has become a common clinical procedure in recent years. The implants are usually made of titanium and are described as either:

- Endosteal — placed **in** the bone. These are manufactured in a variety of shapes — screw, smooth-sided or plate-form, and essentially replace the roots of one or more teeth
- Subperiosteal — placed **on** the bone, under the periosteum and secured in place with screws.

This chapter concentrates on endosteal dental implants which are more commonly used, particularly since P. I. Brånemark's clinical research on the concept of *osseointegration* which he defined as *a direct connection between living bone and a load carrying endosseous implant at the light microscopic level*. There are many different endosteal implant systems available, and it is beyond the scope of this book to discuss all the systems and their various advantages and disadvantages. The Brånemark system, described here, is probably the best known and has been researched over the longest period demonstrating acceptable 20-year success rates. Most currently used implant systems can be viewed as design modifications to this basic concept.

However, whatever the system used, radiology plays an essential role in preoperative treatment planning, postoperative follow-up and success evaluation.

The Brånemark system

Treatment usually involves either a two-stage or a one-stage (non-submerged) surgical procedure followed by the restorative phase. Initially, in the two-stage technique the *fixture* is placed in vital bone ensuring a precision fit. The *cover screw* is screwed into the top of the *fixture* to prevent downgrowth of soft and hard tissue into the internal threaded area. The fixture is then left buried beneath the mucosa for 3–6 months. (It is important during this initial healing period to avoid loading the fixture although early loading protocols are being used in certain clinical circumstances.) The *fixture* is then surgically uncovered, the *cover screw* removed and the *abutment* (the transmucosal component) connected to the *fixture* by the *abutment screw*. An *hexagonal anti-rotation device* is incorporated into the top of the fixture. The *gold cylinder*, an integral part of the final restorative prosthesis, is finally connected to the abutment by the *gold screw*. A standard Brånemark implant is illustrated in Figure 24.1.

Modifications to this basic design include slightly roughened implant surfaces to improve bone to implant contact and more stable, secure abutment/implant connection systems employing internal connections rather than the classic flat-top hexagon described above. A variety of different abutments and connecting restorative elements are available for different clinical situations.

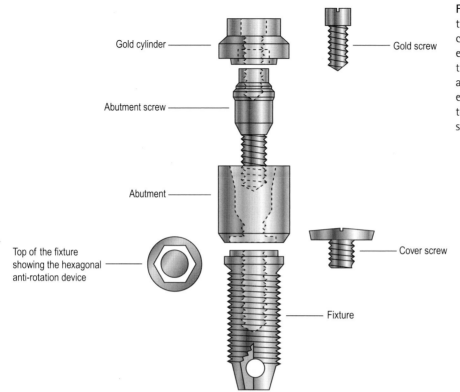

Gold cylinder

Abutment screw

Abutment

Top of the fixture showing the hexagonal anti-rotation device

Gold screw

Cover screw

Fixture

Fig. 24.1 Diagram showing the basic Brånemark system components for a standard endosseous implant. Note: there is a variety of different abutments and restorative elements available that attach to the hexagonal top of the standard fixture.

MAIN INDICATIONS

Replacement of missing teeth in patients with:

- Healthy dentitions which have suffered tooth loss because of trauma
- Free-end saddles
- Developmentally missing teeth
- Remaining teeth not suitable as bridge abutments
- Severe ridge resorption making the wearing of dentures difficult
- Severe gag reflex
- Cleft palates and insufficient remaining teeth to support a denture/obturator
- Reconstruction following radical ablative jaw surgery
- A desire to avoid wearing a removable prosthesis.

TREATMENT PLANNING CONSIDERATIONS

Clinical examination

A thorough clinical examination using study casts, and an overall evaluation of the patient are essential, as good case selection is imperative for the long-term success of implants. A multidisciplinary approach involving surgeons, prosthodontists and dental technicians is often adopted because of the many important factors that need to be taken into account, including:

- The patient's age, general health and motivation
- The condition and position of the remaining teeth (if present), including their occlusion
- The status of the periodontal tissues and the level of oral hygiene
- The condition — quality and quantity — of the edentulous mandibular or maxillary alveolar bone
- The condition of the oral soft tissues.

RADIOGRAPHIC EXAMINATION

Although guidelines have been published by both the American Academy of Oral and Maxillofacial Radiology in 2001 and the European Association for Osseointegraion in 2002, there is still some disagreement on selection criteria in individual clinical situations. In addition, other variables make generalized recommendations difficult. Examples of these include:

- The experience of the operator
- The thoroughness of the clinical examination including the use of ridge-mapping techniques
- The proposed anatomical site.

In 2004 the Faculty of General Dental Practice (UK)'s *Selection Criteria in Dental Radiography* booklet concluded that there is fact only a very small evidence base on which to formulate guidelines for the use of radiographs in implant dentistry.

There are a range of investigations that are suitable in different clinical situations. Clinical choice may well depend on availability of facilities. Investigations include:

- Periapical radiography
- Panoramic radiography
- Cross-sectional linear tomography programmes available with some modern panoramic machines (see Ch. 17)
- Multi-directional (e.g. spiral) cross sectional tomography described in Chapter 16 (see Fig. 24.2)
- Cone beam CT. This recently developed, low dose, digital volume tomographic technique described in Chapter 19 is ideal for implant assessment and is likely to become the imaging

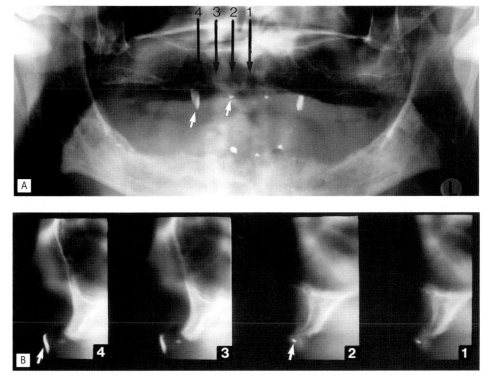

Fig. 24.2 Pre-implant assessment using the Scanora® multidirectional tomographic machine. **A** Panoramic radiograph of an edentulous patient showing various radiopaque localization markers (attached to the denture). **B** 4-mm cross-sectional (transverse) spiral tomographic images of the 321 region. The location of each cross-sectional image is indicated on the panoramic radiograph. The radiopaque markers in the 3 and 1 regions are arrowed on both figures and are in focus on the tomographic slices.

modality of choice (see Figs 24.3 and 24.4). Computer manipulation enables the production of cross-sectional, panoramic and three-dimensional reconstructed images

- Computed tomography (CT). Specific dental computer programmes, designed for implant planning, have been written that are compatible with medical CT. This usually involves about 30 axial scans per jaw, each 1.5 mm thick. This information can then undergo computer manipulation, as with cone beam CT to produce reformatted cross-sectional, panoramic and three-dimensional reconstructed images as shown in Figure 24.5. The radiation dose to the patient is considerably higher when compared to other techniques
- Magnetic resonance (MR). This offers the advantages of not using ionizing radiation and

producing sections in any desired plane without reformatting, as shown in Figure 24.6.

Radiographic information provided

These various radiographic investigations are used to show:

- The position and size of relevant normal anatomical structures, including the:
  - inferior dental canals
  - mental foramina
  - incisive or nasopalatine foramen and canal
  - nasal floor
- The shape and size of the antra, including the position of the antral floor and its relationship to adjacent teeth
- The presence of any underlying disease

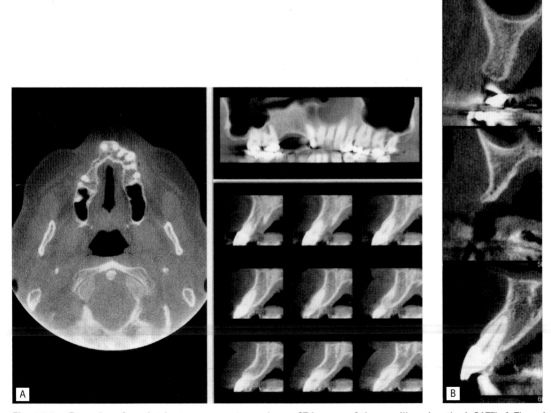

Fig. 24.3   Examples of pre-implant assessment cone beam CT images of the maxilla using the i-CAT™. **A** Three image screens are available simultaneously on the monitor including axial, panoramic and a series of cross-sectional (or trans-axial) images. **B** Three life-size cross-sectional images. (Reproduced with kind permission of Imaging Sciences International, Inc.)

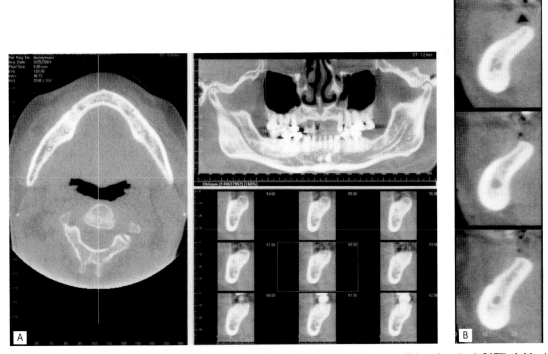

Fig. 24.4   Examples of pre-implant assessment cone beam CT images of the mandible using the i-CAT™. **A** Monitor images and **B** Three life-size cross-sectional images. (Reproduced with kind permission of Imaging Sciences International, Inc.)

- The presence of any retained roots or buried teeth
- The quantity of alveolar crest/basal bone, allowing direct measurements of the height, width and shape
- The quality (density) of the bone, noting:
  - the amount of cortical bone present
  - density of the cancellous bone
  - size of the trabecular spaces.

Important points to note

- Cross-sectional imaging is important to provide information on the width and quality of the alveolar bone and the location of anatomical structures. The choice of imaging modality will obviously depend on the availability of facilities. The more complex the clinical case, the more comprehensive the radiographic assessment needs to be.
- Plastic stents containing radiopaque markers are often required for accurate localization of

cross-sectional images. Gadolinium markers are used with MR (see Fig. 24.6).
- Radiation dose from medical CT imaging is many times greater than from low dose cone beam CT (see Ch. 19) or multidirectional tomography.
- CT and cone beam CT data can be manipulated and reformatted to produce life-size cross-sectional images, three-dimensional images and can provide radiographic density values for cortical and cancellous bone. Both systems are compatible with SIM/Plant specialized software (Columbia Scientific Inc.) which enables simulated implants to be inserted and viewed on a computer to assess size and angulation.
- The magnification on multi directional cross-sectional tomographs varies from one machine to another, but for any particular unit it is fixed and uniform, e.g. Scanora® slices are all magnified by a factor of 1.7.

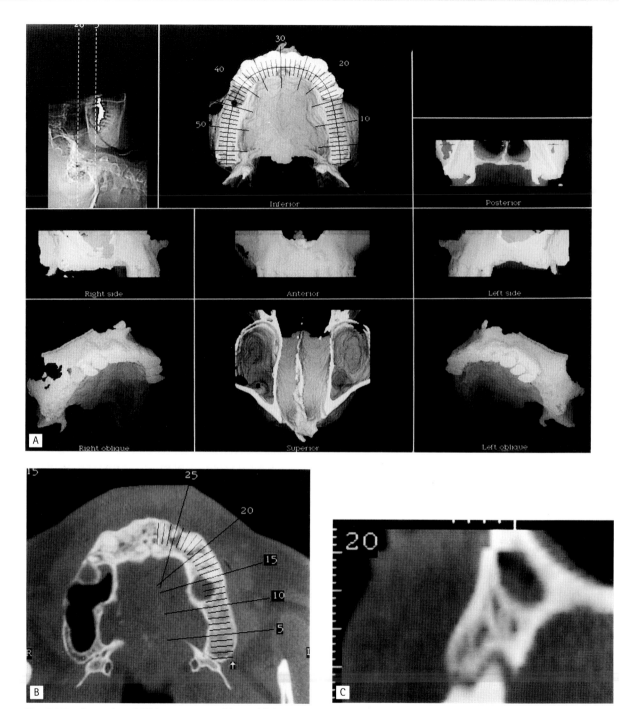

Fig. 24.5 Examples of CT images created by multiplanar reformatting used for pre-implant assessment in the maxilla. **A** Set of three-dimensional reconstructed images. **B** One axial slice showing the position of the various reconstructed cross-sectional images. (Kindly supplied by Dr A. Sidi.) **C** One reconstructed cross-sectional slice – number 20 from the axial slice shown in **B**.

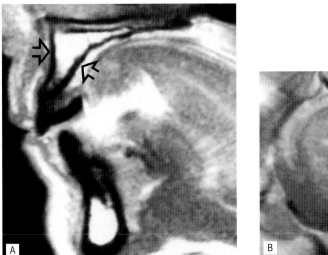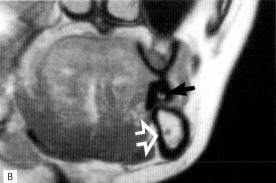

Fig. 24.6A   Sagittal section MR scan showing the buccopalatal width and height of the edentulous anterior maxilla (arrowed). **B** Cross-sectional MR image showing an edentulous left mandible (open arrow) and the stent containing the gadolinium marker (black arrow). The inferior dental canal is clearly evident. (Images kindly supplied by Mr Crawford Gray.)

POSTOPERATIVE EVALUATION AND FOLLOW-UP

Postoperative evaluation can be carried out immediately after surgery and usually after the initial 4–6 months healing period. Further clinical evaluation of the success or otherwise of the implant, including radiographic assessment, should be carried out on an annual basis for the first few years and then bi-annually. Geometrically accurate paralleling technique periapicals (either film-based or digital) are most commonly used. **Note:** The accuracy can be checked by examining the geometric thread pattern of the fixture.

Criteria for success

Ideally, implants should be evaluated against standardized success criteria and not simply assessed for their survival. Several *criteria for success* have been put forward over the years for the different implant systems. Those favoured by the author, and cited frequently in the literature, are those proposed by Albrektsson in 1986. These include:

1. That an individual, unattached implant is immobile when tested clinically.

2. That a radiograph does not demonstrate any evidence of peri-implant radiolucency.
3. That vertical bone loss be less than 0.2 mm annually following the implant's first year of service.
4. That individual implant performance be characterized by an absence of signs and symptoms such as pain, infection, neuropathies, paraesthesia or violation of the inferior dental canal.
5. That, in the context of the above, a success rate of 85% at the end of a 10-year period be the minimum criteria for success.

Radiographic evaluation (see Figs 24.7, 24.8 and 24.9)

Radiographs allow evaluation of criteria 2 and 3, but also are used to assess:

- The position of the fixture in the bone and its relation to nearby anatomical stuctures
- Healing and integration of the fixture in the bone
- The peri-implant bone level and any subsequent vertical bone loss — threaded fixtures allow easy measurement if radiographs are geometrically accurate

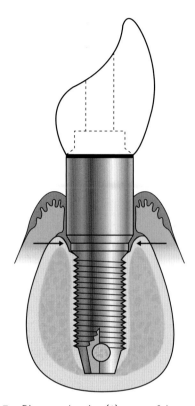

Fig. 24.7 Diagram showing (1) successful osseointegration — the bone/implant interface does not have fibrous tissue interposed, it is a direct contact and attachment between bone and the metallic implant surface, (2) minimal bone loss around the top of the implant, (3) no evidence of peri-implantitis and (4) a close fit of the abutment to the fixture (arrowed). These ideal features apply to the fixture and the surrounding tissues whatever type of abutment and restorative elements are chosen.

- Development of any associated disease, e.g. *perimplantitis*
- The fit of the abutment to the fixture
- The fit of the abutment to the crown/prosthesis
- Possible fracture of the implant/prosthesis.

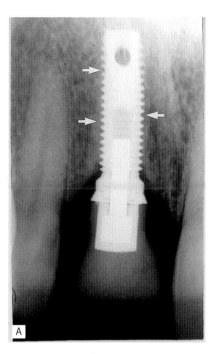

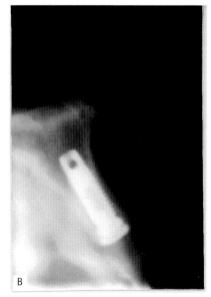

Fig. 24.8A Periapical showing successful osseointegration, 2 years after implant placement. Note the bone/implant interface (arrowed), there is no radiolucency in between. (Kindly supplied by Mr L. Howe.) **B** Cross-sectional spiral tomographic slice in the $\underline{1}$ region immediately after surgery showing the buccopalatal position and angulation of the implant.

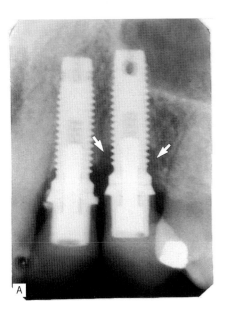

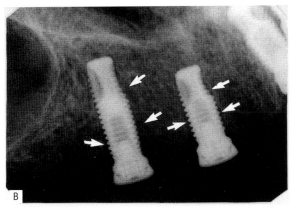

Fig. 24.9A   Periapical showing vertical bone loss (arrowed) around the thread of the implant replacing /4, but virtually no bone loss around the implant replacing /3. **B** Periapical showing unsuccessful osseointegration. Note the radiolucent line between surrounding bone and the implants (arrowed), particularly mesially on the implant replacing 5/ . **C** Periapical showing incorrect seating of the abutment on the fixture (solid arrows) and residual radiolucency from previous periapical area (open arrow). (Examples kindly supplied by Prof R. Palmer, Mr Saravanamuttu and Mr L. Howe.)

FOOTNOTE

The limited nature of the information provided by conventional two-dimensional radiographs on the width or thickness of the alveolar bone cannot be overemphasized. Inadequate clinical and radiographic assessment of possible implant sites, before surgery, may lead to implant failure and more seriously, to temporary or permanent nerve damage and possible litigation.

Chapter 25

Developmental abnormalities

INTRODUCTION

There are many developmental abnormalities that can affect the teeth and facial skeleton. In most cases, clinicians need little more than to be able to recognize these abnormalities — this recognition being based on both the clinical and radiographic findings. Therefore, the bulk of this chapter is designed like an atlas to show examples of some of the more common and important abnormalities that have characteristic radiographic features. A broad classification of the main conditions is also included.

Two important developmental anomalies are often encountered: unerupted mandibular wisdom teeth and malpositioned maxillary canines. These two topics are described in more detail.

CLASSIFICATION OF DEVELOPMENTAL ABNORMALITIES

Developmental anomalies of the maxillofacial region are usually classified into:

- Anomalies of the teeth
- Skeletal anomalies.

Anomalies of the teeth

These include abnormalities in:

- Number
- Structure
- Size
- Shape
- Position.

Abnormalities in number

Missing teeth
- Localized anodontia or hypodontia — usually third molars, upper lateral incisors or second premolars
- Anodontia or hypodontia associated with systemic disease — e.g. Down's syndrome, ectodermal dysplasia.

Additional teeth (hyperdontia)
- Localized hyperdontia
  - Supernumerary teeth
  - Supplemental teeth
- Hyperdontia associated with specific syndromes, e.g. cleidocranial dysplasia, Gardener's syndrome.

Abnormalities in structure

Genetic defects
- Amelogenesis imperfecta
  - Hypoplastic type
  - Hypocalcified type
  - Hypomature type
- Dentinogenesis imperfecta
- Shell teeth
- Regional odontodysplasia (ghost teeth)
- Dentinal dysplasia (rootless teeth).

Acquired defects

- Turner teeth — enamel defects caused by infection from overlying deciduous predecessor
- Congenital syphilis — enamel hypoplastic and altered in shape (see below)
- Severe childhood fevers, e.g. measles — linear enamel defects
- Fluorosis — discolouration or pitting of the enamel
- Discoloration — e.g. tetracycline staining.

Abnormalities in size

- Macrodontia — large teeth
- Microdontia — small teeth, including rudimentary teeth.

Abnormalities in shape

Anomalies affecting whole teeth

- Fusion — two teeth joined together from the fusion of adjacent tooth germs
- Gemination — two teeth joined together but arising from a single tooth germ
- Concrescence — two teeth joined together by cementum
- Dens-in-dente (invaginated odontome) — infolding of the outer surface of a tooth into the interior usually in the cingulum pit region of maxillary lateral incisors.

Anomalies affecting the crowns

- Extra cusps
- Congenital syphilis
  - *Hutchinson's incisors* — crowns small, screwdriver or barrel-shaped, and often notched
  - *Moon's / mulberry molars* — dome-shaped or modular
- Tapering pointed incisors — ectodermal dysplasia.

Anomalies affecting roots and / or pulp canals

- Number — additional roots, e.g. two-rooted incisors, three-rooted premolars or four-rooted molars
- Morphology, including:
  - Bifid roots
  - Excessively curved roots
  - *Dilaceration* — sharp bend in the root direction

- *Taurodontism* — short, stumpy roots and longitudinally enlarged pulp chambers
- Pulp stones — localized or associated with specific syndromes, e.g. Ehlers–Danlos (floppy joint syndrome)
- Cementoma (see odontogenic tumours in Ch. 28).

Odontomes

- Compound odontome — made up of one or more small tooth-like denticles (see Ch. 28)
- Complex odontome — complex mass of disorganized dental tissue (see Ch. 28)
- Enameloma / enamel pearl.

Abnormalities in position

Delayed eruption

- Local causes
  - Loss of space
  - Abnormal crypt position — especially $\overline{8/8}$ and 3/3
  - Overcrowding
  - Additional teeth
  - Retention of deciduous predecessor
  - Dentigerous and eruption cysts
- Systemic causes
  - Metabolic diseases, e.g. cretinism and rickets
  - Developmental disturbances, e.g. cleidocranial dysplasia
  - Hereditary conditions, e.g. gingival fibromatosis and cherubism.

Other positional anomalies

- Transposition, two teeth occupying exchanged positions
- Wandering teeth, movement of unerupted teeth for no apparent reason (distal drift)
- Submersion, second deciduous molars apparently descend into the jaws. Since these teeth do not in fact *submerge*, but rather remain in their original position while the adjacent alveolar bone grows normally, they are now described as being *infraocclusal*.

Skeletal anomalies

These include:

- Abnormalities of the mandible and/or maxilla
- Other rare developmental diseases and syndromes.

Abnormalities of the mandible or maxilla

Micrognathia

- True micrognathia — usually caused by bilateral hypoplasia of the jaw or agenesis of the condyles
- Acquired micrognathia — usually caused by unilateral early ankylosis of the temporomandibular joint.

Macrognathia (prognathism)

- Genetic
- Relative prognathism — mandibular/maxillary disparity
- Acquired, e.g. acromegaly owing to excessive growth hormone from a pituitary tumour.

Other mandibular anomalies

- Condylar hypoplasia
- Condylar hyperplasia
- Bifid condyle
- Coronoid hyperplasia.

Cleft lip and palate

- Cleft lip
  - Unilateral, with or without alveolar ridge
  - Bilateral, with or without alveolar ridge
- Cleft palate
  - Bifid uvula
  - Soft palate only
  - Soft and hard palate
- Clefts of lip and palate (combined defects)
  - Unilateral (left or right)
  - Cleft palate with bilateral cleft lip.

Localized bone defects

- Exostoses (see Ch. 28)
  - Torus palatinus
  - Torus mandibularis
- Idiopathic bone cavities (see Ch. 27)
  - Stafne's bone cavity.

Other rare developmental diseases and syndromes

- Cleidocranial dysplasia (see Ch. 32)
- Gorlin's syndrome (nevoid basal cell carcinoma syndrome) (see Ch. 27)
- Eagle syndrome
- Crouzon syndrome (craniofacial dysostosis)
- Apert syndrome
- Mandibular facial dysostosis (Treacher Collins syndrome).

TYPICAL RADIOGRAPHIC APPEARANCES OF THE MORE COMMON AND IMPORTANT DEVELOPMENTAL ABNORMALITIES

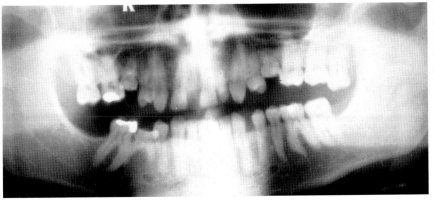

Fig. 25.1 Dental panoramic radiograph showing hypodontia.

$$\frac{8 \quad 5\ 2\ |\ 5}{87\ 5\ \ |\ \ \ 8}$$

are congenitally missing and $\underline{2}$ is rudimentary and peg-shaped.

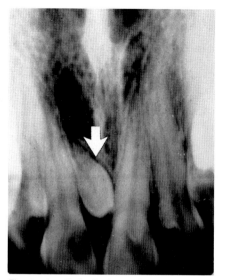

Fig. 25.2 Periapical showing a supernumerary or mesiodens (arrowed) between 1/1.

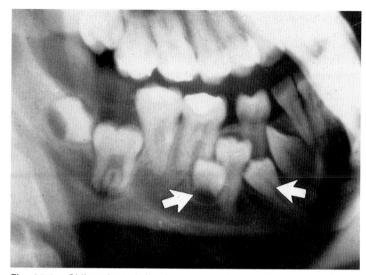

Fig. 25.3 Oblique lateral showing two supplemental lower premolars (arrowed) and a developing 9̄.

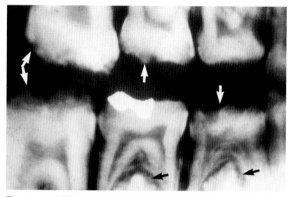

Fig. 25.4 Right bitewing showing the enamel defects of amelogenesis imperfecta (arrowed) in both the deciduous and permanent dentitions.

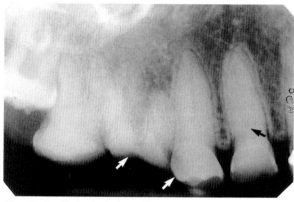

Fig. 25.5 Periapical of maxillary premolars and molars showing the defects of dentinogenesis imperfecta. Note the near obliteration of the pulp chamber (black arrow) and loss of the overlying enamel (white arrows).

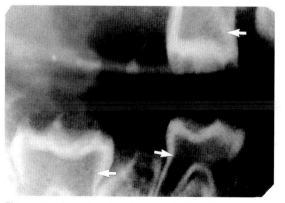

Fig. 25.6 Bitewing showing so-called *shell teeth* – a type of dentinogenesis imperfecta. The enamel is essentially normal but there is almost no dentine and the pulp chambers are very large (arrowed).

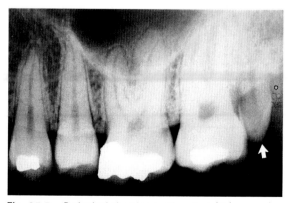

Fig. 25.7 Periapical showing a microdont ⌊8 (arrowed).

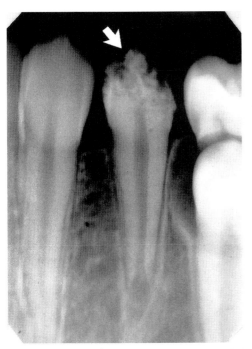

Fig. 25.8 Periapical of 4| showing the typical gnarled enamel defects of a Turner tooth (arrowed), caused by previous infection of the deciduous predecessor.

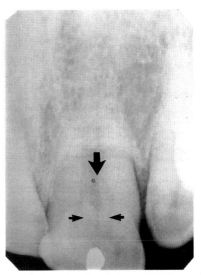

Fig. 25.9 Periapical showing fusion of |12 (arrowed).

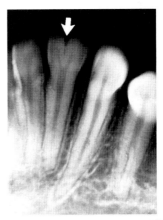

Fig. 25.11 Peripical showing gemination of |1 (arrowed).

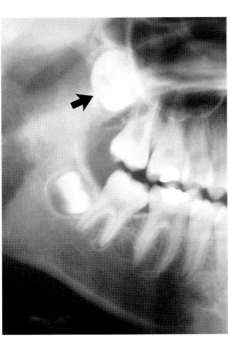

Fig. 25.10 Part of a panoramic radiograph showing a macrodont 8| (arrowed).

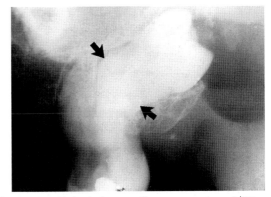

Fig. 25.12 Periapical suggesting concrescence of |78 (arrowed). Note it is not possible to be certain simply from the radiograph that |78 are joined together with cementum.

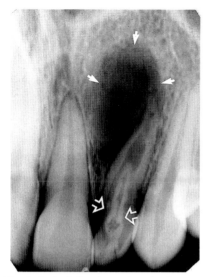

Fig. 25.13 Periapical showing a dens-in-dente or invaginated odontome involving |2 (open arrows). There is an associated periapical area of infection (solid arrows) — a common occurrence with dens-in-dente.

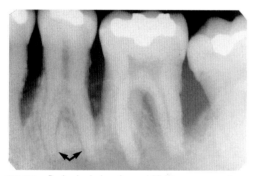

Fig. 25.15 Periapical showing a bifid lower premolar root (arrowed).

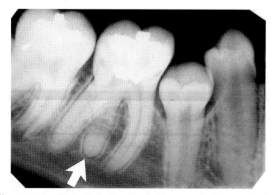

Fig. 25.16 Periapical showing a three-rooted lower first molar (arrowed) (right).

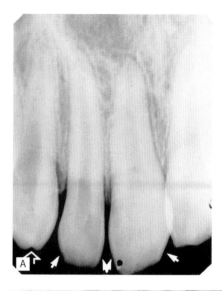

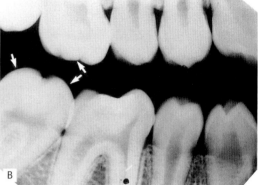

Fig. 25.14 Congenital syphilis. **A** Periapical of maxillary incisors and canine showing Hutchinson's teeth. Note the tapering screwdriver-shaped crowns (solid arrows) and the incisal edge notching (open arrow). **B** Bitewing showing Moon's/mulberry molars. Note the dome-shaped, nodular appearance of the molars (arrowed).

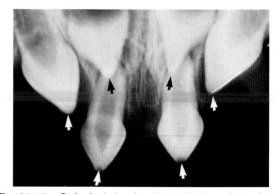

Fig. 25.17 Periapical showing the typical tapering pointed incisor teeth (arrowed) of ectodermal dysplasia.

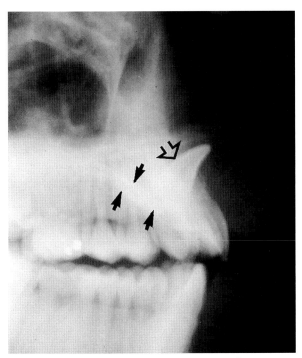

Fig. 25.18 Lateral view showing a dilacerated ⌊1. The crown (open arrow) and the root (solid arrows) are in different planes as a result of the near right angle bend in the root.

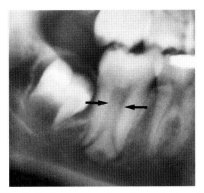

Fig. 25.19 Part of a panoramic radiograph showing a taurodont lower second molar with the typical large pulp chamber (arrowed).

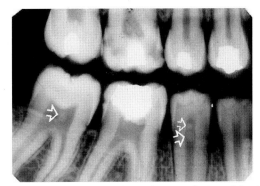

Fig. 25.20 Bitewing showing pulpstones (arrowed) in the pulp chambers of 75⌋ .

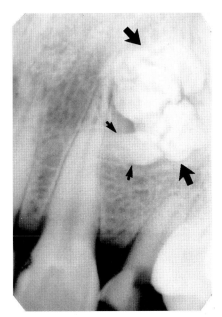

Fig. 25.21 Periapical showing a compound odontome in the anterior maxilla — several small discrete denticles are evident (arrowed) (right).

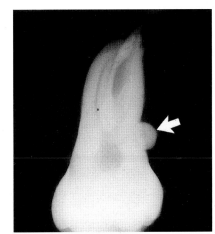

Fig. 25.22 Extracted upper second molar with an almost spherical enameloma (enamel pearl) on its distal aspect (arrowed).

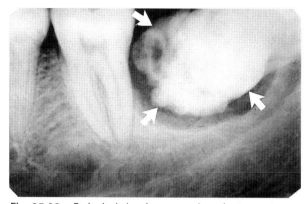

Fig. 25.23 Periapical showing a complex odontome, a disorganized mass of dental tissues in |7 region (arrowed).

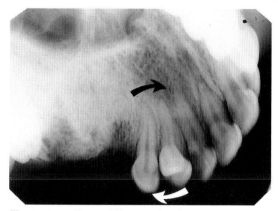

Fig. 25.24 Upper oblique occlusal showing transposition of 43/ to give 34/ (arrowed).

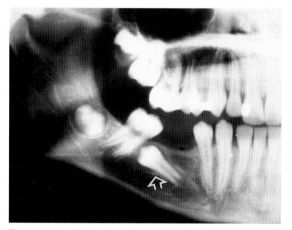

Fig. 25.25 Right side of a panoramic radiograph showing distal drift of a wandering 5| (arrowed).

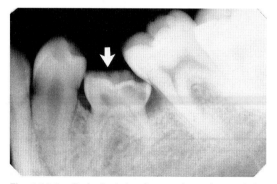

Fig. 25.26 Periapical showing a submerging or *infra-occlusal* |E (arrowed). Note there is no underlying second premolar.

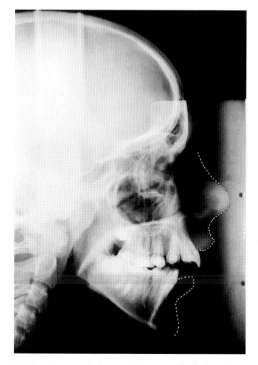

Fig. 25.27 True cephalometric lateral skull showing micrognathia (underdeveloped mandible) in skeletal Class II. The soft tissue profile has been drawn in.

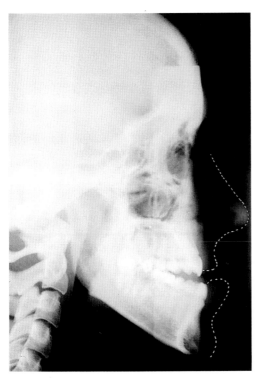

Fig. 25.28 True cephalometric lateral skull showing macrognathia (overgrowth of the mandible) in skeletal Class III. The soft tissue profile has been drawn in.

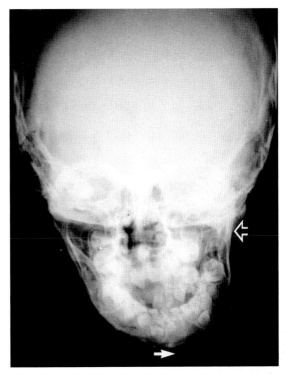

Fig. 25.29 PA skull showing condylar hypoplasia on the left side (open arrow), with a marked deviation of the midline of the mandible to that side (closed arrow).

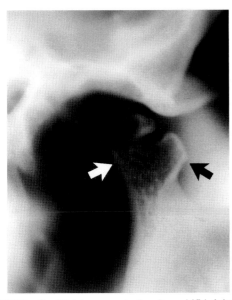

Fig. 25.30 Sagittal tomograph showing a bifid right condyle (arrowed).

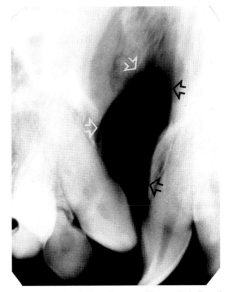

Fig. 25.31 Periapical showing a unilateral cleft palate (arrowed). Note 2| is absent.

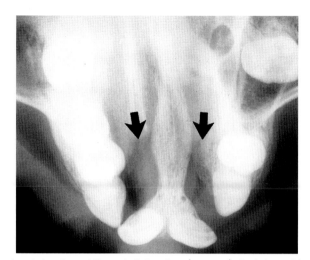

Fig. 25.32 Upper standard occlusal showing a bilateral cleft palate (arrowed). Both lateral incisors are absent.

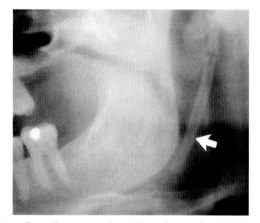

Fig. 25.33 Part of a panoramic radiograph showing a long calcified stylo-hypoid ligament (arrowed), a feature of Eagle's syndrome.

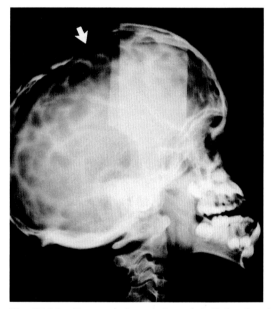

Fig. 25.34 True cephalometic lateral skull showing the typical *copper beaten* appearance of the cranium resulting from craniosynostosis — premature fusion of the cranial sutures. This appearance is seen in both Crouzon's and Apert's syndromes. In this patient, there is also indentation of the anterior fontanelle (arrowed) and the maxilla is hypoplastic.

RADIOGRAPHIC ASSESSMENT OF MANDIBULAR THIRD MOLARS

Clinical symptoms associated with lower wisdom teeth are common, the usual treatment being extraction. Many of the factors that influence that decision and determine the difficulty of the extraction are revealed by the preoperative radiographic assessment.

Radiographic views used

The usual radiographs used include:

- Periapicals
- Dental panoramic radiographs
- Oblique laterals or bimolars.

Periapicals need to be of good *quality*. In particular, the geometric relationship of the third molar to the surrounding structures must be accurate. To satisfy this requirement, modifications to conventional radiographic techniques are often necessary, as described in detail in Chapter 10. If available, cone beam CT, described in Chapter 19, can greatly facilitate this radiographic assessment by providing images in the coronal, axial and sagittal planes.

Radiographic interpretation

The specific features that need to be identified can be divided into those related to:

- The lower third molar itself
- The lower second molar
- The surrounding bone.

Lower third molar assessment

The main features to examine include:

- Angulation
- The crown
- The roots
- The relationship of the apices with the inferior dental (ID) canal
- The depth of the tooth in the alveolar bone
- The buccal or lingual obliquity.

Angulation (see Fig. 25.35)
The third molar could be:

- Mesioangular
- Distoangular
- Horizontal
- Vertical
- Transverse
- Inverted.

The crown
Note in particular:

- The size
- The shape
- The presence and extent of caries
- The presence and severity of resorption.

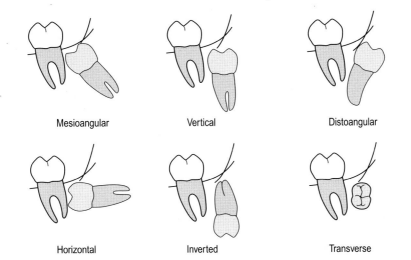

Mesioangular   Vertical   Distoangular

Horizontal   Inverted   Transverse

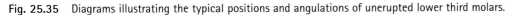

Fig. 25.35 Diagrams illustrating the typical positions and angulations of unerupted lower third molars.

The roots
Note in particular:

- The number
- The shape
- Curvatures, whether they are *favourable* or *unfavourable* (see Fig. 25.36)
- The stage of development.

The relationship of the apices to the ID canal

The apices of the lower third molar often appear close to the ID canal. This apparent closeness is usually due to these structures being super-imposed. However, an *intimate relationship* does sometimes exist. The root may be grooved by the canal, or rarely, included within the developing root, as illustrated in Figure 25.37.

The normal radiographic appearance of the ID canal (two thin, parallel radiopaque lines — the so-called *tramlines*) and the variations that indicate a possible *intimate relationship* are shown in Figure 25.38. These variations include:

- Loss of the tramlines
- Narrowing of the tramlines
- A sudden change in direction of the tramlines

- A radiolucent band evident across the root if the tooth is grooved by or contains the ID bundle.

The depth of the tooth in the alveolar bone

Two main methods are used commonly to assess tooth depth:

- Winter's lines
- Using the roots of the second molar as a guide.

Winter's lines (see Fig. 25.39). In this method, three imaginary lines (traditionally described by number or colour) are drawn on a geometrically accurate periapical radiograph, as follows:

- The first or *white* line is drawn along the occlusal surfaces of the erupted first and second molars.
- The second or *amber* line is drawn along the crest of the interdental bone between the first and second molars, extending distally along the internal oblique ridge, NOT the external oblique ridge. This line indicates the margin of the alveolar bone surrounding the tooth.
- The third or *red* line is a perpendicular dropped from the *white* line to the point of application for an elevator, but is measured from the *amber* line to this point of application. This line

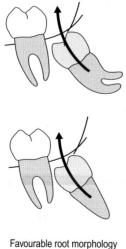

Favourable root morphology

Roots follow the expected line of withdrawal (arrowed)

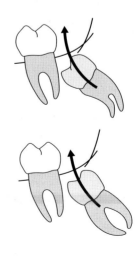

Unfavourable root morphology

Roots oppose the expected line of withdrawal (arrowed)

Fig. 25.36 Diagrams illustrating *favourable* and *unfavourable* root curvatures.

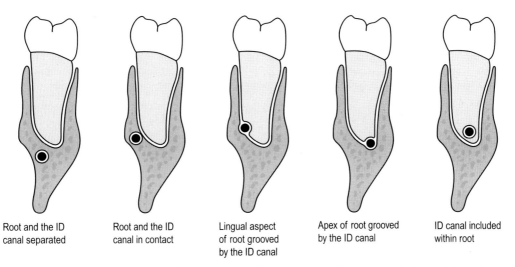

Root and the ID
canal separated

Root and the ID
canal in contact

Lingual aspect
of root grooved
by the ID canal

Apex of root grooved
by the ID canal

ID canal included
within root

Fig. 25.37   Diagrams illustrating the types of intimate relationships that can exist between the lower third molar root and the inferior dental canal.

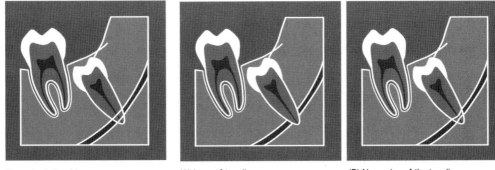

Normal relationship –
root and ID canal separated –
tramlines evident across the root

(A) Loss of tramlines

(B) Narrowing of the tramlines

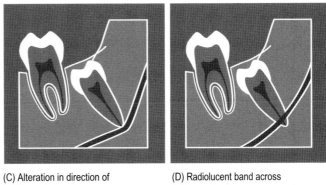

(C) Alteration in direction of
ID canal at root apex

(D) Radiolucent band across
the root

Fig. 25.38   Diagrams illustrating the radiographic appearances of a normal inferior dental canal, and those indicating an intimate relationship between the inferior dental canal and the tooth apex.

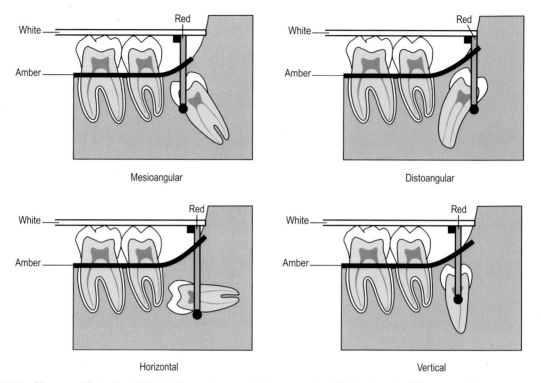

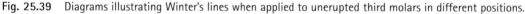

Fig. 25.39 Diagrams illustrating Winter's lines when applied to unerupted third molars in different positions.

measures the depth of the third molar within the mandible. (As a general rule, if the *red* line is 5 mm or more in length, the extraction is considered sufficiently difficult for the tooth to be removed under general anaesthetic or using local anaesthetic and sedation.)

Using the roots of the second molar as a guide (see Fig. 25.40). This method can be summarized as follows:

- The roots of the adjacent second molar are divided horizontally into thirds
- A horizontal line is then drawn from the point of application for an elevator to the second molar
- If the point of application lies opposite the coronal, middle or apical third, the extraction is assessed as being easy, moderate or difficult, respectively.

The buccal or lingual obliquity
- *Buccal obliquity* — the crown of the wisdom tooth is inclined towards the cheek
- *Lingual obliquity* — the crown of the wisdom tooth is inclined towards the tongue.

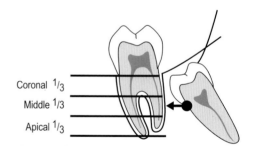

Fig. 25.40 Diagram illustrating the method relating the point of application of an elevator to the roots of the lower second molar to assess the depth of the third molar in the alveolar bone.

The lie of the tooth in the horizontal plane cannot be determined accurately from a periapical radiograph. The views of choice for this assessment include:

- Lower oblique occlusal
- Lower 90° occlusal, centred on the side of interest (see Ch. 12).

Lower second molar assessment

The second molar is assessed to decide the prognosis of the tooth to decide whether the second molar should be extracted instead of, or as well as, the third molar. The main features to examine include:

- The crown
- The roots.

The crown
Note in particular:

- The condition and extent of existing restorations
- The presence of caries
- The presence and severity of resorption.

The roots
Note in particular:

- The number
- The shape, and if it is conical
- The periodontal status
- The condition of the apical tissues.

Assessment of the surrounding bone

The main features to examine include:

- The anteroposterior position of the ascending ramus, to determine access to the tooth and the amount of overlying bone

- The texture and density of the bone
- Evidence of previous pericoronal infection.

All these points relating to the third molar, the second molar and the surrounding tissues are considered together, and a conclusion drawn as to the overall difficulty of the proposed extraction.

Examples of unerupted lower third molars, illustrating some of the more important radiographic features, are shown in Figures 25.41–25.47.

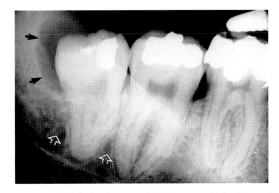

Fig. 25.42 Slightly distoangularly impacted 8̱|. Note the favourable conically shaped roots, the uninterrupted upper tramline of the inferior dental canal (open white arrows) and the radiolucent area distal to the crown (black arrows) caused by the residual follicle.

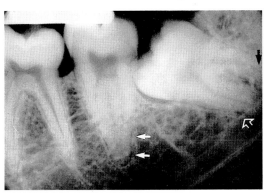

Fig. 25.41 Mesioangularly impacted |8̄. Note the unfavourable root curvatures (black arrow), the uninterrupted upper tramline of the inferior dental canal (open white arrow) and the conically shaped root of |7̄ (solid white arrows).

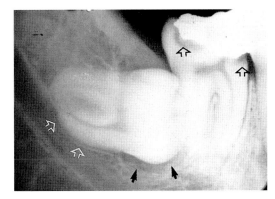

Fig. 25.43 Horizontally impacted 8̱|. Note the pincer-shaped roots and their indentation of the upper margin of the inferior dental canal (open white arrows), radiolucency beneath the crown (solid black arrows) caused by the follicle. In addition, note the carious lesions in 7̱| (open black arrows).

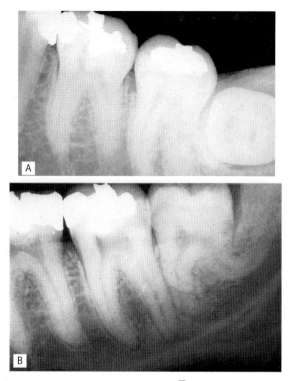

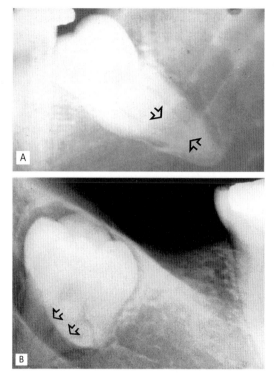

Fig. 25.44 Transversely positioned ⎣8. The crown is viewed end-on. Note that the bucco/lingual obliquity of the tooth cannot be determined from this radiograph. **B** Vertically positioned ⎣8 with very unfavourable root curvatures.

Fig. 25.45 Two radiographs showing some of the radiographic features suggestive of an *intimate relationship* with the inferior dental canal. **A** A radiolucent band is evident across the root (arrowed) and there is a change in direction of the ID canal. **B** A radiolucent band evident across the root and the ID canal is narrowed (arrowed).

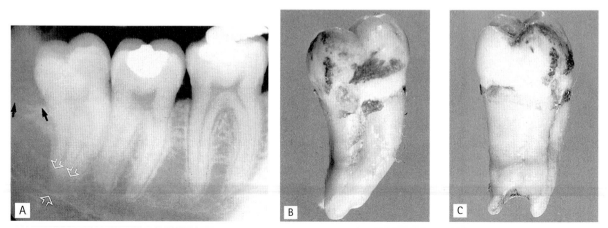

Fig. 25.46A Slightly distoangularly impacted 8⎦. Note the extensive area of bone resorption distal to the crown (black arrows) caused by previous pericoronal infection. There is a radiolucent band across the tooth apex which is also hazy in outline (open white arrows) caused by the inferior dental canal, implying an intimate relationship. **B** The extracted 8⎦ viewed as in the radiograph from the buccal aspect. **C** The extracted tooth viewed from the distal aspect showing clearly the notching of the tooth apex by the inferior dental canal. This explains the radiolucent band across the apex — there is simply less tooth tissue in this zone, because of the position of the inferior dental canal. (Specimen and radiograph kindly supplied by Dr A. Sidi.)

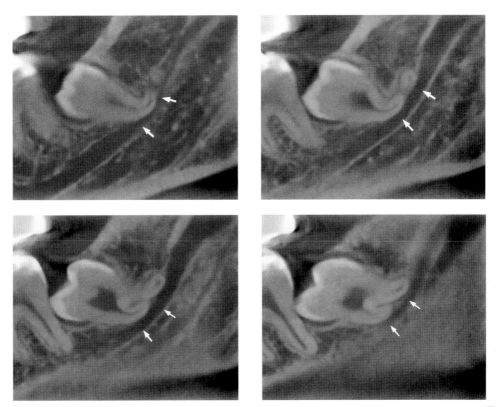

Fig. 25.47 A series of four high resolution 3DAccuitomo™ (J. Morita Company, Japan) cone beam CT images of ⌐8 showing the relationship of the roots to the ID canal (kindly provided by Prof D. Benn).

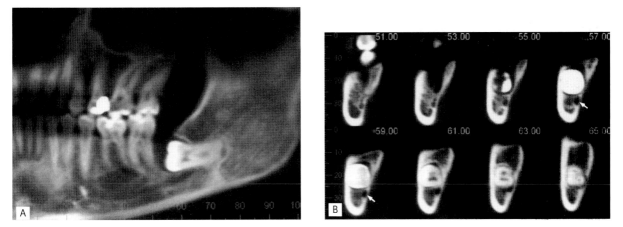

Fig. 25.48 i-CAT™ cone beam CT images of a horizontally unerupted ⌐8, **A** panoramic lateral view and **B** a series of cross-sectional images through the wisdom tooth showing the position of the ID canal clearly. (Reproduced with kind permission of Imaging Sciences International, Inc.)

RADIOGRAPHIC ASSESSMENT OF UNERUPTED MAXILLARY CANINES

The upper canines are often misplaced and fail to erupt as a result of their long path of eruption, the timing of their eruption and the frequency of upper arch overcrowding. Again, many of the factors that influence the treatment of this anomaly can be obtained from the radiographic assessment, the purpose of which is two-fold:

- To determine the size and shape of the canine and any related disease including possible resorption of the adjacent lateral incisor.
- To determine the position of the canine.

Assessment of the canine size and shape and the surrounding tissues

Radiographic views used (see Fig. 25.49)

The usual radiographs used include:

- Periapicals
- Upper standard occlusal
- Panoramic radiograph.

Radiographic interpretation

The specific features that need to be examined relate to:

- The crown
- The root
- Surrounding structures.

The crown
Note in particular:

- Crown size (in relation to the space available in the arch)
- Crown shape
- The presence and severity of resorption
- The presence of any related disease, such as a dentigerous cyst
- The effect on adjacent teeth, such as resorption.

The root
Note in particular:

- Root size
- Root shape
- Stage of development.

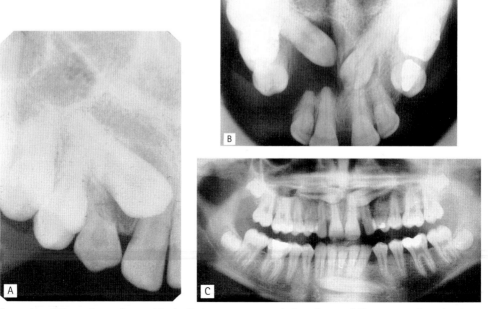

Fig. 25.49 Examples of the radiographs used typically to assess unerupted canines and the surrounding structures.
A Periapical showing unerupted 3| wih retained C.
B Upper standard occlusal showing both upper canines unerupted, a dentigerous cyst associated with 3|, extensive destruction of the alveolar bone and resorption of |3.
C Panoramic radiograph showing unerupted 3/3 and |3.

Assessment of the position of the canine — localization

There are several methods available for localization depending on available facilities. They can be used for canines and other unerupted teeth as well as odontomes and supernumeraries. Although emphasis in this section is on canines, examples of localization of other unerupted developmental anomalies are also shown.

Main localization methods

- Parallax in the horizontal plane
- Parallax in the vertical plane
- Stereoscopic views
- Cross-sectional spiral tomography
- Cone beam CT.

The principle of parallax

Parallax is defined as *the apparent displacement of an object because of different positions of the observer*. In other words, if two objects, in two separate planes, are viewed from two different positions, the objects will appear to move in different directions in relation to one another, from one view to the next, as shown in Figure 25.50.

Using the principle of parallax, if two views of an unerupted canine are taken with the X-ray tubehead in two different positions, the resultant radiographs will show a difference in the position of the unerupted canine relative to the incisors, as follows:

- If the canine is **palatally** positioned, it will appear to have moved in the **same** direction as the X-ray tubehead.
- If the canine is **buccally** positioned, it will appear to have moved in the **opposite** direction to the X-ray tubehead.
- If the unerupted canine is in the **same plane** as the incisors, i.e. in the line of the arch, it will appear **not to have moved** at all.

A useful acronym to remember the movements of parallax is SLOB, standing for:

Same
Lingual
Opposite
Buccal.

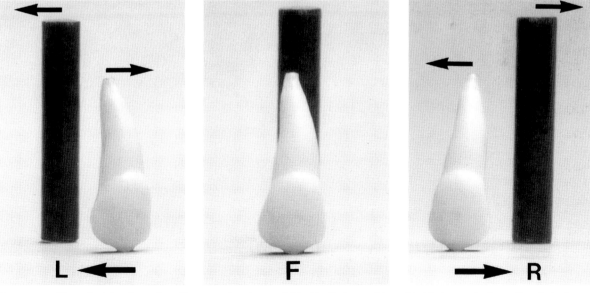

Fig. 25.50   The principle of parallax. Photographs of a small black cylinder positioned behind a tooth. From directly in front (F), the tooth and cylinder are superimposed. With the camera moved to the left (L), the tooth and cylinder are both visible and appear to have moved in different directions. The cylinder, being further away from the camera, appears to have moved in the same direction as the camera, i.e. to the left, while the tooth appears to have moved in the opposite direction. With the camera moved to the right (R) a similar apparent movement of the tooth and cylinder relative to the camera takes place, with the cylinder appearing to have moved to the right and the tooth to the left.

Parallax in the horizontal plane

The movement of the X-ray tubehead is in the horizontal plane, for example:

- 2 periapicals — one centred on the upper central incisor and the other centred on the canine region, as shown in Figure 25.51.

- An upper standard occlusal, centred in the midline plus a periapical or an upper oblique occlusal, centred on the canine region.

Examples are shown in Figures 25.52–25.54.

Note: The advantage of the upper standard occlusal for the initial view is that it shows both sides of the arch and unerupted canines are often bilateral.

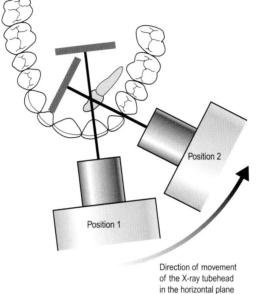

Position 2

Position 1

Direction of movement
of the X-ray tubehead
in the horizontal plane

Fig. 25.51 Diagram showing the two different tubehead positions required for parallax in the horizontal plane: Position (1) centred on the upper central incisor. Position (2) centred on the canine region.

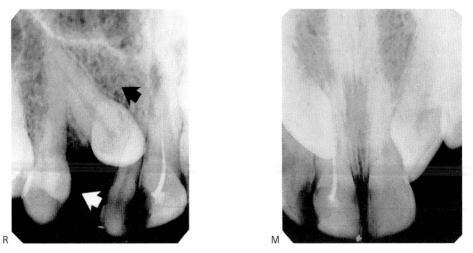

R   M

Fig. 25.52 Two periapicals showing the relative positions of the unerupted 3| to the incisors — M in the midline and R from the right. The X-ray tubehead (white arrow) and the canine (black arrow) appear to have moved in the *same* direction. The canine is thus palatally positioned.

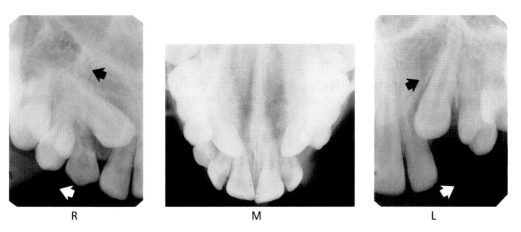

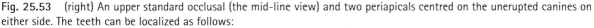

R   M   L

Fig. 25.53 (right) An upper standard occlusal (the mid-line view) and two periapicals centred on the unerupted canines on either side. The teeth can be localized as follows:

1. Examine the midline view radiograph (M), centred on the upper central incisors. The tip of the RIGHT canine appears opposite the root canal of 1| ; the tip of the LEFT canine appears opposite the mesial aspect |2.

2. Examine radiograph (R), the periapical centred on the RIGHT canine region (i.e. the X-ray tubehead has been moved distally in the direction of the white arrow). The tip of the canine appears opposite the mesial aspect of 2| . Therefore, it appears to have moved distally in the direction of the black arrow, i.e. in the *same* direction as the X-ray tubehead was moved.

3. Examine radiograph (L), the periapical centred on the LEFT canine region. The tip of the canine appears opposite the root canal of |2. Again both the X-ray tubehead (white arrow) and the canine (black arrow) appear to have moved in the *same* direction.

Thus the crowns of both the right and left canines are *palatally* positioned in relation to the incisors.

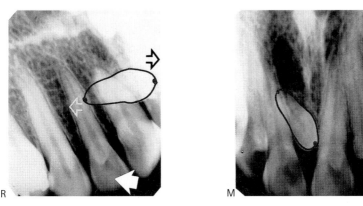

R   M

Fig. 25.54 Two periapicals showing an unerupted mesiodens. It can be localized as follows:

1. Examine the mid-line radiograph (M). The tip of the mesiodens' crown appears opposite the mesial aspect of |1, while its apex appears opposite the root canal of 1| .

2. Examine the periapical centred on the RIGHT canine region (R). The tip of the mesiodens crown appears opposite the root canal of |1, while its apex appears opposite the mesial aspect of 2| .

3. The X-ray tubehead was moved distally in the direction of the large white solid arrow.

4. The crown of the mesiodens appears to have moved mesially (black open arrow), i.e. in the *opposite* direction to the tubehead. It is thus buccally placed.

5. The apex appears to have moved in the *same* direction (white open arrow) as the tubehead and is thus palatally placed. The mesiodens thus lies across the arch, between the central incisors, with its crown buccally positioned and its apex palatally positioned.

Parallax in the vertical plane

The movement of the X-ray tubehead is in the vertical plane, for example:

- A dental panoramic radiograph — the X-ray beam is aimed upwards at 8° to the horizontal
- An upper standard occlusal — the X-ray beam is aimed downwards at 65°–70° to the horizontal, as shown in Figures 25.55 and 25.56.

Note: This combination of views is used frequently in orthodontics, when patients with unerupted canines are usually assessed. Use of these films to their full potential may obviate the need for further films merely to localize the unerupted canines.

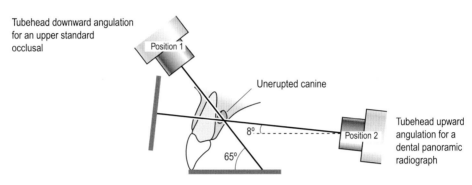

Tubehead downward angulation for an upper standard occlusal

Position 1

Unerupted canine

8°   Position 2   Tubehead upward angulation for a dental panoramic radiograph

65°

Fig. 25.55 Diagram showing the two different tubehead positions when taking a dental panoramic radiograph and an upper standard occlusal, allowing parallax in the vertical plane.

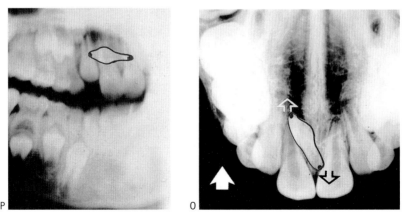

P   O

Fig. 25.56 Part of a dental panoramic radiograph and an upper standard occlusal showing an unerupted mesiodens. It can be localized as follows:

1. Examine the panoramic radiograph (P) taken with the tubehead aimed upwards at 8° to the horizontal. The tip of mesiodens' crown appears opposite the neck of the lateral incisor, while its apex appears opposite the root of ⌊1.

2. Examine the occlusal radiograph (O) taken with the tubehead aimed downwards at 65° to the horizontal. The tip of the mesiodens' crown now appears beyond the apex of 2⌋ , while its apex appears opposite the crown of ⌊1.

3. The X-ray tubehead has moved vertically upwards from view (P) to view (O) in the direction of the solid white arrow.

4. The crown of the mesiodens appears to have moved in the *same* direction (white open arrow) and is thus palatally placed.

5. The apex of the mesiodens appears to have moved in the *opposite* direction (black open arrow), and is thus buccally placed. The mesiodens thus lies across the arch between the central incisors, with its crown palatally positioned and its apex buccally positioned.

Localization using cross-sectional spiral tomography and cone beam CT

Localization of unerupted developmental anomalies using these more modern advanced imaging modalities is straightforward (see Ch 17 and 19), if the facilities are available. They allow visualization of the unerupted abnormality in different planes. There is no need to use the principles of parallax. Two examples are shown in Figures 25.57 and 25.58.

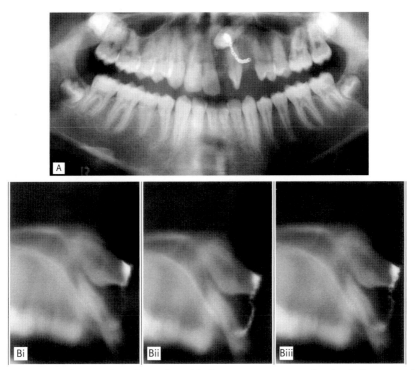

Fig. 25.57   Scanora® images. **A** Panoramic radiograph and **B** three 2 mm cross-sectional spiral tomographs showing the relative positions of bucally placed unerupted left canine (with orthodontic chain attached) and the left lateral incisor. The two teeth are clearly separated and there is no evidence of root resorption of the lateral incisor.

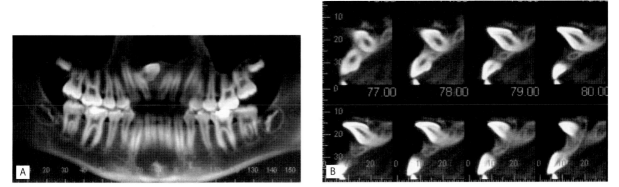

Fig. 25.58   i-CAT™ cone beam CT images of a dilacerated right central incisor, **A** Panoramic view and **B** A series of cross-sectional images through the dilacerated incisor showing clearly the degree of dilaceration and position. (Reproduced with kind permission of Imaging Sciences International, Inc.)

Chapter 26

Radiological differential diagnosis — describing a lesion

INTRODUCTION

Despite the many different conditions that can affect the jaws, they can present radiographically only as areas of relative *radiolucency* or *radiopacity* compared to the surrounding bone. Even this division based on radiodensity is not clearcut — some lesions fall into **both** categories, but at different stages in their development.

As a result, many of these pathological conditions resemble one another closely. This often creates considerable confusion. Fortunately, the sites where the lesions develop, how they grow and the effects they have on adjacent structures tend to follow recognizable patterns. As mentioned in Chapter 20, it is the recognition of these particular patterns that provides the key to interpretation and the formation of a radiological *differential* diagnosis.

A detailed description helps to identify these patterns and determine the lesion's basic characteristics. For example, it may reveal whether the lesion is a cyst or a tumour, whether it is composed of hard or soft tissue and whether, in the case of a tumour, it is benign or malignant. The resultant list of possible diagnoses in turn often determines the patient management and mode of treatment. The final definitive diagnosis is almost always based on histological examination.

DETAILED DESCRIPTION OF A LESION

Initial mention should be made of the patient's age and ethnic background, followed by a systematic description of the lesion which should include comments on its:

- Site or anatomical position
- Size
- Shape
- Outline/edge or periphery
- Relative radiodensity and internal structure
- Effect on adjacent surrounding structures
- Time present, if known.

Site or anatomical position

This should be stated precisely, for example the lesion(s) could be:

- Localized to the mandible, affecting:
    - the anterior region
    - the body — above or below the inferior dental canal, or related to the teeth
    - the angle
    - the ramus
    - the condylar process
    - the coronoid process
    - both sides (bilateral)
    - several sites
- Localized to the maxilla, affecting:
    - the anterior region
    - the posterior region
    - both sides (bilateral)
    - several sites
- Generalized, affecting:
    - both jaws
    - and/or other bones — multiple lesions may also affect the:
        * cranial vault
        * long bones
        * cervical spine

- Originating from a point or epicentre relative to surrounding structures, e.g.:
  - in bone or soft tissue
  - above or below the inferior dental canal
  - in or outside the inferior dental canal
  - in or outside the maxillary antrum
  - inside or outside a tooth follicle
  - at a tooth root apex.

In the mandible, so-called *odontogenic lesions* develop above the inferior dental canal, while *non-odontogenic lesions* develop above, within or below the canal. Thus some conditions have a predilection for certain areas whilst others develop in one site only. For example, radicular dental cysts develop at the apices of non-vital teeth, while so-called fissural bone cysts develop only in the midline. The site or anatomical position of a lesion may therefore provide the initial clue as to its identity.

Size

Conventionally, the lesion is sized in one of two ways including:

- Measuring the dimensions in centimetres
- Describing the boundaries, i.e. the lesion extends from … to … in one dimension and extends from … to … in the other dimension, as shown in Figure 26.1.

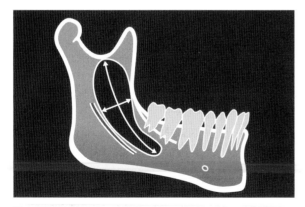

Fig. 26.1 Diagram showing the radiographic appearance of a radiolucent lesion at the angle of the mandible illustrating how to size a lesion, e.g. 'It extends from the mesial aspect of ⁊| up to the sigmoid notch, and from the anterior border of the ramus down to the ID canal', or 'It is approximately 6 cm × 2 cm'.

The size of a lesion is not a particularly helpful differentiating feature as both benign and malignant lesions may present when large or small. However, a few conditions have little or no growth potential and are therefore almost always small (e.g. 2–3 cm), such as Stafne's idiopathic bone cavity, whilst tumours, such as ameloblastoma can grow, if untreated, to an enormous size (10 cm or more). Thus the size of a lesion, while not being specific, may still give some idea of the type of underlying condition.

Shape

Conventionally, the shape of the lesion is described using one or more of the following terms (see Fig. 26.2):

- Unilocular
- Multilocular
- Pseudolocular
- Round
- Oval
- Scalloped or undulating
- Irregular.

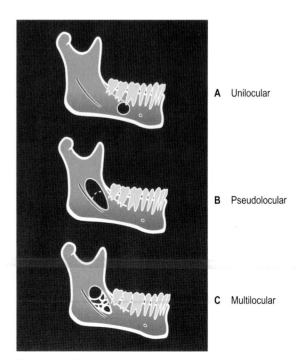

A Unilocular

B Pseudolocular

C Multilocular

Fig. 26.2 Diagrams showing the radiographic appearance of the various shapes of lesions.

The shape of a lesion is one of the more useful and specific characteristics that contribute to the radiological diagnosis. For example, the radicular dental cyst is round and unilocular while the giant cell lesions tend to be multilocular. An irregular shape suggests either irregular growth, such as the solitary bone cyst which typically arches up to extend between the roots of the teeth, or destruction indicating either an inflammatory or malignant lesion.

Outline / edge or periphery

The outline or periphery of lesions is described conventionally as being discrete and well defined or non-discrete and poorly defined and as having various additional characteristics (see Fig. 26.3).

Discrete or well-defined outlines, which may also be:

- Smooth
- Punched-out, i.e. showing no peripheral bone reaction
- Corticated, i.e. having a thick or thin surrounding radiopaque (white) cortex

- Sclerotic, i.e. having a non-uniform radiopaque boundary
- Encapsulated, i.e. surrounded by a radiolucent (black) line which may be complete or partial.

Non-discrete or poorly defined outlines, which may:

- Blend in with normal anatomy and show a gradual change between trabecular patterns
- Show signs of invasion and appear ragged or *moth-eaten*.

The outline or periphery provides information about the nature of the lesion, for example, whether it is benign or malignant and what the speed of growth or development appears to be. The more benign and slow growing the lesion is, the more likely it is to have a well-defined corticated outline. The malignant, more rapidly growing lesions tend to have poorly defined margins because the speed of bone destruction outstrips any bony repair.

Unfortunately, when a lesion such as a cyst becomes acutely infected, the normal outline can often be obliterated and the appearance may suggest a different, more sinister condition.

Relative radiodensity and internal structure

The radiodensity of the lesion should be assessed relative to the surrounding tissues. Radiolucent lesions are only evident within otherwise hard (radiopaque) tissues as a result of a decrease in mineralization, resorption of mineralized tissue or a decrease in thickness. As stated in Chapter 2, the amount of photoelectric absorption and hence opaque/whiteness of a structure is $\propto Z^3$. The atomic number (Z) of bone is approximately 12 (Z^3 = 1728), whereas the atomic number of soft tissue is approximately 7 (Z^3 = 343). A soft-tissue lesion replacing bone will therefore appear radiolucent.

Radiopaque lesions are evident in bone because of an increase in mineralization, increase in thickness, or superimposition on some other structure. They are also evident following calcification in soft tissues (see Ch. 28), having replaced air in the maxillary antra (see Ch. 29) or as a result of an increase in thickness of either normal or abnormal soft tissue.

Thus, relative to the surrounding tissues, the radiodensity of the lesion could be:

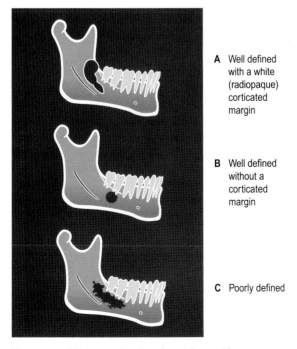

A Well defined with a white (radiopaque) corticated margin

B Well defined without a corticated margin

C Poorly defined

Fig. 26.3 Diagrams showing the radiographic appearance of different lesion outlines or edges.

- Uniformly radiolucent
- Radiolucent with patchy opacities within (mixed)
- Radiopaque.

The relative radiodensity also helps in the differentiating process by highlighting the **internal structure** of partially or completely radiopaque lesions. The alternatives include:

- Fine bone trabeculae, e.g. *ground glass* appearance
- Thick, coarse trabeculae with enlarged trabecular spaces, e.g. *honeycomb* appearance
- Haphazard sclerotic bone, e.g. *cottonwool* patches
- Homogeneous dense cortical bone
- Discrete bony septa, which could be:
  - thin or coarse
  - straight or curved
  - prominent or faint
- Cementum — oval or round amorphous calcification
- Identifiable dental tissue — enamel and/or dentine
- No specific pattern.

Effects on adjacent surrounding structures

The following structures need to be checked (see Fig. 26.4):

The teeth — there may be evidence of:

- Resorption, which is a feature of long-standing, benign but locally aggressive lesions, chronic inflammatory lesions, and malignancy
- Displacement
- Delayed eruption
- Disrupted development, resulting in abnormal shape and/or density
- Loss of associated lamina dura
- Increase in the width of the periodontal ligament space
- Alteration in the size of the pulp chamber
- Hypercementosis.

Surrounding bone — there may be evidence of:

- Expansion:
  - Buccal
  - Lingual
  - In other directions
- Displacement or involvement of surrounding structures, including the:

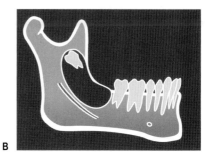

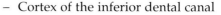

Fig. 26.4 Diagrams showing the radiographic appearance of some of the typical effects that a lesion can have on adjacent structures. **A** Expansion, displacement of ID canal, tooth and bone resorption. **B** Tooth displacement.

  - Cortex of the inferior dental canal
  - Mental foramen
  - Lower border cortex of the mandible
  - Floor of the antrum
  - Floor of the nasal cavity
  - Orbits
- Ragged destruction
- Increased density (sclerosis)
- Subperiosteal new bone formation
- An increase in the normal width of the inferior dental canal
- Irregular bone remodelling, resulting in an abnormal shape or unusual overall bone pattern.

Surrounding soft tissues — there may be evidence of invasion of the soft tissues producing a soft tissue mass.

Knowing what effects on adjacent surrounding structures a lesion is having, provides information about the nature of the lesion and its mode of growth. For example, the more dangerous the lesion, the more damaging and destructive its effects, and the faster its growth. Some lesions grow and expand in particular ways, such as the odontogenic keratocyst (keratocystic odontogenic tumour) which tends to infiltrate the cancellous bone and grow along the body of the mandible and produces little buccal or lingual expansion, whilst an ameloblastoma in the same site tends to expand and infiltrate in all directions.

Time present

The length of time the lesion has been present — days, weeks or years — should be determined, if possible. Unfortunately, this information is not always available. The patient may not be aware of the lesion and there may be no records of when it first became evident. If sequential radiographs are available, they can be very useful in providing information on the speed of growth, or development, of a lesion. This in turn may provide a clue about the nature of the lesion because slow-growing lesions tend to be benign, whilst fast-growing, aggressive lesions are usually malignant.

FOOTNOTE

This methodical, systematic description of the features of a lesion forms the basis of the step-by-step differential diagnostic process and is used throughout Chapters 27 and 28. As is shown later, several of the same features are shared by different conditions. Thus, no one feature alone gives enough information to provide the diagnosis. All the features should be considered carefully to determine their relevance and importance.

Chapter 27

Differential diagnosis of radiolucent lesions of the jaws

INTRODUCTION

This chapter is designed to simplify the process of arriving at a *radiological differential diagnosis* when confronted with a radiolucency of unknown cause on a plain radiograph. This process requires clinicians to follow a methodical step-by-step approach and to know the **typical** features of the various possibilities. Such a step-by-step guide is suggested and summarized in Figure 27.1. Although most lesions are still detected using plain radiographs, this process can be greatly facilitated in many cases if advanced imaging modalities, described in Chapter 19, such as computed tomography (CT), cone beam CT or magnetic resonance (MR) are available.

Unfortunately, most of the lesions encountered share several similar features and often individual conditions can present in many different ways. Thus the summary of features for the more important conditions included in this chapter is an attempt to unravel some of the inevitable confusion. Also, for simplicity, the frequency with which the various lesions present has been divided arbitrarily into common, uncommon and rare. It is hoped and intended, that the reader should expand on this short-notes style framework by referring to the suggested reading list.

Step-by-step guide

Step I

Systematically describe the radiolucency (as outlined in Ch. 26) including its:

- Site or anatomical position
- Size
- Shape
- Outline/edge or periphery
- Relative radiodensity
- Effects on adjacent surrounding structures
- Time present — if known.

Step II

Decide whether or not the radiolucency is:

1. A normal anatomical feature
- In the mandible, e.g.:
  - Mental foramen
  - ID canal
  - Sparse trabecular pattern
  - Developing tooth crypt
- In the maxilla, e.g.:
  - Antrum
  - Nasal fossa
  - Nasopalatine fossa.

2. Artefactual

These radiolucencies are dependent largely on the type of radiograph being examined, but examples include:

- Radiolucency as a result of overexposure
- Superimposed radiolucent air shadows.

3. Pathological

If pathological, the radiolucency could be:

- Congenital
- Developmental
- Acquired.

Step III

If the pathological radiolucency is *acquired*, decide within which of the following main disease categories it may be placed:

- Infection localized to the apical tissues
  - acute
  - chronic
- Infection spreading within the jaw
  - osteomyelitis
  - osteoradionecrosis
- Traumatic lesions
- Cysts
- Tumours or tumour-like lesions
- Bone-related lesions:
  - giant cell lesions
  - osseous dysplasias
  - other lesions.

Step IV

Consider the classification and subdivision of cysts and other similar radiolucencies within each of the other main disease categories, as shown in Table 27.1. This resultant list includes most of the more likely diagnostic possibilities for the unknown radiolucent lesion.

Step V

Compare the radiological features of the unknown radiolucency with the **typical** radiological features of these possible conditions. Then construct a list showing, in order of likelihood, all the conditions that the lesion might be. This list forms the *radiological differential diagnosis*.

Infection is described elsewhere (apical, Ch. 22, spreading, Ch. 32) and trauma is described in Chapter 30. The rest of this chapter is devoted principally to differentiating between the different cysts — the most common of the remaining categories — and the other lesions which often present as very similar radiolucencies.

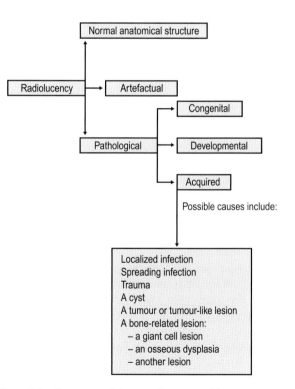

Fig. 27.1 Summary of the step-by-step guide to producing a differential diagnosis.

Table 27.1 Classification of the main cysts and tumours and other bone-related conditions that can present as a cyst-like radiolucency (based broadly on the 2005 WHO Classification)

Cysts	
Odontogenic	Radicular (dental) cyst
	Residual radicular cyst
	Lateral periodontal cyst
	Dentigerous cyst
	Odontogenic keratocyst (keratocystic odontogenic tumour)
Non-odontogenic	Nasopalatine duct / incisive canal cyst
	Bone cysts (see bone-related lesions)
Tumours and tumour-like lesions	
Benign odontogenic	Ameloblastoma
(epithelial with mature, fibrous stroma without	Squamous odontogenic tumour
odontogenic ectomesenchyme)	Calcifying epithelial odontogenic tumour (Pindborg tumour)
	Adenomatoid odontogenic tumour
	Keratocystic odontogenic tumour (odontogenic keratocyst)
Benign odontogenic	Ameloblastic fibroma
(epithelial with odontogenic ectomesenchyme, with	Ameloblastic fibro-odontoma
or without hard tissue formation)	Calcifying cystic odontogenic tumour (calcifying odontogenic cyst)
Benign odontogenic	Odontogenic fibroma
(Mesenchymal and/or odontogenic ectomesenchyme	Odontogenic myxoma
with or witout odontogenic epithelium)	
Malignant odontogenic	Odontogenic carcinoma
	Odontogenic sarcoma
Non-odontogenic intrinsic primary bone tumours	Benign — Fibroma
	— Chondroma
	— Central haemangioma
	— Neurofibroma
	Malignant — Osteosarcoma
	— Fibrosarcoma
	— Chondrosarcoma
Extrinsic primary tumours involving bone	Squamous cell carcinoma
Secondary metastatic bone tumours	
Lymphoreticular tumours of bone	Multiple myeloma
	Large cell lymphoma
	Burkitt's lymphoma
	Ewing's tumour
Langerhans cell disease	Eosinophilic granuloma
(Histiocystosis X)	Hand–Schüller–Christian disease
	Letterer–Siwe disease
Bone-related lesions	
Giant cell lesions	Central giant cell lesion (granuloma)
	Brown tumour in hyperparathyroidism
	Cherubism
	Aneurysmal bone cyst
Osseous dysplasias	Periapical osseous dysplasia
(Fibro-cemento-osseous lesions)	Focal osseous dysplasia
(early stages)	Florid osseous dysplasia
	Familial gigantiform cementoma
Other lesions	Ossifying fibroma
	Fibrous dysplasia
	Simple bone cyst
	Stafne's bone cavity

TYPICAL RADIOGRAPHIC FEATURES OF CYSTS

Inflammatory odontogenic cysts

Radicular (dental) cyst (Fig. 27.2)

This inflammatory cyst develops from the epithelial remnants of Hertwig's root sheath — the cell rests of Malassez.

- *Age*: Usually adults, 20–50 year-olds.
- *Frequency*: Most common of all jaw cysts (about 70%).
- *Site*: Apex of any non-vital tooth, particularly upper lateral incisors.
- *Size*: 1.5–3 cm in diameter (if smaller the radiographic distinction between cyst and granuloma cannot usually be made).
- *Shape*: — Round
   — Unilocular.

- *Outline*: — Smooth
   — Well defined
   — Well corticated if long-standing (unless infected) and continuous with the lamina dura of the associated tooth.
- *Radiodensity*: Uniformly radiolucent.
- *Effects*: — Adjacent teeth — displaced, rarely resorbed
   — Buccal expansion
   — Displacement of the antrum.

Note: The term *buccal bifurcation cyst* is used to describe an inflammatory odontogenic cyst which develops on the side of a molar tooth in relation to a buccal enamel spur or pearl.

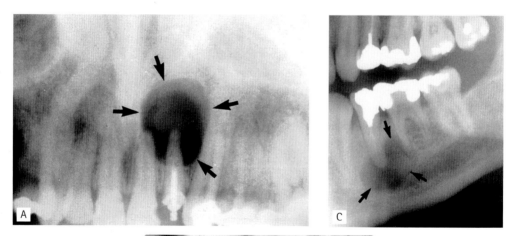

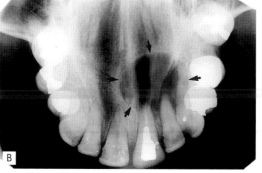

Fig. 27.2A Static panoramic (Panoral) radiograph showing a typical radicular (dental) cyst (arrowed) associated with the non-vital |2. **B** Upper standard occlusal showing a large radicular cyst associated with the root-filled |1. **C** Part of a panoramic radiograph showing a typical unilocular radicular cyst associated with the non-vital |5.

Residual radicular cyst (Fig. 27.3)

This term refers to a radicular (dental) cyst remaining after the causative tooth has been extracted.

- *Age*: Adults, over 20 years old.
- *Site*: Apical regions of the tooth-bearing portion of the jaws.
- *Size*: Variable, usually 2–3 cm in diameter.
- *Shape*: — Round
  - — Unilocular.
- *Outline*: — Smooth
  - — Well defined
  - — Usually well corticated.
- *Radiodensity*: Uniformly radiolucent.
- *Effects*: — Adjacent teeth displaced, rarely resorbed
  - — Buccal expansion
  - — Displacement of the antrum.

Developmental odontogenic cysts

Lateral periodontal cyst (Fig. 27.4)

The diagnosis of this rare developmental cyst should be reserved for a cyst in the lateral periodontal region that is not an inflammatory cyst or an atypical odontogenic keratocyst. It is thought to develop from either the cell rests of the dental lamina or from remains of the reduced enamel epithelium on the lateral surface of the root.

- *Age*: Adults over 30 years old.
- *Frequency*: Rare.
- *Site*: Lateral surface of the roots of vital teeth in the lower canine/premolar region or upper lateral incisor region.
- *Size*: Small, less than 1 cm in diameter.
- *Shape*: — Unilocular, very occasionally multilocular
  - — Round.
- *Outline*: — Smooth
  - — Well defined and corticated.
- *Radiodensity*: Uniformly radiolucent.
- *Effects*: — Adjacent teeth — displaced if cyst becomes large, rarely resorbed
  - — Buccal expansion if large.

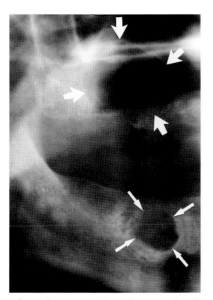

Fig. 27.3 Part of a panoramic radiograph showing two residual radicular cysts (arrowed), one in the maxilla and one in the mandible.

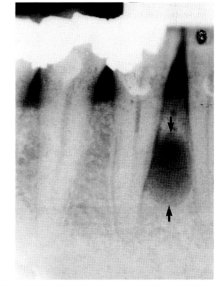

Fig. 27.4 Periapical showing a typically small lateral periodontal cyst (arrowed) between the 3̲ and 4̲. Although the adjacent premolar was restored, it was vital and symptom free. (Kindly provided by Mr N. Drage.)

Dentigerous (follicular) cyst (Fig. 27.5)

This cyst develops from the remnants of the reduced enamel epithelium after the tooth has formed.

- *Age*: Usually adolescents or young adults, 20–40 year-olds, occasionally the elderly.
- *Frequency*: About 20% of all cysts.
- *Site*: Associated with the crown of an unerupted and displaced tooth, typically teeth where eruption is impeded, e.g. 3|3 and 8|8.
- *Size*: Very variable, cyst suspected if follicular space exceeds 3 mm but may grow to several centimetres in diameter and extend up into the ramus.
- *Shape*: — Round or oval, typically enveloping the crown symmetrically
  — Unilocular
  — 3 varieties are described depending on the cyst/crown relationship:
    (i)   central
    (ii)   lateral
    (iii) circumferential.
- *Outline*: — Smooth
  — Well defined
  — Often well corticated.
- *Radiodensity*: Uniformly radiolucent.
- *Effects*: — Associated tooth unerupted and displaced
  — Adjacent teeth:
    Displaced
    Resorbed in about 50%
    Enveloped by large cysts
  — Buccal or medial expansion, can be extensive with large cysts causing facial asymmetry and displacement of the antrum.

Note: The term *eruption* cyst is used to describe a dentigerous cyst when it is in the soft tissues overlying the unerupted tooth.

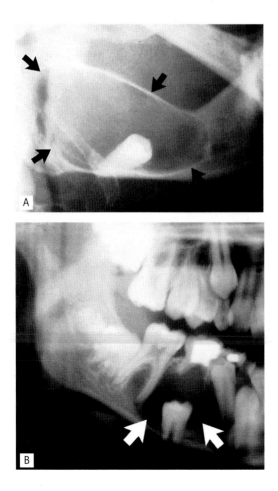

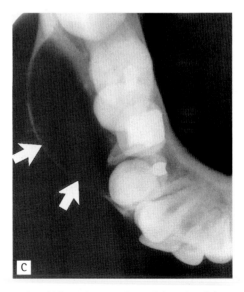

Fig. 27.5A   Oblique lateral of the right side of the mandible showing a typical circumferential dentigerous cyst (arrowed) associated with the unerupted and displaced 8|. **B** Part of a panoramic radiograph showing a unilocular central dentigerous cyst (arrowed) associated with the unerupted and inferiorly displaced 5|. **C** Right side of a lower 90° occlusal of the same patient showing the typical buccal expansion (arrowed).

Odontogenic keratocyst (keratocystic odontogenic tumour) (Fig. 27.6)

Somewhat controversially in 2005 the WHO Working Group recommended that the *odontogenic keratocyst* be renamed the *keratocystic odontogenic tumour* as they felt this name better reflected its neoplastic nature. The WHO now define this lesion as a benign uni- or multicystic intraosseous tumour of odontogenic origin with a histologically characteristic lining of parakeratinized stratified squamous epithelium with a potentially aggressive, infiltrative behaviour. It is believed to develop from the epithelium of the dental lamina — the cell rests of Serres — instead of the normal tooth which is therefore typically missing from the series. Lesions are typically solitary but multiple odontogenic keratocysts are a feature of *nevoid basal cell carcinoma syndrome* (Gorlin's syndrome), which also includes multiple basal cell carcinomas, and skeletal anomalies, e.g. bifid ribs and calcification of the falx cerebri.

- *Age*: Very variable, peak incidence between second and third decades.
- *Frequency*: Rare.
- *Site*: — Posterior body/angle of the mandible extending into the ramus
  — Anterior maxilla in canine region.
- *Size*: Variable, but often large in the mandible.
- *Shape*: — Oval, extending along the body of the mandible with little mediolateral expansion
  — Pseudolocular or multilocular.
- *Outline*: — Smooth and scalloped
  — Well defined and corticated.
- *Radiodensity*: Uniformly radiolucent.
- *Effects*: — Adjacent teeth — minimal displacement, rarely resorbed
  — Extensive expansion within the cancellous bone.
  — May cause cortical perforation.
  — May include crown of $\overline{8|8}$. by enfolding so resembling a dentigerous cyst.

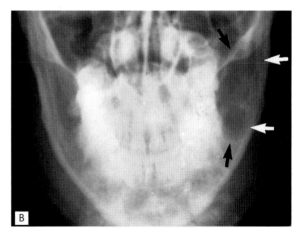

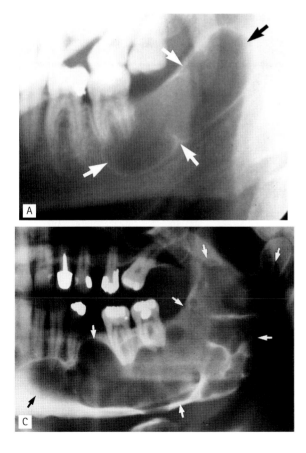

Fig. 27.6A Oblique lateral of the left side of the mandible showing a typically extensive pseudolocular odontogenic keratocyst (arrowed) which has apparently developed instead of $\overline{|8}$. B PA jaws of the same patient showing that it has caused minimal mediolateral expansion (arrowed).
C Left side of a panoramic radiograph showing a very large multilocular odontogenic keratocyst (arrowed) occupying almost all the left side of the mandible.

Non-odontogenic cysts

Nasopalatine duct / incisive canal cyst (Fig. 27.7)

This cyst develops from epithelial remnants of the nasopalatine duct or incisive canal.

- *Age*: Variable, but most frequently detected in middle age (40–60 year-olds).
- *Frequency*: Most common of all non-odontogenic cysts, affecting about 1% of total population.
- *Site*: Midline, anterior maxilla just posterior to the upper central incisors.
- *Size*: Variable, but usually from 6 mm to several centimetres in diameter.
- *Shape*: — Round or oval (superimposition of the nasal septum or anterior nasal spine may cause the cyst to appear heart-shaped or resemble an inverted tear drop)
  — Unilocular.

- *Outline*: — Smooth
  — Well defined
  — Well corticated (unless infected).
- *Radiodensity*: Uniformly radiolucent but radiopaque shadows sometimes superimposed.
- *Effects*: — Adjacent teeth — distal displacement, rarely resorbed
  — Palatal expansion (only identifiable if extensive).

Note: Differentiation is sometimes required between a nasopalatine duct cyst and a large normal nasopalatine foramen. Several features need to be considered including:

- Size — if over 6 mm, a cyst is more likely
- Shape — foramina are usually oval or irregular
- Outline — foramina are usually well defined laterally but not all the way round
- Relative radiodensity — a cyst tends to be more radiolucent having resorbed bone.

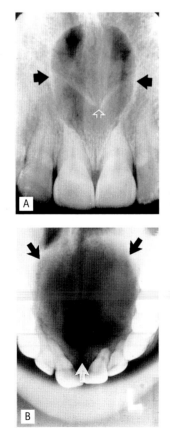

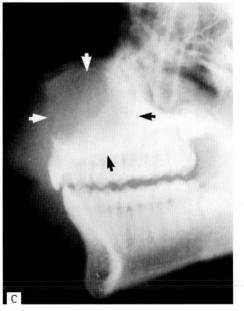

Fig. 27.7A Periapical showing a typical nasopalatine duct cyst (solid arrows) in the midline between the upper central incisors. Note the superimposed shadow of the anterior nasal spine (open white arrows). **B** Upper occlusal showing a very extensive nasopalatine duct cyst (arrowed) occupying nearly the entire palate. **C** Lateral view of the same patient showing the expansion of the cyst into the nasal cavity and palate (arrowed).

Bone cysts or pseudocysts

Despite their names — *simple bone cyst* and *aneurysmal bone cyst* — these entities are no longer categorized as cysts. In the new WHO Classification they come under the heading of *bone-related lesions*. They more commonly affect the skeleton and only relatively rarely affect the jaws.

Simple (solitary) bone cyst (Fig. 27.8)

Defined as an intra-osseous pseudocyst, devoid of an epithelial lining and either empty or filled with serous or sanguinous fluid. The aetiology is unknown.

- *Age*: Children or young adults, peak incidence in second decade.
- *Frequency*: Rare.
- *Site*: — Mandible, particularly anteriorly and in the premolar/molar region.
- *Size*: Variable, up to several centimetres in diameter.

- *Shape*: — Unilocular
  - — Irregular, but the upper border arches up between the roots of the teeth.
- *Outline*: — Smooth and undulating
  - — Moderately well defined
  - — Moderately well or poorly corticated.
- *Radiodensity*: Uniformly radiolucent.
- *Effects*: — Adjacent teeth — minimal or no displacement, very rarely resorbed
  - — Minimal or no expansion of the jaw.

Aneurysmal bone cyst (see Fig. 27.21)

This rare lesion is defined as an expansile osteolytic lesion, often multilocular with histologically blood filled spaces separated by fibrous septa containing osteoclast type giant cells and reactive bone. It is categorized as a *giant cell lesion* and described later.

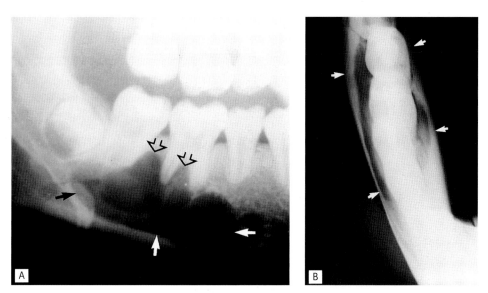

Fig. 27.8A Oblique lateral of the right side of the mandible of a teenager showing a typical solitary bone cyst (solid arrows) in the body of the mandible. Note the upper border arching up between the roots of the molar teeth (open arrows). **B** Oblique lower occlusal of the same patient showing no apparent buccolingual expansion (arrowed).

TYPICAL RADIOGRAPHIC FEATURES OF TUMOURS AND TUMOUR-LIKE LESIONS

Odontogenic tumours

Ameloblastoma (Fig. 27.9)

An aggressive but non-metastasizing tumour originating from remnants of the odontogenic epithelium of the enamel organ or dental lamina. Four main types include:

- Solid/multicystic type
- Extra-osseous/peripheral type
- Desmoplastic type
- Unicystic type.

Solid/multicystic ameloblastoma
- *Age*: Adults 30–60 years old.
- *Frequency*: Rare, but still the most common odontogenic tumour.
- *Site*: — 80% posterior body/angle/ramus of mandible
  — Anterior mandible in black Africans.
- *Size*: Very variable depending on the age of the lesion, may become very large if neglected and cause gross facial asymmetry.
- *Shape*: — Multilocular, distinct septa dividing the lesion into compartments with large, apparently discrete areas centrally and with smaller areas on the periphery

  — Occasionally unilocular in early stages
  — Rarely *honeycomb* or *soap-bubble* appearance or multicystic.
- *Outline*: — Smooth and scalloped
  — Well defined
  — Well corticated.
- *Radiodensity*: Radiolucent with internal radiopaque septa.
- *Effects*: — Adjacent teeth displaced, loosened, often resorbed
  — Extensive expansion in all dimensions
  — Maxillary lesions can extend into the paranasal sinuses, orbit or base of the skull.

Unicystic ameloblastoma
Accounts for 5–15% of all ameloblastomas and is found equally in the mandible and the maxilla. It usually presents as a unilocular radiolucency associated with the crown of an unerupted tooth (peak age: 16 years), or as a unilocular radiolucency at the apices of teeth, resembling a radicular cyst (peak age: 35 years).

Note: Since different ameloblastomas can mimic a large variety of other radiolucent lesions, this possibility must always be borne in mind when formulating a radiological differential diagnosis.

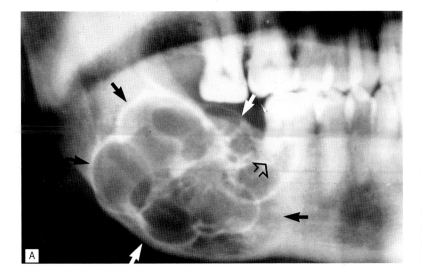

Fig. 27.9A Part of a panoramic radiograph showing the typical multilocular appearance of a large ameloblastoma at the angle of the mandible, with extensive expansion (solid arrows) and resorption of adjacent teeth (open arrow).

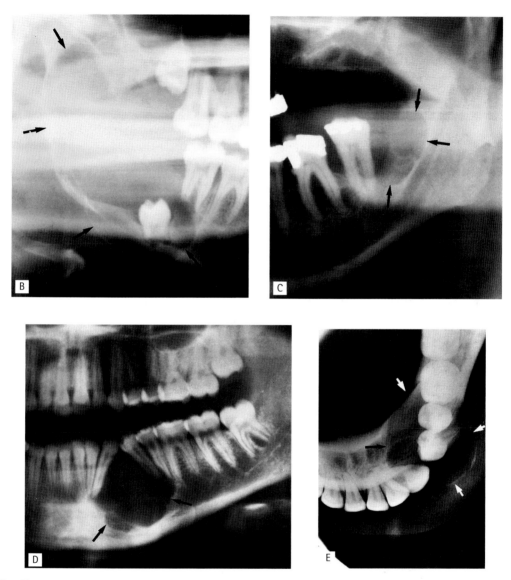

Fig. 27.9B Right side of a panoramic radiograph showing a very extensive ameloblastoma (arrowed) with a less multilocular appearance but still causing considerable expansion and displacement of $\overline{8|}$. **C** Left side of a panoramic radiograph showing bilocular ameloblastoma (arrowed) distal to the molar. **D** Part of a panoramic radiograph showing an ameloblastoma in a more unusual anterior position causing displacement of the adjacent teeth. **E** Lower occlusal of the same patient showing the bucolingual extent of the lesion (arrowed).

Ameloblastic fibroma (Fig. 27.10)

A rare, benign, mixed odontogenic tumour originating from both the odontogenic epithelium and the connective tissue of the developing tooth germ. Histologically, it consists of odontogenic ectomesenchyme resembling dental papilla and epithelial strands and rests resembling dental lamina and enamel organ. Radiographically these tumours closely resemble ameloblastomas but develop in a younger age group.

- *Age*: Children and adolescents — mean age 14 years.
- *Frequency*: Rare.

- *Site*: Posterior mandible (usually) or maxillary premolar/ molar region.
- *Size*: Variable.
- *Shape*: — Multilocular
    — Unilocular in the early stages.
- *Outline*: — Smooth
    — Well defined
    — Well corticated.
- *Radiodensity*: Radiolucent with internal radiopaque septa if multilocular.
- *Effects*: — Adjacent teeth displaced
    — Buccal/lingual expansion of the jaw
    — 50% associated with an unerupted or malpositioned tooth.

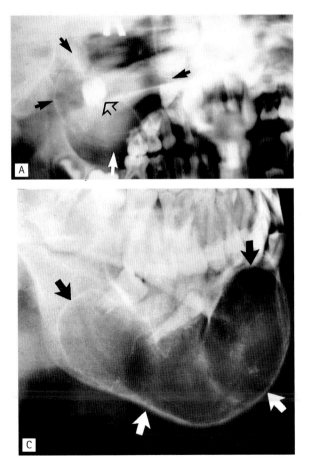

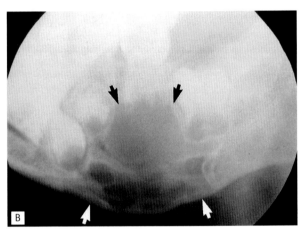

Fig. 27.10A Part of a panoramic radiograph of a 4-year-old showing a large ameloblastic fibroma in the right maxilla, causing marked expansion (solid arrows) and displacement of the developing first molar (open arrow). (Kindly provided by Mrs J. E. Brown.) **B** Oblique lateral of another small child showing a multilocular ameloblastic fibroma (arrowed) in the left body of the mandible causing displacement of the developing premolars and expansion of the lower border.
C Oblique lateral showing a very extensive ameloblastic fibroma (arrowed) of the right side in a 17-year-old.

Other epithelial odontogenic tumours

The other more important epithelial odontogenic tumours, with or without odontogenic ectomesenchyme, that can present as a radiolucency include:

- Calcifying epithelial odontogenic tumour (CEOT) or Pindborg tumour
- Ameloblastic fibro-odontoma
- Adenomatoid odontogenic tumour (AOT)
- Calcifying cystic odontogenic tumour (calcifying odontogenic cyst).

However, as the name of a couple of them suggests, these lesions often develop internal calcifications and more typically present as lesions of variable radiopacity. They are therefore described in detail with appropriate examples in Chapter 28. A brief summary of each is outlined below.

Calcifying epithelial odontogenic tumour (CEOT), Pindborg tumour

This rare odontogenic tumour usually presents in the premolar/molar region of the mandible in 20–60 year-old adults. They can be either unilocular or multilocular, but tend to remain relatively small although they can cause expansion of surrounding cortical bone. They are often associated with an unerupted tooth particularly $\overline{8 \mid 8}$. The outline of the lesion tends to be of variable definition and cortication but is frequently scalloped. They are often radiolucent in their early stages; then numerous scattered radiopacities usually become evident within the lesion, often most prominent around the crown of any associated unerupted tooth. This appearance is sometimes described as *driven snow*. Adjacent teeth can be either displaced and/or resorbed (see Fig. 28.8).

Ameloblastic fibro-odontoma

These rare, unilocular or multilocular odontogenic tumours resemble closely ameloblastic fibromas (see Fig. 27.10), and also affect children. However, they are often associated with an unerupted tooth and usually contain enamel or dentine, either as multiple small opacities or as a solid mass (see Fig. 28.9).

Adenomatoid odontogenic tumour (AOT)

Another rare odontogenic tumour, but unusually the most frequent site affected, is the anterior maxilla in the incisor/canine region. Young adults are usually affected. The lesion tends to be unilocular, round or oval, and often surrounds an entire unerupted tooth. When radiolucent in their early stages, they can closely resemble a dentigerous cyst. However, as the lesion matures, small opacities (*snowflakes*) within the central radiolucency may be seen peripherally. Adjacent teeth are often displaced as the lesion expands but are rarely resorbed (see Fig. 28.10).

Calcifying cystic odontogenic tumour (calcifying odontogenic cyst or Gorlin's cyst)

The new name of this lesion reflects its classification by the WHO as an odontogenic tumour. It presents typically anteriorly in either the mandible or the maxilla as a unilocular, well-defined, well-corticated radiolucency resembling any other odontogenic cyst. It can affect any age group having been reported in patients from 5–92 years old. One third of cases are associated with an unerupted tooth or odontome. As the lesion matures, a variable amount of calcified material, of tooth-like density, becomes evident scattered throughout the radiolucency. The opacities can range from small flecks to large masses. Adjacent teeth are usually displaced and/or resorbed (see Fig. 28.11).

Odontogenic fibroma (Fig. 27.11)

Controversy still exists as to the concept and definition of the odontogenic fibroma as a distinct lesion. The WHO classify it separately and describe it as a rare neoplasm characterized histologically by varying amounts of inactive looking odontogenic epithelium embedded in a mature fibrous stroma. Two sub-types are described, thought to develop from different parts of the tooth germ:

- Epithelium-poor originating from the dental follicle
- Epithelium-rich originating from the periodontal ligament.

Typically lesions present as cyst-like well defined, unilocular radiolucencies with dense corticated margin. Rarely calcified material may develop internally and adjacent teeth may be displaced.

Odontogenic myxoma (Fig. 27.12)

An intra-osseous neoplasm characterized histologically by stellate and spindle-shaped cells embedded in an abundant myxoid or mucoid extracellular matrix originating from the odontogenic connective tissue fibroblasts of the developing tooth germ.

- *Age*: Young adults — most diagnosed in the 2nd–4th decades.
- *Frequency*: Rare, but the third most common odontogenic tumour.
- *Site*: Posterior mandible or posterior maxilla.
- *Size*: Variable, but may become very large if untreated.

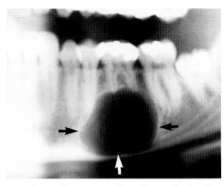

Fig. 27.11   Part of a panoramic radiograph showing a round, unilocular, well-defined radiolucency (arrowed) at the apex of |6 which was clinically vital. Histopathology confirmed an odontogenic fibroma.

- *Shape*:   — Multilocular (*honeycomb* or *soap-bubble*)
            — Occasionally unilocular.
- *Outline*:   — Smooth and often scalloped
              — Well defined with variable cortication.
- *Radiodensity*: Radiolucent with fine internal radiopaque septa or trabeculae often arranged at right angles to one another, producing an appearance sometimes described as resembling the *strings of a tennis racket* or the letters *X* and *Y*.
- *Effects*:   —Adjacent teeth displaced and loosened, occasionally resorbed
              — May be associated with a missing or unerupted tooth
              — Extensive buccal and lingual expansion with possible cortical perforation when large.

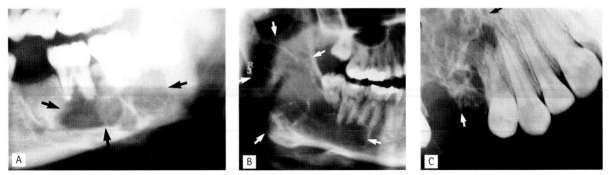

Fig. 27.12A   Left side of a panoramic radiograph showing the typical multilocular appearance of an odontogein myxoma (arrowed) in the body of the mandible. B Right side of a panoramic radiograph showing an extensive odontogenic myxoma (arrowed) with final internal septa. C Part of an upper oblique occusal showing a multilocular almost *honeycomb* appearance of an odontogenic myxoma (arrowed) in the maxilla.

Radiolucent non-odontogenic tumours

Intrinsic primary benign bone tumours

Central haemangioma (Fig. 27.13)

This is a rare, benign tumour that occasionally affects the jaws, particularly the mandible. It is usually regarded as a developmental malformation (hamartoma) of the blood vessels in the marrow spaces, rather than a true neoplasm.

Central haemangioma can present at any age but is usually discovered in adolescents. It can produce a **very** variable radiographic appearance. These variations are important because of the life-threatening nature of the lesion; they include:

- Most commonly a multilocular, expanding lesion which may be associated with displacement and resorption of associated teeth. The size and number of locules can vary considerably, and, if numerous, can present with a *honeycomb* appearance.
- A moderately well-defined zone of radiolucency within which the trabecular spaces are enlarged and the trabeculae themselves are coarse and thick and are said to be arranged like a *hub* or the *spokes of a wheel*.
- Rarely, a relatively well-defined, round, cyst-like radiolucency — not distinctive in any way.
- Large lesions may cause cortical expansion, occasionally producing the *sunray* or *sunburst* appearance.

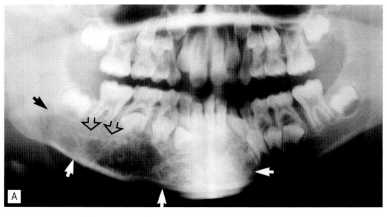

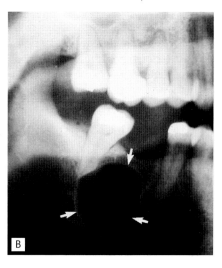

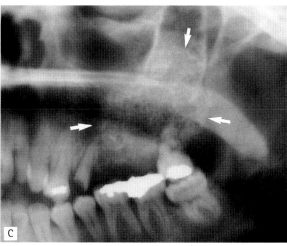

Fig. 27.13A   Part of a panoramic radiograph of an 8-year-old showing a large central haemangioma occupying most of the body of the mandible (solid arrows). The typical *honeycomb* appearance is evident on the right (open arrows) and there is evidence of root resorption. B Part of a panoramic radiograph showing a unilocular cyst-like haemangioma (arrowed). (Kindly provided by Mr K. Hussain.) These two examples highlight the very variable appearance of this important lesion. C Left side of a panoramic radiograph showing the multilocular *honeycomb* appearance of a large haemangioma in the posterior maxilla (arrowed).

Intrinsic primary malignant bone tumours

Osteosarcoma (Fig. 27.14)

Rare, rapidly destructive malignant tumour of bone. From a radiological viewpoint, there are three main types:

- Osteolytic — no neoplastic bone formation.
- Osteosclerotic — neoplastic osteoid and bone formed.
- Mixed lytic and sclerotic — patches of neoplastic bone formed.

- *Age*: Young adults under 30 years old.
- *Frequency*: Rare, but the most common primary malignant bone tumour.
- *Site*: Usually the mandible.
- *Size*:⎫
- *Shape*:⎪ All very variable
- *Outline*:⎬ depending on the type of
- *Radiodensity*:⎪ lesion (lytic or sclerotic)
- *Effects*:⎭ and how long it has been present.

Early features:

- Non-specific, poorly defined radiolucent area around one or more teeth.
- Widening of the periodontal ligament space.

Later features:

- Osteolytic lesion:
  - Unilocular, ragged area of radiolucency
  - Poorly defined, *moth-eaten* outline
  - So-called *spiking* resorption and/or loosening of associated teeth.
- Osteosclerotic and mixed lesions:
  - Poorly defined radiolucent area
  - Variable internal radiopacity with obliteration of the normal trabecular pattern
  - Perforation and expansion of the cortical margins by stretching the periosteum, producing the classic, but rare *sun ray* or *sunburst* appearance (see Ch. 28)
  - *Spiking* resorption and/or loosening of associated teeth
  - Distortion of the alveolar ridge.

Fibrosarcoma and chondrosarcoma

Both of these primary malignant tumours of bone are rare and produce the irregular, poorly defined radiolucent areas often indicative of the rapid bone destruction of malignancy.

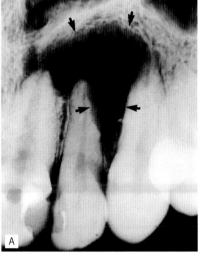

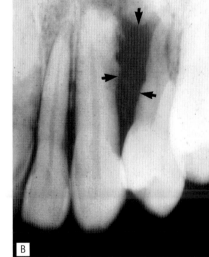

Fig. 27.14A Periapical of ⌊1,2,3 showing a poorly defined ragged area of radiolucency (arrowed) with resorption of the lateral aspect of ⌊2 root. Biposy revealed an osteolytic osteosarcoma. **B** Periapical showing a similar smaller poorly defined area of bone destruction between ⌊3,4 (arrowed) which was again shown to be an osteosarcoma.

Extrinsic primary malignant tumours involving bone

Squamous cell carcinoma (Fig. 27.15)

Squamous cell carcinomas of the oral mucosa directly overlying bone, in their latter stages, often invade the underlying bone to produce a destructive radiolucency.

- *Age*: Adults over 50 years old.
- *Frequency*: Rare, but the most common oral malignant tumour.
- *Site*: Mandible, or maxilla if originating in the antrum.

- *Size*: Variable.
- *Shape*: Irregular area of bone destruction often initially saucer-shaped.
- *Outline*: — Irregular and *moth-eaten*
    — Poorly defined
    — Not corticated.
- *Radiodensity*: Radiolucent, radiodensity dependent on degree of destruction.
- *Effects*: — Adjacent teeth may be displaced, loosened and/or resorbed or left *floating in space*
    — Destruction of surrounding bone may lead to pathological fracture.

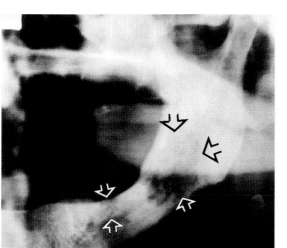

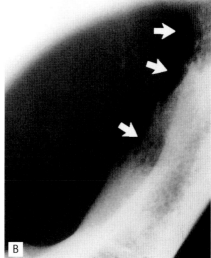

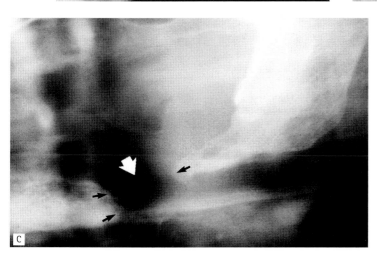

Fig. 27.15A Part of a panoramic radiograph of a patient who presented with a large squamous cell carcinoma on the left ventral surface of his tongue and the floor of his mouth. The radiograph shows two areas of poorly defined radiolucency (arrowed) with a ragged or *moth-eaten* appearance. **B** Left side of a lower 90° occlusal of the same patient showing the bony destruction (arrowed) of the lingual surface of the mandible as the soft tissue tumour invades the bone. **C** Part of a panoramic radiograph of another patient who presented with a very large squamous cell carcinoma of the floor of the mouth that had penetrated through the mandible (white arrow) causing a pathological fracture. The ragged bone edges are marked with the black arrows.

Secondary (metastatic) bone tumours (Fig. 27.16)

Carcinomas from the bronchus, breast, prostate, kidney and thyroid sometimes metastasize to the jaws and produce the typical destructive radiolucency of a malignant lesion (see Ch. 22).

- *Age*: Adults over 40 years old.
- *Frequency*: Rare, but the second most common malignant tumours of the jaws.
- *Site*: Usually centrally in the mandible, molar and premolar regions, occasionally at the apex of a tooth.
- *Size*: Variable, dependent on the length of time the lesion has been present.

- *Shape*: Irregular area or areas of bone destruction.
- *Outline*: — Irregular and *moth-eaten*
  — Poorly defined, not corticated.
- *Radiodensity*: Radiolucent, but some carcinomas from the prostate and breast may be osteogenic and show areas of bone production/sclerosis.
- *Effects*: — Adjacent teeth may be displaced, loosened and/or resorbed
  — Destruction of surrounding bone
  — Involvement of overlying soft tissues.

Note: The radiographic appearance, while strongly indicating a destructive malignant lesion, does not enable the distinction between a primary or secondary tumour to be made.

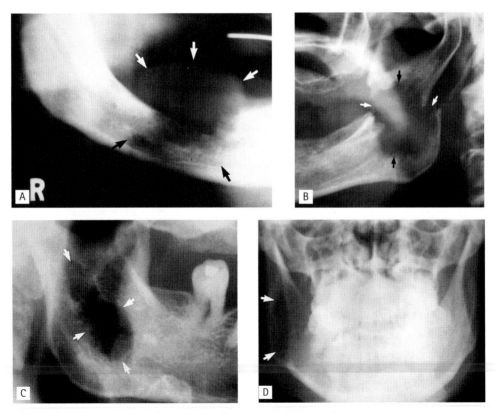

Fig. 27.16A Right side of a panoramic radiograph showing the typical destructive, *moth-eaten* radiolucency of a malignant lesion (black arrows). Overlying soft tissue involvement is also evident (white arrows). Subsequent investigation showed this to be a secondary metastatic tumour from the breast. **B** Left side of a panoramic radiograph showing a large irregular destructive secondary metastatic tumour in the ascending ramus (black arrows). There is an associated pathological fracture (white arrows). **C** Left side of a panoramic radiograph and **D** PA jaws of the same patient showing a poorly defined radiolucent secondary metastatic deposit, from the lung, presenting centrally in the ramus (arrowed).

Lymphoreticular tumours of bone (Fig. 27.17)

Multiple myeloma (Fig. 27.17)

Multifocal proliferation of the plasma cell series within the bone marrow, resulting in over-production of immunoglobulins.

- *Age*: Adults, middle-aged.
- *Frequency*: Uncommon.
- *Site*: Multiple lesions affecting:
  — Skull vault
  — Posterior parts of the mandible
  — Other parts of the skeleton.
- *Size:* Variable, individual lesions may be several centimetres in diameter.
- *Shape:* — Round
  — Unilocular, though multifocal.
- *Outline:* — Punched-out
  — Well defined, not corticated.

- *Radiodensity:* Radiolucent.
- *Effects:* Enlargement and/or coalescence of lesions may lead to pathological fracture.

Others

- Large cell (anaplastic) lymphoma — adults under 40 years
- Burkitt's (African) lymphoma — children (see Fig. 27.17C)
- Ewing's tumour — adults under 40 years.

These lymphoreticular tumours are rare and apart from the age group predilection (shown above), they present in a similar, relatively non-specific manner. Radiographically they usually present as expansile, destructive, poorly defined, radiolucent areas — suggestive of malignant disease.

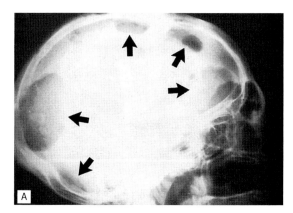

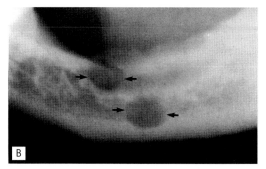

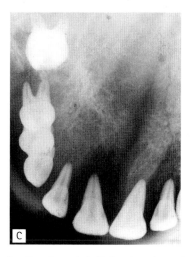

Fig. 27.17A   True lateral skull showing the typical multiple punched-out lesions (arrowed) of the skull vault of multiple myeloma. **B** Oblique lateral of the left side showing two similar lesions in the mandible (arrowed). **C** Upper oblique occlusal showing the typical appearance of destructive malignancy of Burkitt's lymphoma. Almost all normal anatomical structures have been destroyed.

Langerhans cell disease (histiocytosis X)

Langerhans cell disease is used as a broad grouping of three different clinical manifestations of the same disease. All three manifestations produce tumour-like lesions in bone, caused by proliferation of Langerhans cells and eosinophilic leucocytes:

- *Solitary eosinophilic granuloma* — localized to the skeleton, affecting adolescents and young adults (see Fig. 27.18)
- *Multifocal eosinophilic granuloma* (Hand–Schüller–Christian disease) — chronic and wide-spread, begins in childhood but may not be fully developed until early adulthood, 20–30 years
- *Letterer–Siwe disease* — acute or subacute and widespread, affecting children under three years old.

Radiographically, the bone lesions (in whatever parts of the skeleton are affected) are similar in all three diseases.

- *Frequency*: Rare.
- *Site*: Multiple lesions (in multifocal eosinophilic granuloma and Letterer–Siwe disease only) throughout the skeleton, occasionally solitary lesion, affecting:
    - Skull vault
    - Mandible or maxilla, posteriorly in the alveolar process.
- *Size*: Small, 1–2 cm in diameter.
- *Shape*: — Unilocular
    — Round.
- *Outline*: — Smooth
    — Relatively well defined
    — Not corticated, appears punched-out.
- *Radiodensity*: Radiolucent.
- *Effects*: — Adjacent teeth — not resorbed, but the periodontal bone support is sometimes destroyed so that they appear to be *floating* or *standing in space*
    — No expansion of the surrounding bone.

Note: Appearance not suggestive of malignant disease.

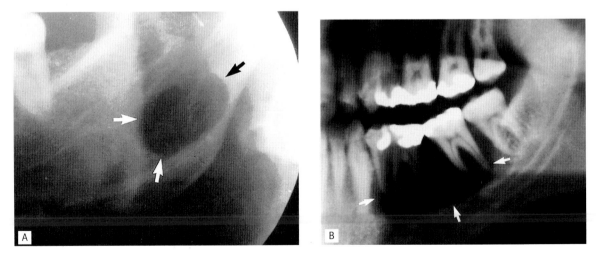

Fig. 27.18A Oblique lateral of the left side of the mandible showing a well-defined, unilocular, punched-out, radiolucency (arrowed) beneath the inferior dental canal and therefore non-odontogenic, which proved to be an eosinophilic granuloma. **B** Left side of a panoramic radiograph showing an extensive punched-out destructive eosinophilic granuloma (arrowed) causing the $\overline{6,7}$ to appear to be *floating in space*. (Kindly provided by Dr J. Luker.)

TYPICAL RADIOGRAPHIC FEATURES OF BONE-RELATED LESIONS

Giant cell lesions

Central giant cell lesion (granuloma) (Fig. 27.19)

A relatively rare lozalized, benign but sometimes aggressive osteolytic proliferation consisting histiologically of fibrous tissue with haemorrhage and haemosiderin deposits, presence of osteoclast-like giant cells and reactive bone formation producing an expansile radiolucent lesion.

- *Age*: All ages can be affected but usually young adolescents and adults under 30 years old. One third of cases reported in patients under 20.
- *Frequency*: Rare.
- *Site*: Mandible — all parts particularly premolar/molar region and anteriorly often crossing the midline.

- *Shape*: Multilocular, may be unilocular in early stages.
- *Outline*: — Smooth and scalloped
  — Well-defined
  — Generally not well corticated.
- *Radiodensity*: Radiolucent, larger lesions have thin internal septa or trabeculae producing the multilocular, or sometimes *honeycomb* appearance.
- *Effects*: — Adjacent teeth often displaced, sometimes resorbed
  — Surrounding buccal and lingual bone expanded unevenly producing the scalloped border.

Based on their clinical and radiological effects on adjacent structures, central giant cell lesions are sometimes subdivided into two categories:

- *Non-aggressive*, which exhibit slow-growing, benign behaviour
- *Aggressive*, which show the typical features of rapidly growing, destructive lesions.

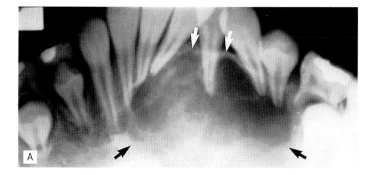

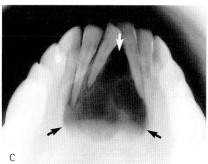

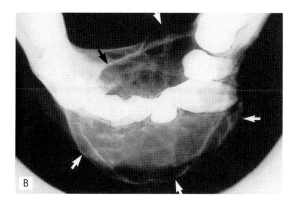

Fig. 27.19 Typical appearance of central giant cell lesion. **A** Anterior portion of a static panoramic showing the multilocular appearance, expansion (arrowed) and considerable displacement of the adjacent teeth. **B** Lower 90° occlusal showing the gross buccal and lingual expansion (arrowed) and the scalloped cortical border. **C** Lower 45° occlusal of another patient showing the appearance of a similar but much smaller central giant cell lesion (arrowed).

Brown tumours in hyperparathyroidism

The general radiological features of hyper-parathyroidism are discussed in detail in Chapter 32. A few patients with this disease, in addition to the generalized decrease in bone density, also develop circumscribed, cyst-like radiolucencies. Histologically and radiologically these individual lesions (so-called *brown tumours*) are indistinguishable from central giant cell lesions (see earlier).

Cherubism (Fig. 27.20)

This rare disease of the jaws is inherited, usually as an autosomal dominant, but some cases appear spontaneously. Radiologically the lesions resemble closely other giant cell-containing lesions.

- *Age*: Children, 2–6 years old.
- *Frequency*: Rare.
- *Site*: — Angle/posterior mandible — bilateral
  — Occasionally posterior maxilla — also bilateral.

- *Size*: Variable, up to several centimetres in diameter, and may fill the whole jaw.
- *Shape*: — Multilocular
  — Bilateral lesions typically symmetrical.
- *Outline*: — Smooth
  — Well defined
  — Well corticated.
- *Radiodensity*: Radiolucent with internal radiopaque septa producing a multilocular appearance.
- *Effects*: — Adjacent teeth — gross displacement of deciduous and permanent teeth, occasionally resorbed, deciduous teeth sometimes exfoliated early
  — Extensive buccal/lingual expansion
  — Encroachment on the antra by maxillary lesions.

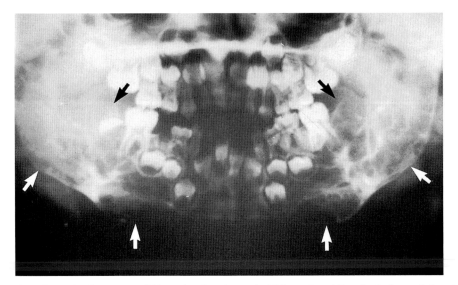

Fig. 27.20   Panoramic radiograph of a 5-year-old boy showing the typical bilateral multilocular lesions of cherubism affecting the mandible (arrowed).

Aneurysmal bone cyst (Fig. 27.21)

As stated earlier, despite its name this rare lesion is categorized as a *giant cell lesion* and is defined as an expansile osteolytic lesion, often multilocular with histologically blood-filled spaces separated by fibrous septa containing osteoclast-type giant cells and reactive bone.

- *Age*: Adolescents and young adults under 30 years old. Peak incidence in the second decade.
- *Frequency*: Rare.
- *Site*: — Body/posterior mandible including the ramus but very rarely the condyle
  — Maxilla occasionally.

- *Shape*: — Unilocular or multilocular
  — Faint internal trabeculation may produce a *soap-bubble* appearance.
- *Outline*: — Smooth
  — Moderately well defined
  — Peripheral cortex usually retained even when large.
- *Radiodensity*: Radiolucent with evidence of faint, random internal trabeculations.
- *Effects*: — Adjacent teeth — displaced, rarely resorbed
  — Buccal and lingual expansion of the cortex, often marked and described as *ballooning* or *blow-out*
  — Rarely cortical perforation.

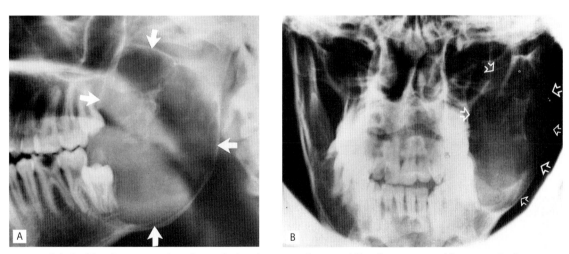

Fig. 27.21 **A** Left side of a panoramic radiograph showing a very large multilocular aneurysmal bone cyst in the ramus (arrowed). Note the marked expansion and the displacement of 8|. **B** PA jaws of the same patient showing *ballooning* expansion (arrowed).

Bone-related lesions — osseous dysplasias

The 2005 WHO Classication, shown in Table 27.1, now categorizes *fibro-cemento-osseous lesions* as *osseous dysplasias* and includes four conditions:

- Periapical osseous dysplasia
- Focal osseous dysplasia
- Florid osseous dysplasia
- Familial gigantiform cementoma.

They are all skeletal disorders in which bone is replaced by fibrous tissue which in turn is replaced by bone or mineralized tissue to a varying degree as the lesions age. Thus, in their early stages all the osseous dysplasias can present as cyst-like radiolucencies, although they are only sometimes seen clinically at this stage. It is more common to see them in their later stages when they present as mixed radiolucent/radiopaque lesions with varying degrees of opacity. Two radiolucent examples are shown here (Figs 27.22 and 27.23). The more radiopaque lesions are discussed and illustrated in Chapter 28.

Periapical osseous dysplasia (Fig. 27.22)

- *Age*: Middle-aged adults (typically black women).
- *Frequency*: Rare.
- *Site*: Apices of vital lower incisor teeth.
- *Size*: Small, usually only up to 5–6 mm in diameter.
- *Shape*: — Round, unilocular
  — Often multiple.
- *Outline*: — Variable but usually poorly defined
  — Not corticated.
- *Radiodensity*: — Early stage — radiolucent
  — Intermediate stage — radiolucent with patchy opacity within the radiolucency
  — Late stage — densely radiopaque but surrounded by a thin radiolucent line.
- *Effects*: — Adjacent teeth — not displaced, not resorbed, typically vital, with intact periodontal ligament space, but lamina dura may be discontinuous
  — No expansion of the jaw.

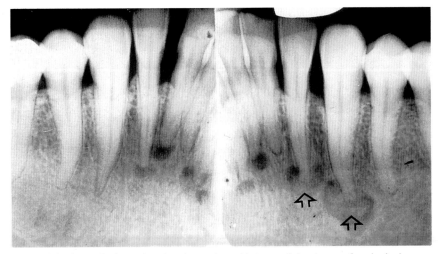

Fig. 27.22 Periapicals of the lower incisors showing the early and intermediate stages of periapical osseous dysplasia. Several, small, discrete radiolucencies are evident at the apices. The more mature lesions at the apices 23 show evidence of internal calcification (open arrows).

Florid osseous dysplasia (Fig. 27.23)

- **Age**: Middle-aged adults (typically black women).
- **Frequency**: Rare.
- **Site**: Widespread, often in all four quadrants (dentulous and edentulous) but associated with the apices of the teeth if present.
- **Size**: Variable, but individual lesions up to 2 cm in diameter.
- **Shape**: — Multiple
            — Round, but frequently coalesce.
- **Outline**: — Smooth but lobular
            — Moderately well defined but irregular
            — Occasionally corticated.
- **Radiodensity**: — Early stage — multiple radiolucencies
            — Intermediate stage —multiple radiolucencies with gradually increasing patchy internal opacities

            — Late stage — multiple irregular dense radiopacities with individual lesions, sometimes surrounded by a thin radiolucent line.
- **Effects**: — Adjacent teeth — not displaced, not resorbed, typically vital
            — Occasionally may cause expansion or enlargement of the affected jaw
            — Can be associated with low grade osteomyelitis.

Other bone-related lesions

The other bone-related lesions that could present as a radiolucency include:

- Fibrous dysplasia (see Ch. 28 as more commonly mixed radiodensity)
- Ossifying fibroma (see Ch. 28 as more commonly mixed radiodensity)
- Simple bone cyst (see earlier)
- Stafne's bone cavity.

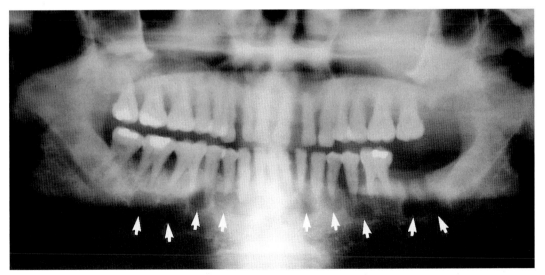

Fig. 27.23 Panoramic radiograph showing multiple radiolucent lesions (arrowed) in the mandible of early stage florid osseous dysplasia.

Stafne's bone cavity (Fig. 27.24)

A bone cavity or depression on the lingual aspect of the mandible near the lower border, frequently said to contain aberrant salivary gland tissue.

- *Age*: Adults.
- *Frequency*: Rare.

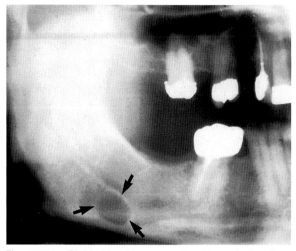

Fig. 27.24 Right side of a panoramic radiograph showing the typical cyst-like appearance of Stafne's bone cavity at the angle of the mandible, below the inferior dental canal (arrowed).

- *Site*: Angle of the mandible, below the inferior dental canal but above or involving the lower border.
- *Size*: 1–2 cm in diameter, size does not usually alter with age.
- *Shape*: — Round
         — Unilocular.
- *Outline*: — Well defined
         — Variable cortication.
- *Radiodensity*: Uniformly radiolucent.
- *Effects*: — No effect on nearby teeth
         — No expansion
         — Lingual depression not usually detectable clinically.

FOOTNOTE

In view of this large number of radiolucent conditions, an ordered, systematic approach when producing a differential diagnosis is essential. Although the old adage that common things are commonly seen applies aptly to radiology, clinicians always have to be prepared for the possibility that they may be dealing with one of the rare, and perhaps sinister conditions.

For revision purposes, Table 27.2 summarizes those lesions which present typically as unilocular or multilocular radiolucencies.

Table 27.2 Summary of the main unilocular and multilocular radiolucent lesions

Typically unilocular lesions	Typically multilocular or pseudolocular lesions
Radicular (dental) cyst	Odontogenic keratocyst
Residual radicular cyst	(keratocystic odontogenic tumour)
Dentigerous cyst	Ameloblastoma
Lateral periodontal cyst	Ameloblastic fibroma
Nasopalatine duct cyst	Calcifying epithelial odontogenic tumour
Simple (solitary) bone cyst	Odontogenic myxoma
Calcifying epithelial odontogenic tumour	Haemangioma
Calcifying cystic odontogenic tumour	Giant cell lesions:
Adenomatoid odontogenic tumour	— Central giant cell lesion
Odontogenic fibroma	— Brown tumour
Primary bone tumours	— Cherubism
Haemangioma	— Aneurysmal bone cyst
Secondary (metastatic) tumours	
Multiple myeloma	
Eosinophilic granuloma	
Osseous dysplasias (early stages)	
Stafne's bone cavity	

Chapter 28

Differential diagnosis of lesions of variable radiopacity in the jaws

As explained in Chapter 26, a variety of conditions that can affect the jaws are *radiopaque* relative to the surrounding bone, although the degree of opacity can be very variable. A step-by-step guide, similar to that suggested for radiolucent lesions in Chapter 27, is outlined to emphasize the importance of a methodical approach when producing a differential diagnosis. The suggested approach is summarized in Figure 28.1. Although most lesions are still detected using plain radiographs, this process can be greatly facilitated in many cases if advanced imaging modalities, described in Chapter 19, such as computed tomography (CT), cone beam CT or magnetic resonance (MR) are available.

Step I

Describe the variable radiopacity noting in particular:

- Site or anatomical position — is the opacity actually within bone or is it within the surrounding soft tissues and thus superimposed on the bone? To localize the opacity, two radiographs are usually required ideally at right angles to one another.
- Size.
- Shape.
- Outline or periphery — a particularly useful differentiating feature, since if the opacity is surrounded by a thin radiolucent line, it is invariably of dental tissue origin.
- Relative radiodensity.

- Effects on adjacent surrounding structures.
- Time present, if known.

Step II

Decide whether the variable radiopacity is:

1. A normal anatomical feature
- In the mandible, e.g.:
  - An area of dense bone sometimes referred to as a dense bone island
  - A bony prominence such as the external oblique ridge, mylohyoid line or genial tubercles
  - Another overlying bone such as the hyoid bone.

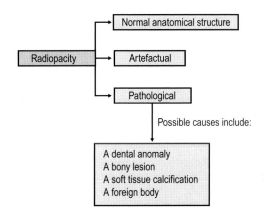

Fig. 28.1 Step-by-step guide to the differential diagnosis of radiopacities.

- In the maxilla, e.g.:
  - Another overlying bone such as the zygoma or anterior nasal spine
  - Another overlying structure such as the nasal cartilages or soft palate.

2. Artefactual

These depend largely on the type of radiograph, but examples include:

- Real or ghost earring shadows — seen on dental panoramic radiographs (see Ch. 17)
- Fixer solution splashes
- Objects or scratches on intensifying screens.

3. Pathological

Step III

If the radiopacity is *pathological*, decide within which of the following major categories it should be placed:

- Abnormalities of the teeth
- Conditions affecting the bone
- Superimposed soft tissue calcifications
- Foreign bodies.

Step IV

Consider the subdivisions of these pathological categories. A typical list is shown in Table 28.1.

Step V

Compare the radiological features of the unknown opacity with the typical radiological features of these possible conditions. Then construct a list showing, in order of likelihood, all the conditions that the lesion might be. As mentioned in Chapter 27, this list forms the *radiological differential diagnosis*.

The typical radiographic features of the important radiopacities are described below using a similar style to that adopted in Chapter 27. It must be emphasized that this is a **simplified** approach and that most lesions can produce a variety of appearances.

Table 28.1 Classification of the more common lesions that can present as variable radiopacities in the jaws

Abnormalities of the teeth	
Unerupted and misplaced teeth including supernumeraries	
Odontomes — compound	
— complex (see odontogenic tumours)	
Root remnants	
Hypercementosis	

Conditions of variable radiopacity affecting the bone	
Developmental	Exostoses including tori — mandibular or palatal
Inflammatory	Low grade chronic infection — sclerosing osteitis
	Osteomyelitis — sequestra; involucrum formation
Tumours	
Odontogenic (*late stages*)	Calcifying epithelial odontogenic tumour (CEOT)
	Ameloblastic fibro-odontoma
	Adenomatoid odontogenic tumour (AOT)
	Calcifying cystic odontogenic tumour (calcifying odontogenic cyst)
	Cementoblastoma
	Odontomes — compound
	Odontomes — complex
Non-odontogenic	Benign — Osteoma
	— Chondroma
	Malignant — Osteosarcoma
	— Osteogenic secondary metastases
Bone-related lesions	
Osseous dysplasias (*Fibro-cemento-osseous lesions*) (*late stages*)	Periapical osseous dysplasia
	Focal osseous dysplasia
	Florid osseous dysplasia
	Familial gigantiform cementoma
Other lesions	Ossifying fibroma
	Fibrous dysplasia
Bone diseases	Paget's disease of bone
	Osteopetrosis

Superimposed soft tissue calcifications	
Salivary calculi	
Calcified lymph nodes	
Calcified tonsils	
Phleboliths	
Calcified acne scars	

Foreign bodies	
Intra-bony	
Within the soft tissues	
On or overlying the skin	

TYPICAL RADIOGRAPHIC FEATURES OF ABNORMALITIES OF THE TEETH

Unerupted or misplaced teeth including supernumeraries (Fig. 28.2)

Radiopacities caused by unerupted or misplaced teeth and supernumeraries are readily identifiable as such radiographically, by their characteristic shape and radiodensity.

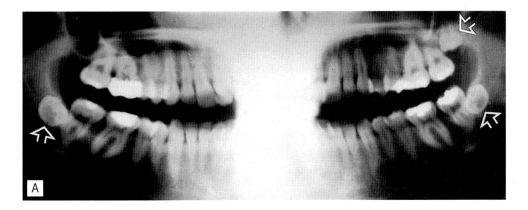

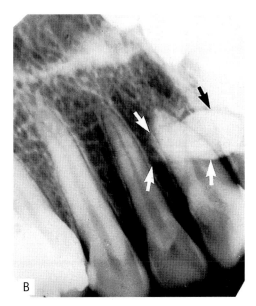

Fig. 28.2   Examples of opacities caused by unerupted teeth. **A** Panoramic radiograph showing the typical appearance of unerupted and misplaced wisdom teeth (arrowed) — $\overline{8|8}$ are positioned transversely. **B** Periapical showing a conically shaped mesiodens (arrowed) overlying 21/1. Density, shape and outline confirm that the opacity is composed of dental tissue.

Odontomes

Although both compound and complex odontomes are more accurately classified as epithelial odontogenic tumours with odontogenic ectomesenchyme showing dental hard tissue formation (WHO Classification 2005), they are often also described as dental developmental anomalies (see Ch. 25).

Compound odontome

This odontome is made up of several small tooth-like denticles. The miniature tooth shapes are of dental tissue radiodensity, with a surrounding radiolucent line, and are easily identified radiographically (Fig. 28.3).

Complex odontome

This odontome is made up of an irregular, confused mass of dental tissues bearing no resemblance in shape to a tooth. The enamel content provides the dense radiopacity, suggestive of dental tissue and again the mass is surrounded by a radiolucent line (Fig. 28.4).

Root remnants (Fig. 28.5)

Deciduous and permanent root remnants remaining in the alveolar bone, following attempted extraction, are common. The site, shape and density make radiographic identification relatively simple. Additional diagnostic radiographic features include the surrounding radiolucent line of the periodontal ligament shadow and sometimes evidence of a root canal.

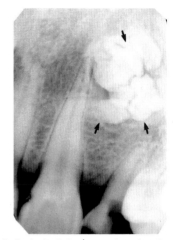

Fig. 28.3 Periapical of the |12 region showing a radiopaque compound odontome (arrowed), consisting of small denticles.

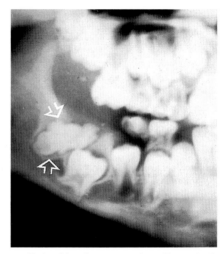

Fig. 28.4 Right side of a panoramic radiograph showing the typical irregular, densely radiopaque mass of a complex odontome in the position of 7| (arrowed). It is preventing the eruption of 6|. The opacity shows the characteristic surrounding radiolucent line, confirming its dental tissue origin.

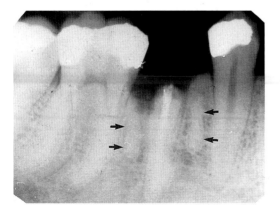

Fig. 28.5 Periapical showing opacities (arrowed) either side of 5| root caused by the root remnants of the deciduous E|. Note that their radiodensity is equivalent to the adjacent roots and their surrounding radiolucent line.

Hypercementosis (Fig. 28.6)

The formation of excessive amounts of cementum, usually around the apical portion of the root, is common. The cause is unknown, but it is sometimes seen in Paget's disease of bone and is then typically craggy and irregular. Diagnostically hypercementosis is not a problem — the resultant opacity being part of the tooth root and producing an alteration to the root outline.

TYPICAL RADIOGRAPHIC FEATURES OF CONDITIONS OF VARIABLE OPACITY AFFECTING BONE

Developmental

Exostoses, including tori (mandibular or palatal)

Exostoses are small, irregular overgrowths of bone sometimes developing on the surface of the alveolar bone. They consist primarily of compact bone and produce an ill-defined radiopacity when superimposed over the bulk of the alveolar bone. Usually two views are required to establish the exact site (see Fig. 28.7).

Specific exostoses develop in particular sites and are often bilateral:

- *Torus mandibularis* — lingual aspects of the mandible, in the premolar/molar region
- *Torus palatinus* — either side of the midline towards the posterior part of the hard palate.

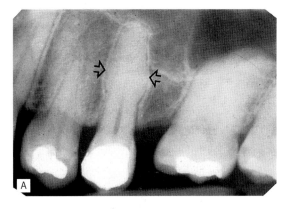

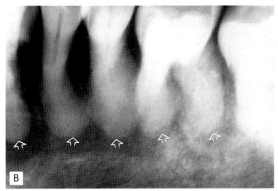

Fig. 28.6A Periapical showing early hypercementosis affecting |5 (arrowed). **B** Periapical showing marked hypercementosis (arrowed) associated with Paget's disease of bone. Note also the abnormal *orange peel* appearance of the bone.

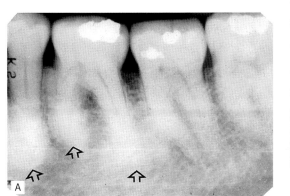

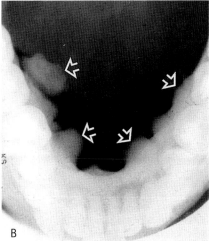

Fig. 28.7A Periapical of |5678 showing ill-defined areas of radiopacity (arrowed) overlying the teeth. **B** Lower 90° occlusal of the same patient showing the large irregular exostoses (mandibular tori) on the lingual aspect of the mandible (arrowed).

Tumours

Calcifying epithelial odontogenic tumour (CEOT or Pindborg tumour) (Fig. 28.8)

Defined by the WHO as a locally invasive epithelial odontogenic neoplasm, characterized histologically by amyloid material that may become calcified.

- *Age*: 20–60 year-old adults.
- *Frequency*: Rare — approximately 1% of all odontogenic tumours.
- *Site*: —Molar/premolar region of the mandible.
  —Maxilla occasionally.
- *Shape*: — Unilocular or multilocular
  — Usually round
  — Often associated with an unerupted tooth, particularly $\overline{8\,|\,8}$.

- *Outline*: — Variable definition, frequently scalloped
  — Variable cortication.
- *Radiodensity*: — Radiolucent in early stages then numerous scattered radiopacities usually become evident within the lesion often most prominent around the crown of any associated unerupted tooth
  — This appearance is sometimes described as *driven snow*.
- *Effects*: — Adjacent teeth sometimes displaced, sometimes resorbed
  — Expansion of the cortical bone.

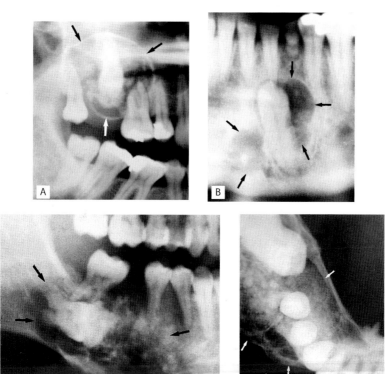

Fig. 28.8A Right side of a panoramic radiograph showing a calcifying epithelial odontogenic tumour in the maxilla (arrowed) associated with the unerupted $\underline{7|}$. There are obvious areas of calcification within the lesion. **B** Part of a panoramic radiograph showing another CEOT (arrowed) associated with the unerupted lower left canine, with only faint internal calcification. **C** Right side of a panoramic radiograph showing a poorly defined calcifying epithelial odontogenic tumour (arrowed) associated with the unerupted molar. **D** Lower 90° occlusal of the same patient showing the expansive, multilocular nature of the lesion and the discrete internal calcifications.

Ameloblastic fibro-odontoma (Fig. 28.9)

These rare, unilocular or multilocular odontogenic tumours resemble closely ameloblastic fibromas (see Fig. 25.10), and also affect children. However, they are often associated with an unempted tooth and usually contain enamel or dentine, either as multiple, small opacities or as a solid mass.

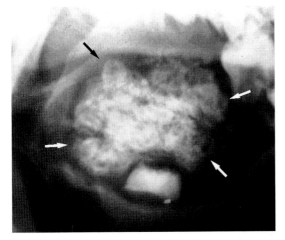

Fig. 28.9   Oblique lateral showing a large expansive ameloblastic fibro-odontoma (arrowed) in the mandible of a 5-year-old. The internal calcification is comparable to tooth tissue and histopathology confirmed the presence of enamel and dentine. Note the unerupted tooth.

Adenomatoid odontogenic tumour (AOT) (Fig. 28.10)

Described by the WHO as being composed of odontogenic epithelium embedded in a mature connective tissue stroma and characterized by slow but progressive growth.

- *Age*: Variable, but 90% develop before the age of 30 with most diagnosed in the second decade.
- *Frequency*: Rare — approximately 2–7% of all odontogenic tumours.
- *Site*: — Anterior maxilla — incisor/canine region
  — Occasionally anterior mandible.
- *Shape*: — Unilocular
  — Usually round or oval
  — Often surrounds an entire unerupted tooth.
- *Outline*: — Smooth and well defined
  — Well corticated.
- *Radiodensity*: — Initially radiolucent, but small opacities (*snowflakes*) within the central radiolucency may be seen peripherally as the lesion matures.
- *Effects*: — Adjacent teeth displaced, rarely resorbed
  — Associated tooth often unerupted
  — Buccal/palatal expansion.

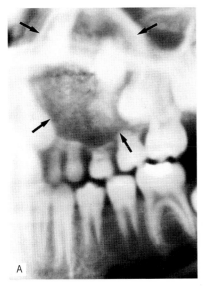

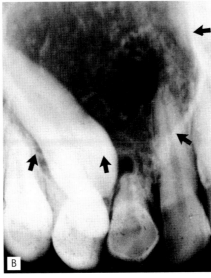

Fig. 28.10A   Part of a panoramic radiograph showing a monolocular adenomatoid odontogenic tumour in the anterior maxilla (arrowed) surrounding the unerupted ⌊3. Internal calcification is evident. **B** Periapical of the anterior maxilla showing another adenomatoid odontogenic tumour (arrowed) with internal calcification, associated with an unerupted canine. (Reproduced from *A Radiological Atlas of Diseases of the Teeth and Jaws* with kind permission from the authors R.M. Browne, H.D. Edmondson and P.G.J. Rout.)

A   B

Calcifying cystic odontogenic tumour (calcifying odontogenic cyst or Gorlin's cyst) (Fig. 28.11)

As stated earlier, the new name of this lesion reflects its classification by the WHO as an odontogenic tumour, who described it as a benign cystic neoplasm of odontogenic origin characterized histologically by ameloblastoma-like epithelium with ghost cells that may calcify. It presents typically anteriorly in either the mandible or the maxilla as a unilocular, well-defined, well-corticated radiolucency resembling other odontogenic cysts, but, as it develops, a variable amount of calcified material becomes evident, scattered throughout the radiolucency. The opacities can range from small flecks to large masses.

- *Age*: Variable, reported in patients between 5–92 years old.
- *Frequency*: Rare.
- *Site*: Mandible or maxilla — anterior or premolar regions, one third associated with an unerupted tooth or odontome.
- *Size*: Usually small, up to 4 cm in diameter.
- *Shape*: Variable, but usually unilocular.
- *Outline*: — Smooth, well defined
  — Well corticated.
- *Radiodensity*: — Initially radiolucent but in more advanced stages contains a variable amount of calcified radiopaque material of tooth-like density.
- *Effects*: — Adjacent teeth usually displaced, causing root divergence, and/or resorbed
  — Bony expansion.

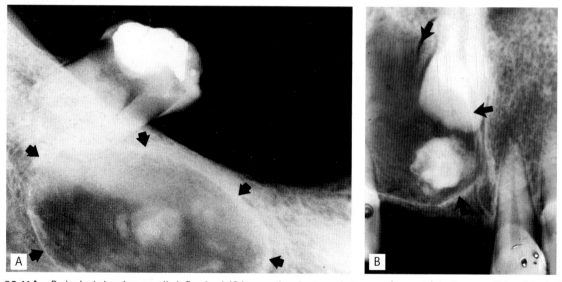

Fig. 28.11A Periapical showing a well-defined calcifying cystic odontogenic tumour (arrowed) in the mandible with obvious areas of internal calcification. **B** Periapical showing a calcifying cystic odontogenic tumour (arrowed) in the anterior maxilla. The central incisor is unerupted and there is internal calcification of tooth-like density.

Cementoblastoma (Fig. 28.12)

As indicated in Table 27.1, the cementoblastoma is classified by the WHO as an odontogenic tumour which is characterized by the formation of cementum-like tissue in connection with the root of a tooth.

- *Age*: Reported in patients between 8–44 years old, with a mean age of 20.
- *Frequency*: Rare.
- *Site*: Apex of mandibular first permanent molars, occasionally premolars. Exceptionally associated with the primary dentition.
- *Size*: Variable, but up to 2–3 cm in diameter.

- *Shape*: — Round or irregular, sometimes described as resembling a *golf ball*
  — Attached to a tooth root.
- *Outline*: — Well defined.
- *Radiodensity*: — Radiopaque but often surrounded by a thin radiolucent line owing to an outer zone of osteoid.
  — Often surrounded by a diffuse area of sclerotic bone.
- *Effects*: — Attached to the tooth root which is usually obscured as a result of resorption and fusion to the tooth
  — If large, may cause localized expansion of the cortical plates.

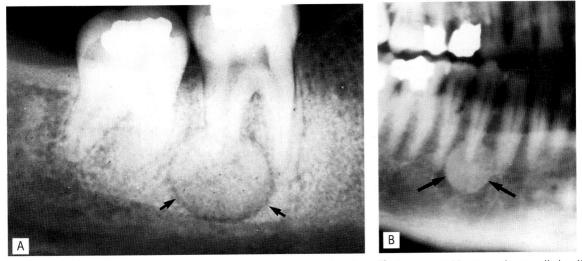

Fig. 28.12A Periapical showing the typical radiopaque mass at the apex of the 6̄| of a cementoblastoma, the so-called *golf ball* appearance. The mass is attached to the root and has a thin radiolucent line around it (arrowed). **B** Part of a panoramic radiograph showing a radiopaque cementoblastoma at the apex of 4̄| (arrowed).

Osteomas (Fig. 28.13)

Osteomas of the jaws may be located in the medullary bone (*endosteal osteoma*) or arise on the surface of the bone as a pedunculated mass (*periosteal osteoma*). They are usually detected in young adults and are typically asymptomatic, solitary lesions. Multiple jaw osteomas are a feature of the rare inherited condition *Gardner's syndrome*.

There are two main types:

- Compact — consisting of dense lamellae of bone and including the so-called *ivory osteoma* occasionally seen in the frontal sinus (see Ch. 29).
- Cancellous — consisting of trabeculae of bone.

Both tumours are uncommon. The type of bone making up the tumour determines the degree of radiopacity.

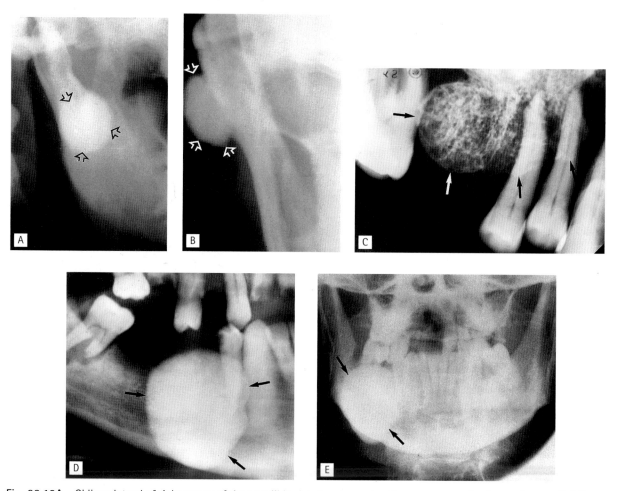

Fig. 28.13A   Oblique lateral of right ramus of the mandible showing a round radiopaque compact osteoma (arrowed). **B** Part of a PA jaws of the same patient showing the lesion (arrowed) arising from the lateral surface of the mandible confirming a periosteal osteoma. **C** Periapical showing a periosteal cancellous osteoma (arrowed). **D** Part of a panoramic radiograph and **E** PA jaws of the same patient showing a very large endosteal compact osteoma (arrowed) in the body of the mandible.

Osteosarcoma (Fig. 28.14)

Rare, rapidly destructive malignant tumour of bone. From a radiological viewpoint, there are three main types:

- Osteolytic — no neoplastic bone formation.
- Osteosclerotic — neoplastic osteoid and bone formed.
- Mixed lytic and sclerotic — patches of neoplastic bone formed.

Early features:

- Non-specific, poorly defined radiolucent area around one or more teeth.
- Widening of the periodontal ligament space.

Later features:

- Osteolytic lesion:
  - Unilocular, ragged area of radiolucency
  - Poorly defined, *moth-eaten outline*
  - So-called *spiking* resorption and/or loosening of associated teeth.
- Osteosclerotic and mixed lesions:
  - Poorly defined radiolucent area
  - Variable internal radiopacity with obliteration of the normal trabecular pattern
  - Perforation and expansion of the cortical margins by stretching the periosteum, producing the classical, but rare *sun ray* or *sunburst* appearance.

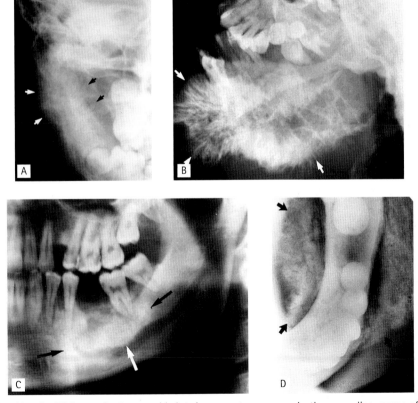

Fig. 28.14A   Right side of a PA jaws of a 7-year-old showing an osteosarcoma in the ascending ramus of the mandible. The *sunray* or *sunburst* appearance is evident medially and laterally (arrowed). **B** Oblique lateral showing a very extensive osteogenic osteosarcoma of the mandible with obvious *sunray* or *sunburst* bone formation. **C** Left side of a panoramic radiograph showing an irregular, poorly defined area of radiopacity (arrowed) in the body of the mandible. **D** Lower 90° occlusal of the same patient showing extensive buccal and lingual abnormal bone formation (arrowed) of another osteogenic osteosarcoma.

Osseous dysplasias

Periapical osseous dysplasia (Fig. 28.15)

- *Age*: Middle-aged adults (typically black women).
- *Frequency*: Rare.
- *Site*: Apices of several lower incisor teeth.
- *Size*: Small, usually only up to 5–6 mm in diameter.
- *Shape*: — Round, unilocular
  — Often multiple.
- *Outline*: — Variable but usually poorly defined and not corticated.
- *Radiodensity*: — Early stage—radiolucent
  — Intermediate stage — radiolucent with patchy opacity within the radiolucency
  — Late stage — densely radiopaque but surrounded by a thin radiolucent line.
- *Effects*: — Adjacent teeth:
  — not displaced or resorbed
  — typically vital, with intact periodontal ligament space, but lamina dura may be discontinous
  — No expansion of the jaw.

Focal osseous dysplasia (Fig. 28.16)

This usually solitary fibrocemento-osseous lesion occupies a portion of the spectrum between the periapical and florid cemento-osseous dysplasias.

- *Age*: Adults between 40 and 50 years old (typically white women).
- *Frequency*: Uncommon.
- *Site*: Any areas of the jaws (dentulous or edentulous), but mainly posterior mandible, and often in extraction sites.
- *Size*: Small, less than 1.5 cm in diameter.
- *Shape*: Round, unilocular.
- *Outline*: — Well defined but irregular
  — Not corticated.
- *Radiodensity*: — Early stage — radiolucent
  — Intermediate stage — radiolucent with patchy opacity within the radiolucency
  — Late stage — densely radiopaque but often surrounded by a thin radiolucent line.
- *Effects*: — Adjacent teeth:
  — not displaced
  — not resorbed
  — typically vital, with intact periodontal ligament space, but lamina dura may be discontinuous
  — No expansion of the jaw.

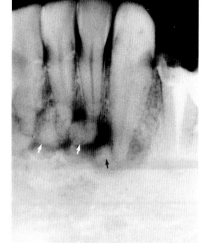

Fig. 28.15 Periapical showing the latter stage of periapical osseous dysplasia. The developing internal calcification is arrowed.

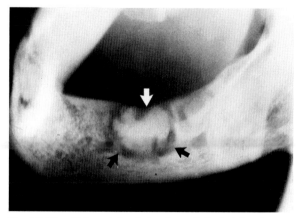

Fig. 28.16 Oblique lateral showing relatively late-stage focal osseous dysplasia in the region of the /6̄ extraction site (arrowed). An appreciable amount of internal calcification is evident.

Florid osseous dysplasia (Fig. 28.17)

- *Age*: Middle-aged adults (typically black women).
- *Frequency*: Rare.
- *Site*: Widespread, often in all four quadrants (dentulous and edentulous) but associated with the apices of the teeth if present.
- *Size*: Variable, but individual lesions up to 2–3 cm in diameter.
- *Shape*: — Multiple
  - — Round, but frequently coalesce.
- *Outline*: — Smooth but lobular
  - — Moderately well defined but irregular
  - — Occasionally corticated.
- *Radiodensity*: — Early stage — multiple radiolucencies
  - — Intermediate stage — multiple radiolucencies with gradually increasing patchy internal opacities
  - — Late stage — multiple irregular dense radiopacities within individual lesions sometimes surrounded by a thin radiolucent line.
- *Effects*: — Adjacent teeth:
  - — not displaced
  - — not resorbed
  - — typically vital
  - — Occasionally may cause expansion or enlargement of the affected jaw
  - — Can be associated with low grade sclerosing osteomyelitis.

Familial gigantiform cementoma

This is a rare familial osseous dysplasia. It is inherited as an autosomal dominant condition and confined almost exclusively to young, 10–20 year-old whites. The lesions characteristically show relatively rapid growth, causing marked facial deformity.

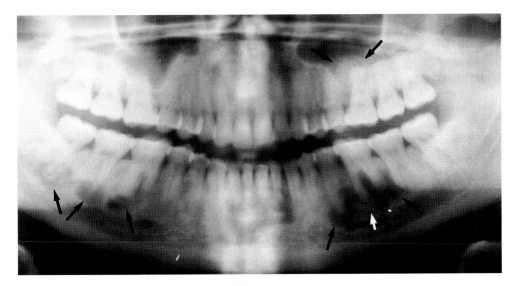

Fig. 28.17 Panoramic radiograph showing the multiple lesions (arrowed) of variable radiodensity of florid osseous dysplasia.

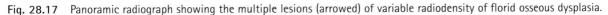

Bone-related lesions

As shown in Table 27.1, the WHO classify a number of different conditions under the general heading *bone-related*. Two of these can present as mixed radiolucent/radiopaque lesions in the jaws including:

- Fibrous dysplasia
- Ossifying fibroma.

Fibrous dysplasia (Fig. 28.18)

Fibrous dysplasia is described by the WHO as a genetically-based sporadic disease of bone affecting single or multiple bones. The jaws and other bones in the skull can be affected as well as other bones in the skeleton. The general radiological features of fibrous dysplasia are covered in Chapter 32.

The radiographic features of jaw lesions include:

- **Age**: 10–20 year-old adolescents.
- **Site**: Maxilla — usually posteriorly, more commonly than the mandible. Maxillary lesions may spread to involve adjacent bones such as the zygoma, sphenoid, occiput and base of skull.
- **Size**: Variable and difficult to define.
- **Shape**: Round.
- **Outline**: — Poorly defined with the margins merging imperceptibly with adjacent normal bone
  — Not corticated.
- **Radiodensity**: — Initially radiolucent (but rarely seen clinically at this stage)
  — Gradually becomes opaque to produce the typical *ground glass, orange peel* and *finger print* appearances resulting from superimposition of many fine, poorly-calcified bone trabeculae arranged in a disorganized fashion
  — Continuing to become more opaque with age.
- **Effects**: — Adjacent teeth:
  — sometimes displaced but rarely resorbed
  — loss of associated lamina dura
  — Buccal and lingual alveolar expansion
  — Encroachment on, or obliteration of, the antrum
  — Involvement of adjacent bones including the base of the skull.

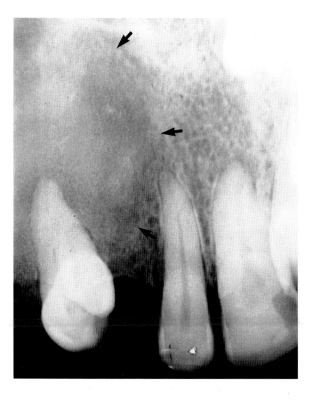

Fig. 28.18 Periapical of the upper right maxilla showing the generalized radiolucency with the fine internal trabeculation of monostostic fibrous dysplasia, giving a *ground glass* appearance. The almost imperceptible junction between abnormal and normal bone is arrowed.

Ossifying fibroma (Fig. 28.19)

This lesion has previously been called *cementifing fibroma* and *cemento-ossifying fibroma* but the 2005 WHO classification uses the term *ossifying fibroma* which is described as a well-demarcated lesion composed histologically of fibrocellular tissue and mineralizing material of varying appearance.

- *Age*: Variable, but usually in the 2nd–4th decades (particularly women).
- *Frequency*: Rare.
- *Site*: Usually posterior mandible, but different variants can affect the maxilla and paranasal sinuses.
- *Size*: Variable, may grow to several cm in diameter and cause facial asymmetry.
- *Shape*: — Round
  — Unilocular.
- *Outline*: — Smooth, well defined

- — When opaque usually surrounded by a thin encapsulating radiolucent line
- — Usually corticated and circumscribed.
- *Radiodensity*: — Early stage — radiolucent
  — Intermediate stage — radiolucent with gradually increasing internal radiopaque calcified patches
  — Late stage — radiopaque zones coalesce to form a densely radiopaque mass with or without a radiolucent periphery.
- *Effects*: — Adjacent teeth:
  — often displaced
  — occasionally resorbed
  — Expansion of the surrounding bone in all dimensions often demonstrating a *downward bowing* of the mandibular lower border cortex.

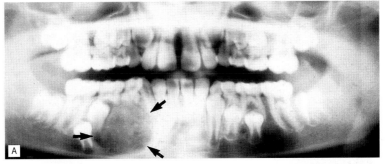

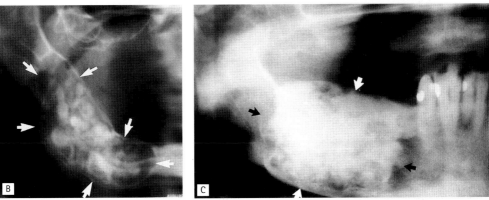

Fig. 28.19A Part of a panoramic radiograph of a 9-year-old showing an intermediate stage ossifying fibroma, with fine internal calcifications evident, in the right body of the mandible (arrowed). There is also displacement of the unerupted lower premolars and permanent canine. **B** Part of panoramic radiograph showing a large ossifying fibroma (arrowed) occupying most of the body of the mandible with considerable internal calcification. **C** Right side of a panoramic radiograph showing a large mature radiopaque ossifying fibroma (arrowed).

Other important bone conditions

Paget's disease of bone and osteopetrosis, two generalized conditions that can cause an overall increase in bone radiopacity, are discussed in detail in Chapter 32.

TYPICAL RADIOGRAPHIC FEATURES OF SOFT TISSUE CALCIFICATIONS

A variety of radiopaque calcifications within the overlying soft tissues can present radiographically. Differential diagnosis is relatively straightforward once the **site** of the opacity has been determined.

Radiopaque salivary calculi (see Ch. 33)

Submandibular gland calculi (Fig. 28.20) are often radiopaque and develop within the main duct or in the gland itself. Those in the main duct can be superimposed on the alveolar bone producing an opacity apparently within the bone. Stones in the gland present usually below the lower border of the mandible.

Calcified lymph nodes (Fig. 28.21)

Calcification of lymphoid tissue is relatively common following chronic infection (e.g. tuberculosis), especially in older patients.

- *Nodes involved*: Submandibular or cervical chain, single or multiple.
- *Site*: Behind or below the angle of the mandible.
- *Appearance*: Irregular heterogeneous opaque mass, said to resemble a *mass of coral*.

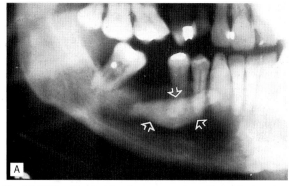
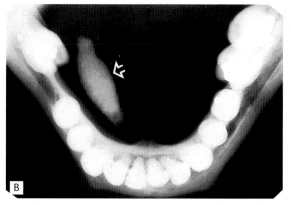

Fig. 28.20A   Right side of a panoramic radiograph showing a large radiopacity in the lower premolar region (arrowed). **B** Lower 90° occlusal of the same patient showing the opacity to be a large stone in the right submandibular duct.

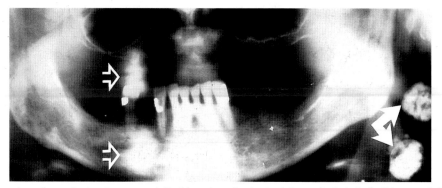

Fig. 28.21 Panoramic radiograph showing two calcified lymph nodes in the left cervical chain (solid arrows). Note also the *ghost* shadows of the lymph nodes on the right premolar/canine region (open arrows).

Calcified tonsils (Fig. 28.22)

Calcification of the tonsillar lymphoid tissue is sometimes seen as an incidental finding on dental panoramic radiographs, especially in elderly patients. Areas of calcification appear as small irregular opaque masses overlying the superior aspect of the ramus of the mandible; they are often bilateral.

Phleboliths (Fig. 28.23)

Phleboliths are calcifications of thrombi within veins and are occasionally seen in haemangiomas. If the radiograph shows the calcified blood vessel end-on, the phlebolith has a characteristic *target* appearance — radiopaque around the periphery and radiolucent in the centre.

Calcified acne scars

Occasionally calcification can develop in the scars of severe acne producing multiple small radiopacities in the area involved. If acne calcification is suspected radiographically, the diagnosis can be confirmed by clinical examination.

TYPICAL RADIOGRAPHIC FEATURES OF FOREIGN BODIES

A variety of foreign bodies can produce radiopacities. The appearance depends obviously on the nature of the foreign body, its density and its location. Figure 28.24 shows a selection of foreign bodies.

FOOTNOTE

It is worth repeating that the radiodensity of many of the lesions mentioned in this chapter changes as they mature. During their early stages of development, there may be no evidence of internal calcification, making radiological differential diagnosis more difficult. For revision purposes Table 28.2 summarizes the main lesions of variable radiodensity which can develop internal radiopaque calcifications and so present with mixed radiolucent/radiopaque appearances.

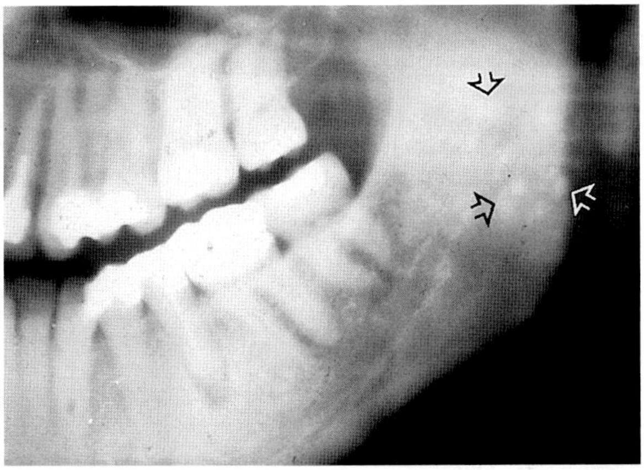

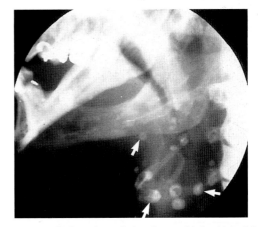

Fig. 28.22 Left side of a panoramic radiograph showing the typical appearance of tonsillar calcifications (arrowed) overlying the ramus of the mandible.

Fig. 28.23 Oblique lateral showing multiple phleboliths (arrowed) associated with a haemangioma. Note the typical *target* appearance of some of the calcifications.

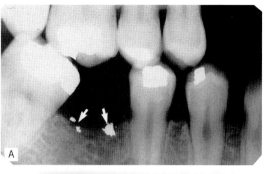

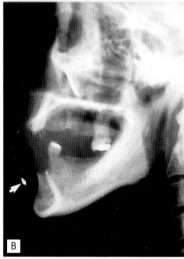

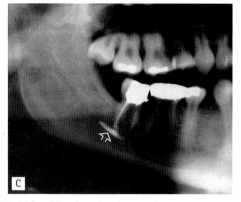

Table 28.2   Summary of the main lesions that can present with variable radiodensity by developing internal radiopaque calcifications

Tumours
   Calcifying epithelial odontogenic tumour (CEOT)
   Ameloblastic fibro-odontoma
   Adenomatoid odontogenic tumour (AOT)
   Calcifying cystic odontogenic tumour
   Cementoblastoma
   Chondroma
   Osteoma
   Osteogenic osteosarcoma
Osseous dysplasias
   Periapical osseous dysplasia
   Focal osseous dysplasia
   Florid osseous dysplasia
   Familial gigantiform cementoma
Bone-related lesions
   Fibrous dysplasia
   Ossifying fibroma

Fig. 28.24A   Bitewing showing amalgam remnants (arrowed), dislodged and left behind after an extraction. If evident clinically, they are referred to as *amalgam tattoos*. **B** True lateral skull showing a radiopaque foriegn body (arrowed) in the lower lip. **C** Right side of a panoramic radiograph showing radiopaque root canal sealant (arrowed) in the inferior dental canal.

Chapter 29

The maxillary antra

INTRODUCTION

The maxillary antra, because of their close proximity to the upper teeth, are the most important of the paranasal sinuses in dentistry. Nowadays the imaging modalities of choice to investigate possible disease within the antra are computed tomography (CT), cone beam CT and magnetic resonance (MR) (see Ch. 19). However, as the antra are often imaged on conventional dental radiographs, as well as on certain skull views, clinicians still need to know:

- The anatomy of the antra, including their shape, size, normal variations and related structures.
- How the antra are represented normally on conventional dental and skull radiographs and how these radiographs are assessed.
- The radiographic features of disease.

Similar radiographic changes can be seen in the other paranasal sinuses — frontal, ethmoidal and sphenoidal. They are of less clinical relevance in dentistry and are discussed only briefly.

NORMAL ANATOMY

The maxillary antrum or sinus is an approximately pyramidal cavity. It contains air, is lined by mucoperiosteum with a pseudostratified ciliated columnar epithelium and occupies most of the body of the maxillary bone. It is present at birth, but at that stage it is little more than a slit-like out-pouching of the nasal cavity. It grows rapidly by a process known as pneumatization during the eruption of the deciduous teeth and reaches about half its adult size by three years of age. The final size of the antra (like the other air sinuses) is very variable.

Pneumatization in adulthood causes further changes in antral shape and size. The cavity often enlarges downwards into the alveolar process or laterally into the body of the zygoma. The internal surface can be smooth or ridged with prominent bony septa. The lateral wall contains canals or grooves for the nerves and blood vessels supplying the upper posterior teeth.

The main anatomical parts of the antra (see Fig. 29.1) can be divided into:

- A central air-filled cavity
- A roof or upper border, bounded by the orbit
- A medial wall, bounded by the nasal cavity
- A posterior wall, related to the pterygopalatine fossa
- A lateral wall, related to the zygoma and cheek
- An anterior wall, related to the cheek
- A floor, related to the apices of the upper posterior teeth.

NORMAL APPEARANCE OF THE ANTRA ON CONVENTIONAL RADIOGRAPHS

An antrum appears radiographically as a radiolucent cavity in the maxilla, with well-defined, dense, corticated radiopaque margins or walls. In general, the larger the cavity the more radiolucent it will appear. The internal bony septa and blood vessel canals in the walls all produce their own shadows. The thin epithelial lining is not normally seen. The different parts of the antra shown on conventional dental and skull radiographs are summarized in Table 29.1. Typical normal radiographic appearances are shown in Figures 29.2–29.4. In addition a suggested systematic approach to viewing the antra on the 0° OM is shown in Figure 29.4.

Fig. 29.1 Diagrams of a left antrum showing the basic shape and various walls and margins. **A** From the front. **B** From the side.

Table 29.1 Summary of the different parts of the antra shown on conventional dental and skull radiographs

Area of antrum shown	Radiographic projection
Floor	Periapical
	Upper oblique occlusal
	Panoramic
Main antral cavity	0° OM
	True lateral skull
Lower aspect of antral cavity	Periapical
	Upper oblique occlusal
	Panoramic
Posterior wall	Panoramic
	True lateral skull
Anteromedial wall	Panoramic
	True lateral skull
Lateral wall	0° OM
Roof	0° OM
Relationship with upper posterior teeth	Periapical
	Upper oblique occlusal
	Panoramic

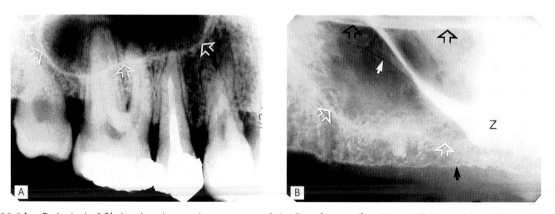

Fig. 29.2A Periapical of 8| showing the usual appearance of the floor (arrowed) and base of the antral cavity in relation to the upper posterior teeth in a dentate adult. **B** Periapical of 8| showing the various normal anatomical structures evident in an edentulous adult. These include: the floor of the antrum (white open arrows), the floor of the nasal cavity (black open arrows), the inferior surface of the alveolar ridge (black solid arrows), radiolucent neurovascular channels in the antral wall (solid white arrow) and the zygomatic buttress (Z).

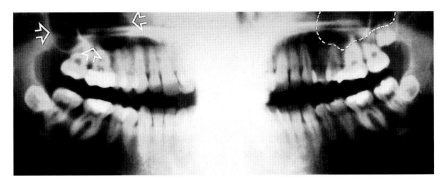

Fig. 29.3 Panoramic radiograph showing the usual appearance of the antral floor, medial and posterior walls. These have been drawn in on the patient's LEFT side and are arrowed on the RIGHT side.

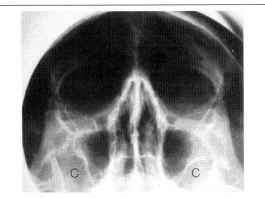

General overview of the entire film

1 Check the positioning of the patient's head, noting particularly :-
 • Any rotation or asymmetry
 • Adequate backward tilting of the head to throw the shadows of the petrous parts of the temporal bones below the antra

2 Check the exposure factors

3 Stand back and view the film from a distance (1–2 m)

The antra

4 Compare the antral shadows on both sides — they should be radiolucent

5 Compare the radiodensity of the antrum on each side with the radiodensity of the soft tissue shadow lateral to it (marked C on the radiograph above). The antra should be more radiolucent since they contain air.

6 Check the integrity and shape of the roof and lateral walls

7 Check the medial wall — this is the least well-defined zone and hence the most difficult to interpret

Fig. 29.4 Standard occipitomental (0° OM) showing the normal radiolucent appearance of the antral cavities together with a suggested systematic approach for examining the antra. Note: Swelling of the soft tissues of the cheek overlying an antrum may cause that antrum to appear opaque when compared to the other side, but it will still be radiolucent when compared with the adjacent cheek shadow.

ANTRAL DISEASE

The major pathological conditions that can affect the antra, directly or indirectly, include:

- Infection/inflammation
  - Acute sinusitis
  - Chronic sinusitis.
- Trauma
  - Oro-antral communication
  - Fractures of the maxillofacial skeleton
  - Foreign bodies within the antrum.
- Cysts
  - Intrinsic
  - Extrinsic.
- Tumours
  - Intrinsic
  - Extrinsic.
- Other bone abnormalities (see Ch. 32)
  - Fibrous dysplasia
  - Paget's disease of bone
  - Osteopetrosis.

These various disease entities can result in the following radiological changes:

- Total or partial opacity/obliteration of the main antral cavity
- Alteration in the integrity of the antral walls, including discontinuity as a result of a fracture or destruction by an intrinsic or extrinsic tumour
- Alteration in the antral outline, including expansion or compression caused by an intrinsic or extrinsic lesion or disease process
- The presence of a foreign body within the antrum.

INVESTIGATION AND APPEARANCE OF DISEASE WITHIN THE ANTRA

Various imaging modalities can be used to investigate possible disease within the antra, depending on their availability. These include:

- Computed tomography (CT) — currently recommended by the Royal College of Radiologists in the UK
- Cone beam CT
- Magnetic resonance (MR)
- Multidirectional (spiral) tomography
- Dental panoramic radiography
- Intraoral periapical/occlusal radiography
- Skull radiography
  - 0° occipitomental
  - True lateral.

Appearances of antral diseases using various imaging modalities are shown in Figures 29.5–29.23.

Infection / inflammation

Acute sinusitis

Acute sinusitis is most commonly caused by an upper respiratory tract infection, particularly the common cold. The effects on the antrum include:

- Thickening of the antral mucosal lining
- Increase in secretions
- Formation of pus.

Acute sinusitis can be diagnosed and treated clinically. As a result, the Royal College of Radiologists in the UK in their booklet *Making Best Use of a Department of Clinical Radiology* 5th ed (2003) recommend that radiological imaging is not necessary.

Chronic sinusitis (Figs 29.5–29.9)

Important causes
- Prolonged antral infection (10 days).
- Trauma, including roots or teeth displaced into the antrum or the formation of an oro-antral communication.
- Apical infection associated with an upper posterior tooth (rare).

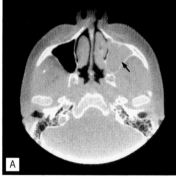
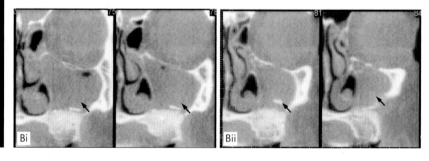
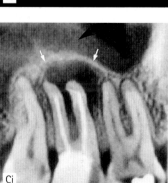
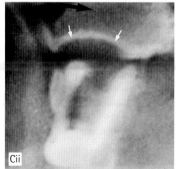

Fig. 29.5 Examples of antral infection/inflammation shown using cone beam CT. **A** Axial scan and **B** series of coronal images showing total opacity of the antrum on one side (arrowed). (Reproduced with kind permission of Imaging Sciences International, Inc.) **C** (i) Sagittal and (ii) coronal images showing apical infection associated with 7| that has resulted in re-modelling of the antral floor creating the *antral halo* appearance (white arrows), with associated mucosal thickening (black arrows) (kindly provided by Prof D. Benn).

Typical effects on the antrum

- Some shrinkage of the thickened mucosal lining from the acute phase.
- Continued formation of secretions and pus.
- Sometimes mucosal polyp formation.
- Sometimes thickening of the antral walls.
- Destruction and remodelling of the antral floor associated with an infected tooth apex.

Main radiological features

- Total/partial opacity within the antral cavity.

- Fluid level — usually in the base of antral cavity with a characteristic meniscus shape.
- Round, domed opacity produced by a mucosal polyp.
- Occasionally an increase in the bony antral walls.
- Typical inflammatory changes if infected teeth are involved — this may lead to resorption and remodelling to produce the appearance described as *antral halo* (see also Ch. 22).
- Evidence of a foreign body (if applicable).

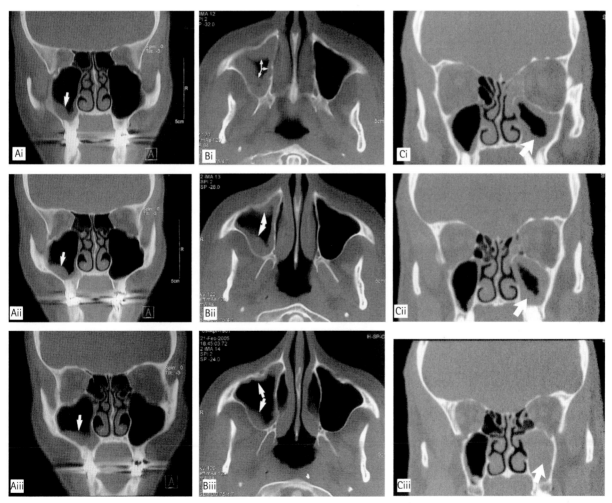

Fig. 29.6 Various appearances of the effects of chronic sinusitis shown on CT. **A** Contiguous coronal CT scans showing mucosal thickening in the base of the antrum (arrowed). **B** Contiguous axial CT scans showing mucosal thickening on the medial and lateral walls of the antrum (arrowed) (kindly provided by Drs J. Kabala and J. Luker). **C** Contiguous coronal CT scans showing mucosal thickening and total opacity of the antrum (arrowed).

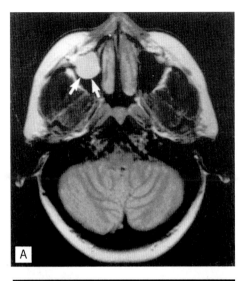

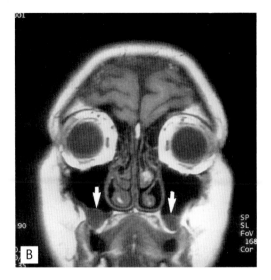

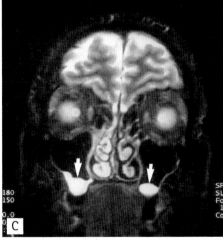

Fig. 29.7 Various appearances of the effects of chronic sinusitis shown on MR. **A** Axial MR scan showing a round antral mucous retention cyst (arrowed) arising from the anterolateral wall. **B** T1-weighted and **C** T2-weighted coronal MR images of the same patient with bilateral mucosal retention cysts (arrowed) (kindly provided by Drs J. Kabala and J. Luker).

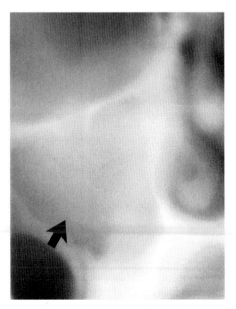

Fig. 29.8 A 2 mm-thick Scanora® spiral tomographic cross-sectional image showing a totally opaque chronically infected right antrum (arrowed).

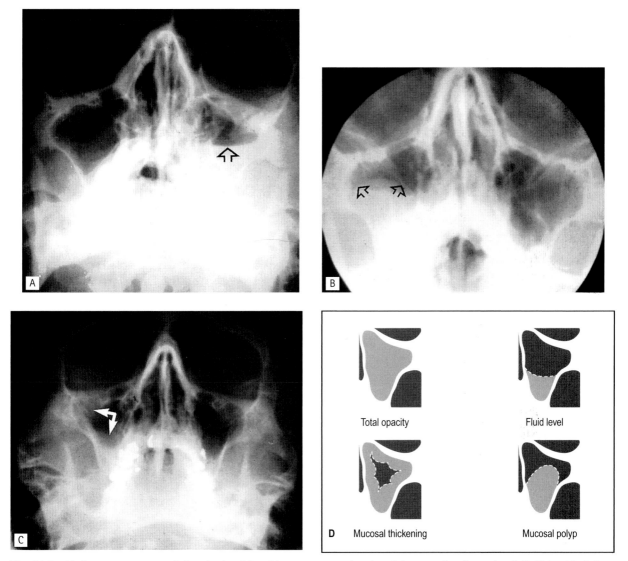

Fig. 29.9 Various appearances of chronic sinusitis evident on conventional occipitomental radiographs. **A** Fluid level in left antrum (arrowed) — note the shape of the meniscus. **B** Round, domed antral polyp in the base of the right antrum (arrowed). **C** Mucosal thickening on the inner aspects of the lateral walls of the right antrum (arrowed). **D** Simplified line diagrams of the left antrum (as depicted on a 0° OM) illustrating the various appearances.

Trauma

Oro-antral communication

Important causes
- Extraction of closely related upper posterior teeth can remove part of the antral floor or fracture the tuberosity.
- Inappropriate or incorrect use of elevators during root or tooth removal — may also cause the root, or rarely the tooth, to be displaced into the antrum.

Main radiographic features
- Break in the continuity of the floor may be evident (see Fig. 29.10) — however, the diagnosis of an oro-antral communication is made clinically, not radiographically, since the defect in the floor of the antrum may not be evident on the two-dimensional radiograph.
- Characteristic features of acute or chronic sinusitis (see earlier) owing to the ingress of bacteria.
- Evidence of the displaced root or tooth — a second view of the antrum with the head in a different position may be required to ascertain the exact location of the displaced object.

Fractures of the maxillo-facial skeleton

Fractures are discussed in detail in Chapter 30 and only a brief summary is shown below.

Important sites possibly involving the antra
- Le Fort I
- Le Fort II
- Le Fort III
- Zygomatic complex
- Naso-ethmoidal complex
- Orbit
  - Rim
  - Blow-out
- Dento-alveolar.

Main radiographic features
- Break in the continuity of one or more of the antral walls depending on the type of fracture.
- Total opacity or fluid level within the antral cavity caused by haemorrhage (see Figs 29.11 and 29.12).
- Features of sinusitis if subsequent infection develops (this is in fact surprisingly rare).
- The orbital blow-out fracture classically produces a tear-drop-shaped opacity in the upper part of the antrum, the *hanging drop* appearance, caused

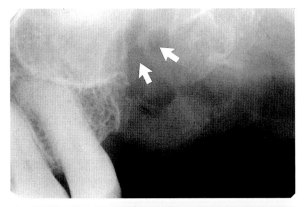

Fig. 29.10 Periapical of |Q showing a discontinuity of the antral floor (arrowed) following the extraction of the molar tooth that resulted in a clinical oro-antral communication. Note this break in continuity of the floor is not always evident in cases of oro-antral communication.

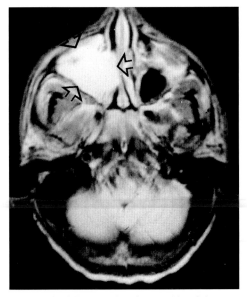

Fig. 29.11 Axial MR scan showing a white right antrum (arrowed) that was filled with blood following a middle third facial fracture. (Kindly supplied by Mrs J. E. Brown.)

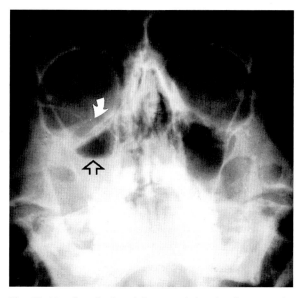

Fig. 29.12   Standard occipitomental showing fracture of the right zygomatic complex with a break in the antral roof (white arrow). The right antrum shows a definite fluid level as a result of blood in the antrum (open arrow).

by herniation of the orbital contents downwards into the antrum following collapse of the antral roof (see Fig. 29.13). The infraorbital margin remains intact. See also Figure 30.30.

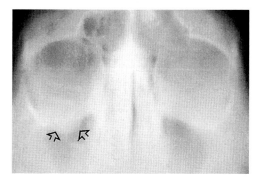

Fig. 29.13   Coronal section tomograph of a patient with an orbital blow-out fracture of the right orbital floor/antral roof showing the downward herniated contents of the orbit into the antrum (arrowed), the so-called *hanging drop* appearance.

Foreign bodies in the antrum

Important causes
- Displaced root fragments or teeth.
- Excess root canal filling material forced through the apex of an upper posterior tooth during endodontics.
- Antrolith — calcification within the antrum.
- Foreign material pushed into the antrum through an existing oro-antral communication.

Main radiographic features
- The presence, position and often the nature of the foreign body.
- Occasionally associated sinusitis.

Cysts

The more important cysts that can affect the antra include:

- Intrinsic — mucosal retention cyst
- Extrinsic — odontogenic cysts, e.g.:
  - Radicular (dental) cysts ⎫ associated with
  - Residual cysts ⎬ upper posterior
  - Dentigerous cysts ⎭ teeth.

Mucosal retention cyst

Cause
The cause is unknown, but is presumably due to blockage of a mucus-secreting cell in the antral lining.

Main radiographic features (see Figs 29.7 and 29.9B)
- Incidental finding.
- Well-defined, round, dome-shaped opacity within the antrum varying in size from a tiny lesion to one completely filling the antrum.
- Usually no evidence of thickening of the remainder of the epithelial lining.
- Usually no alteration of the antral outline
- Occasionally bilateral (see Fig. 29.14).

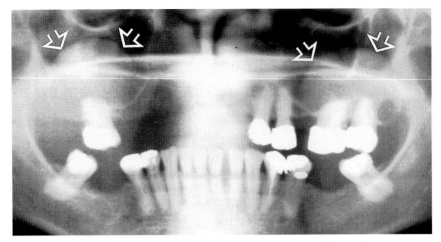

Fig. 29.14 Panoramic radiograph showing bilateral antral mucosal retention cysts (arrowed).

Odontogenic cysts

These cysts are extrinsic to the antra developing in the alveolar bone beneath the antral floor.

Main radiographic features of a small cyst

- Round, dome-shaped opacity in the base of the antrum with a well-defined, radiopaque corticated margin to the edge of the meniscus, i.e. the odontogenic cyst has a bony margin and so can be differentiated from the soft tissue mucosal retention cyst or antral polyp (see Figs 29.15 and 29.16).
- Lateral expansion of the alveolar bone.

- Sometimes displacement of the associated tooth.

Main radiographic features of a large cyst

- Total opacity of the antral region owing to complete compression of the antral cavity.
- Loss of antral outline.
- Sometimes displacement of the associated tooth (see Figs 29.17 and 29.18).

Note: Subsequent marsupialization or decompression of the cyst will usually result in the reformation of the antral cavity.

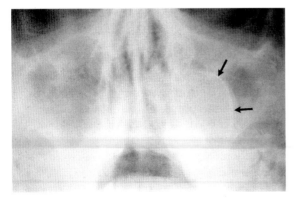

Fig. 29.15 Occipitomental showing the well-defined, round, domed opacity on the left side caused by a radicular (dental) cyst arising from |3. The radiopaque (white) corticated margin to the top of the meniscus (the displaced antral floor) is arrowed.

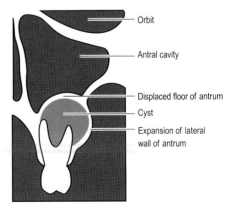

Fig. 29.16 Simplified line diagram illustrating the essential radiographic features of a small odontogenic cyst and its effects on the antrum (as depicted on an 0° OM).

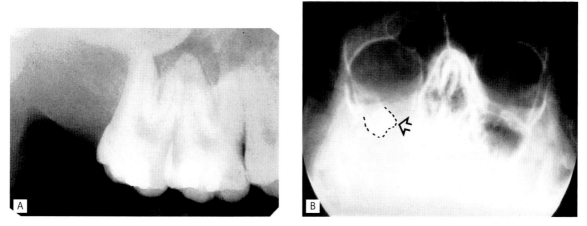

Fig. 29.17 Large dentigerous cyst associated with 8]. **A** Periapical of the upper right posterior teeth. Note the lack of antral floor outline and absence of 8]. **B** Occipitomental of the same patient showing total opacity of the right antral region with no evidence of the lateral antral margin. The displaced upper wisdom tooth is evident underneath the orbit (outlined and arrowed).

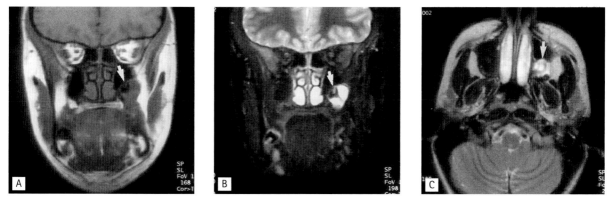

Fig. 29.18 MR images of a dentigerous associated with an unerupted displaced third molar expanding into the antrum. **A** T1-weighted coronal image showing the cyst and unerupted tooth (arrowed). **B** T2-weighted coronal image — the cyst fluid appears white (arrowed). **C** T2-weighted axial showing the cyst (arrowed) (kindly provided by Drs J. Kabala and J. Luker).

Tumours

Benign intrinsic tumours

These are all rare but can include:
- *Papilloma* — this produces, radiographically, a well-defined, non-specific, soft tissue opacity within the antrum
- *Osteoma* — this produces, radiographically, a well-defined, round or lobulated, homogeneous, densely opaque mass within the antrum. The osteoma is most common in the frontal sinus.

Malignant intrinsic tumours

Squamous cell carcinoma and adenocarcinoma — these uncommon but important tumours produce a rapidly growing, aggressive soft tissue mass within the antrum causing destruction of one or more of the antral walls.

Main radiographic features of a small early lesion
- Non-specific, well-defined, round soft tissue opacity within the antrum.
- Variable destruction of the bony antral walls.

Main radiographic features of a large well-established lesion

- Total opacity of the antral cavity (see Fig. 29.19) — in the absence of symptoms suggesting infection, or a history of trauma, a totally opaque antrum is a cause for serious concern and further investigation is necessary.
- Destruction of one or more of the antral walls (see Fig. 29.20) and invasion of surrounding hard and soft tissues—hence the need for CT.
- Occasional displacement or resorption of teeth.

Extrinsic tumours

Any tumour that can affect the maxilla — whether benign or malignant — can have an effect on the antra with the typical associated bony changes.

All are uncommon but three of the more important tumours are:

- Ameloblastoma
- Osteosarcoma
- Squamous cell carcinoma.

The main radiographic features of concern are those indicating malignancy and include:

- Total/partial opacity of the antral cavity
- Destruction of one or more of the walls of the antrum
- Expansion of the maxilla
- Occasional displacement or resorption and loosening of the adjacent teeth (Figs 29.21–29.23).

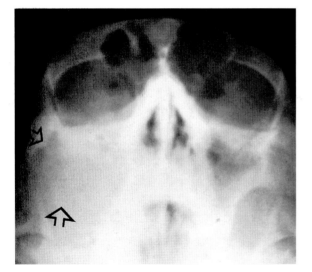

Fig. 29.19 Occipitomental showing a totally opaque right antrum caused by a large squamous cell carcinoma, with destruction of the lateral antral wall (large arrow) and zygoma (small arrow).

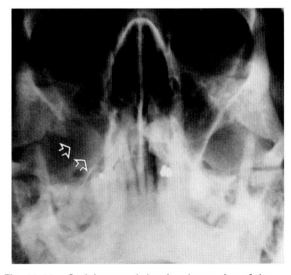

Fig. 29.20 Occipitomental showing destruction of the lateral wall of the right antrum (arrowed) by a squamous cell carcinoma. In this case, there is little evidence of increased opacity within the antrum.

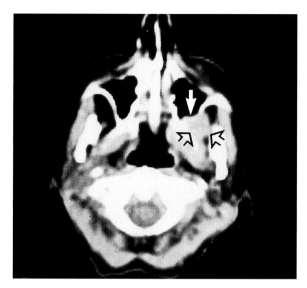

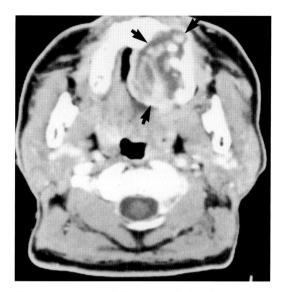

Fig. 29.21   An axial CT scan showing a destructive squamous cell carcinoma (arrowed) in the pterygopalatine fossa invading the posterior antral wall.

Fig. 29.22   An axial CT scan at the level of the antral floor showing a very extensive destructive lesion (arrowed) that proved histologically to be an osteosarcoma.

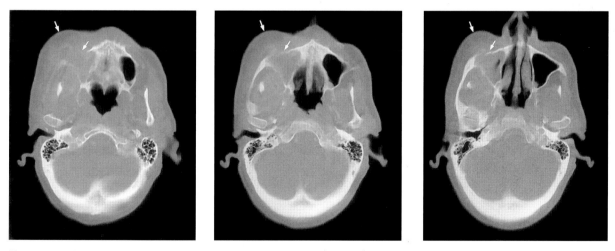

Fig. 29.23   A series of axial CT slices showing a very large mass (arrowed) of a squamous cell carcinoma probably arising in the cheek showing extensive local destruction including the lateral wall of the antrum and extension into the antrum (kindly provided by Drs J. Kabala and J. Luker).

OTHER PARANASAL AIR SINUSES

As mentioned earlier, the frontal, ethmoidal and sphenoidal air sinuses are of limited importance in routine dentistry. Many of the conditions described in relation to the maxillary antra can affect these paranasal sinuses and produce similar effects. Occasionally routine skull radiography reveals unusual abnormalities, such as the *ivory osteoma* in the frontal sinus (see Fig. 29.24). But generally the investigation of choice for the paranasal air sinuses is computed tomography (CT), as shown in Figure 29.25.

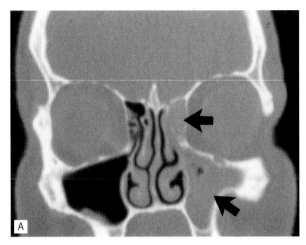

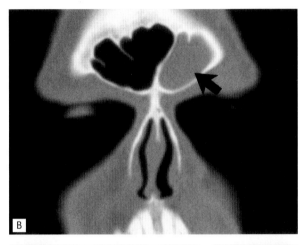

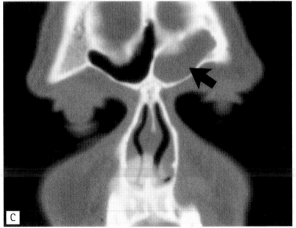

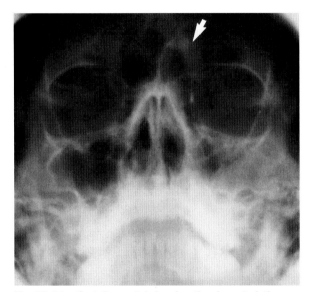

Fig. 29.24 Occipitomental showing the characteristic opacity of a benign ivory osteoma (arrowed) in the frontal sinus.

Fig. 29.25 Three coronal CT scans of the same patient showing, **A**, total opacity of the maxillary, ethmoidal and **B, C** frontal sinuses (arrowed) on one side as a result of acute infection.

Chapter 30

Trauma to the teeth and facial skeleton

INTRODUCTION

Injuries to the teeth and facial skeleton are, unfortunately, common. The type and severity of injuries can vary considerably, from minor damage to the teeth to grossly comminuted fractures of the skull.

Whatever the suspected injury, radiography is an essential requirement both in the initial assessment and in the follow-up appraisal. However, the radiographic examination may be restricted and limited by the general state of the patient and the type and severity of other injuries. For example, severe facial injuries are often associated with intracranial damage and/or cervical spine injuries, the importance of which far outweighs any damage to the teeth and their supporting structures. The radiographic investigation must therefore be tailored to each patient's needs.

This chapter outlines the approach to radiographic investigation of trauma by separating injuries into four distinct categories:

- Injuries to the teeth and their supporting structures
- Fractures of the mandible
- Fractures of the middle third of the facial skeleton
- Other injuries involving:
  - The skull vault
  - The cranial base
  - The cervical spine
  - Intracranial tissues.

INJURIES TO THE TEETH AND THEIR SUPPORTING STRUCTURES

Types of injury

Based broadly on the classification suggested by Andreasen and Andreasen (2001), the different types of dental injuries can be divided into:

- Fractures of the teeth
- Luxation injuries to the teeth
- Fractures of the alveolar bone
- Other injuries.

Fractures of the teeth

These include:

- Coronal fractures:
  - Involving only enamel
  - Involving enamel and dentine
  - Involving enamel, dentine and the pulp
  - Involving enamel, dentine and cementum
  - Involving enamel, dentine, cementum and the pulp.
- Root fractures:
  - Without a coronal fracture
  - With a coronal fracture.

Luxation injuries

These include:

- Concussion
- Subluxation
- Intrusive luxation
- Extrusive luxation
- Lateral luxation
- Avulsion.

Fractures of the alveolar bone

These include:

- Fractures of the socket
- Fractures of the alveolar process
- Fracture of the associated jaw.

Other injuries

These include:

- Displacement of an underlying developing tooth which may become dilacerated as a result
- Soft tissue injuries, such as:
  - Laceration
  - Imbedding of a foreign body
- Iatrogenic injuries, such as:
  - Injuries sustained during extractions, including damage to adjacent teeth and fracture of the associated alveolar bone
  - Perforation of the tooth apex or side of the root during conservative or endodontic treatment
- Swallowing or inhaling an avulsed tooth.

Radiographic investigation

Although the type of injury may be evident clinically, radiographic investigation of all traumatized teeth is needed initially, to assess fully the degree of underlying damage. Radiographs are also required later to assess healing and/or the development of post-trauma complications. The ideal radiographic requirements include:

- Two views of the injured tooth from different angles, ideally at right angles to one another, but more usually with the X-ray tubehead in two different positions in the *vertical* plane. For example in the anterior region:
  - A *periapical* (paralleling technique)
  - An *upper standard occlusal*
- Reproducible views to provide a base-line assessment and to allow subsequent follow-up evaluation
- Views of the chest and/or abdomen if a tooth or foreign body is thought to have been inhaled or swallowed, including:
  - Soft tissue lateral and AP of the larynx and pharynx

  - PA of the chest
  - Right lateral of the chest
  - AP of the abdomen.

Diagnostic information provided

The diagnostic information provided by these radiographs may include:

- The type of injury to the teeth
- The site(s) of fractures
- The degree of displacement of the tooth fragments
- The stage of root development
- The condition of the apical tissues
- The presence, site and displacement of alveolar bone fractures
- The condition of adjacent or underlying teeth
- Evidence of healing
- Post-trauma complications, including:
  - Resorption
  - Infection
  - Cessation of tooth development
- The location of the tooth if swallowed or inhaled.

Radiographic interpretation

The expected radiographic features indicating a fractured root are shown in Figure 30.1 and include:

- A radiolucent line between the fragments
- An alteration in the outline shape of the root and discontinuity of the periodontal ligament shadow.

Examples of injured teeth and some of the more common post-injury complications evident radiographically, are shown in Figures 30.2 and 30.3.

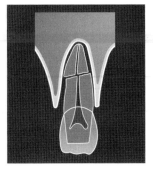

Fig. 30.1 Diagram illustrating the radiographic appearance of a theoretical root fracture showing a radiolucent line between the fragments, alteration in the outline shape of the root and discontinuity of the periodontal ligament shadow.

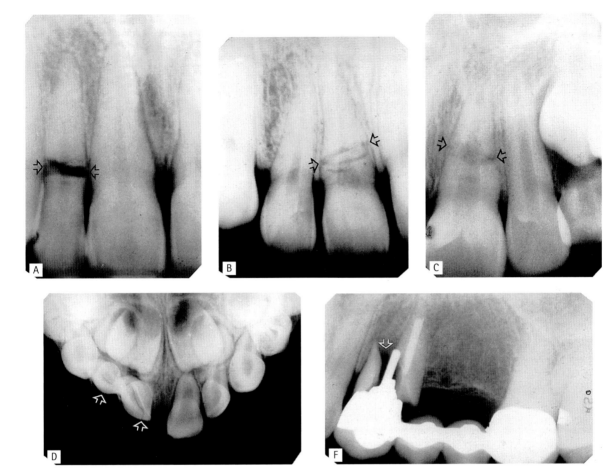

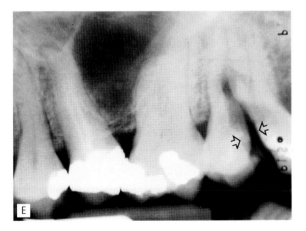

Fig. 30.2 Examples of traumatized teeth and their supporting structures. **A** Root fracture of 2| (arrowed), just beyond the cervical region, with wide separation of the fragments. **B** Root fracture of 1|; three radiolucent lines are evident, but only minimal separation of the fragments and disruption of the root outline (arrowed). **C** Root fracture of |1; a broad radiolucent zone is evident across the root with marked discontinuity in root outline and the periodontal ligament shadow (arrowed). **D** Intrusion and fracture of BA| (arrowed), but with no apparent displacement of the underlying permanent teeth. Intrusion is often associated with fracture of the labial bone (not evident on this view). **E** Vertical fracture of the crown and root of |7 (arrowed). **F** Fracture of |4 root (arrowed) with wide separation of the fragments owing to stresses transmitted through the post.

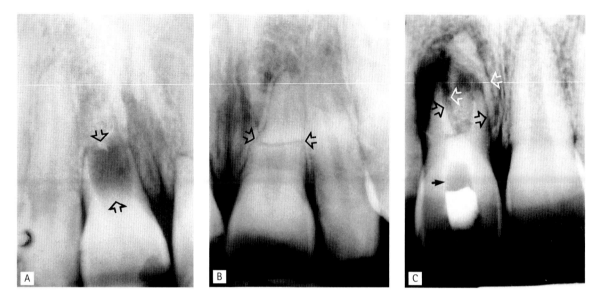

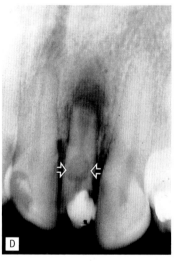

Fig. 30.3 Examples of common post-injury complications. **A** Immature root form following complete cessation of root development after death of 1⌋ at the time of injury (arrowed). **B** ⌊1of the same patient showing a complete, but abnormally shaped, root with (root) fracture (arrowed). The periodontal ligament shadow is continuous. **C** Apical infection and resorption of 1⌋ resulting in separation and displacement of the root fragments (open arrows). A radiopaque calcium hydroxide dressing is evident in the root canal with a radiopaque temporary restoration in the crown. The radiolucent area in between contains cottonwool (solid arrow). **D** Apical infection, external resorption of the apex and extensive internal root resorption (arrowed) of ⌊2, following a coronal fracture involving the pulp. A radiopaque temporary dressing is evident in the crown. **E** Large area of apical infection associated with 1⌋ (open arrows). Root formation of 1⌋ has ceased and the apex is immature. In addition, the 2⌋ (damaged but not killed by the original trauma) shows complete sclerosis of the pulp chamber (solid arrows). **F** Severe dilaceration and non-eruption of ⌊1 (arrowed), following trauma to the deciduous incisors several years previously.

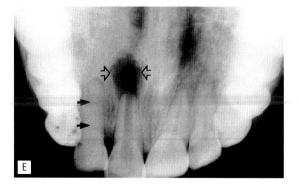

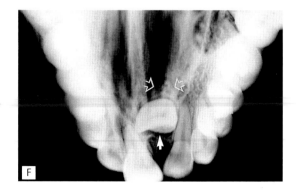

Limitations of radiographic interpretation of fractured roots

Unfortunately, as a result of the inherent limitations of a two-dimensional image, radiographic interpretation of traumatized teeth is not always as straightforward as Figures 30.2 and 30.3 may suggest.

As shown in Figure 30.4 the radiographic appearances can be influenced by:

- The position and severity of the fracture
- The degree of displacement or separation of the fragments
- The position of the film and X-ray tubehead in relation to the fracture line(s).

It is for these reasons that a minimum of two views, from two different angles, is essential.

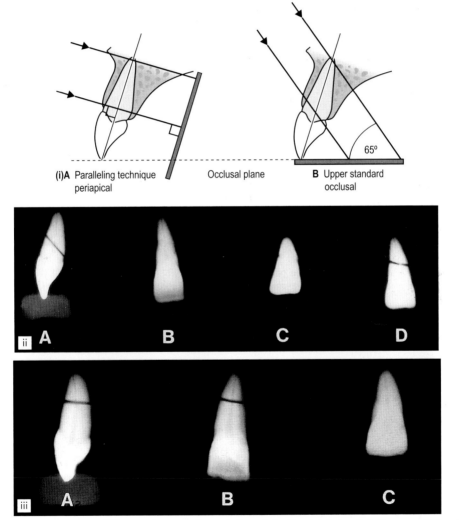

Fig. 30.4(i) Diagram showing the difference in vertical angulation of the X-ray tubehead. **A** For a paralleling technique periapical. **B** An upper standard occlusal of the maxillary incisors. **(ii)** The different radiographic appearances of a tangential root fracture using different projections. **A** From the side showing the direction of the fracture and separation of the fragments. **B** Using a horizontal X-ray beam. **C** Using a steeply angled (75°) X-ray beam. **D** Using an angled (65°) X-ray beam. **(iii)** The different radiographic appearances of a horizontal root fracture. **A** From the side. **B** Using a horizontal X-ray beam. **C** Using an angled (65°) X-ray beam.

SKELETAL FRACTURES

As mentioned earlier, radiographs are an essential part of the initial assessment and follow-up appraisal of all patients with suspected facial fractures. They are crucial in evaluating:

- The presence of fractures
- The site and direction of the fracture line(s)
- The degree of displacement and separation of the bone ends
- The relationship of teeth to the fracture line
- The location of associated foreign bodies in hard and soft tissues
- The presence of coincidental or contributory disease
- The alignment of the bone fragments after treatment
- Healing and the identification of post-trauma complications including infection, non-union or malunion.

FRACTURES OF THE MANDIBLE

Clinicians need to know:

- **Where** the mandible tends to fracture
- **Which** radiographic views are required to show each of the fracture sites
- **What** radiological features indicate the presence of fracture(s)
- **How** to assess the radiographs for possible fractures.

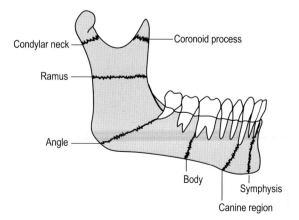

Fig. 30.5 Diagram showing the main fracture sites of the mandible. Although only one side of the jaw is illustrated, mandibular fractures are often bilateral.

Main fracture sites

The main sites where the mandible tends to fracture are shown in Figure 30.5.

Radiographic projections required

Several different views are used to show the various fracture sites. Once again, the ideal minimum requirement in all cases is two views at right angles to one another. When that is not possible, two views at two different angles should be used. In addition, intraoral views (either periapicals or occlusals) are required when fractures are in the tooth-bearing portion of the mandible and teeth are involved in the fracture line. The typical projections that can be used for the different sites are summarized in Table 30.1.

Table 30.1 Summary of the main mandibular fracture sites and the common radiographic projections used for each site

Fracture site	Commonly used radiographs
Angle	Dental panoramic radiograph or oblique lateral Posteroanterior (PA jaws)
Condylar neck	Dental panoramic radiograph or oblique lateral Posteroanterior (PA jaws) (for low neck fractures) Reverse Towne's (for high neck fractures)
Body	Dental panoramic radiograph or oblique lateral Postero anterior (PA jaws) Periapicals of involved teeth Lower 90° occlusal
Canine region	Dental panoramic radiograph or oblique lateral Periapicals of involved teeth True lateral skull
Symphysis	Lower 45° occlusal Lower 90° occlusal
Ramus	Dental panoramic radiograph or oblique lateral Posteroanterior (PA jaws)
Coronoid process	Dental panoramic radiograph or oblique lateral 0° occipitomental (0° OM)

Radiological features of mandibular fractures (Fig. 30.6)

The typical radiographic appearances include:

- Radiolucent line(s) between the bone fragments if they are separated. Note that fractures through the buccal and lingual cortical plates may produce *two* radiolucent lines
- A radiopaque line if the fragments overlie one another
- An alteration in the outline of the bone if the fragments are displaced, producing a step deformity of the lower border or the occlusal plane.

Important points to note
- The extent/severity of any displacement depends on:
  - The direction and strength of the fracturing force
  - The direction of the resultant fracture line
  - The relevant muscles attached to each fragment and their direction of pull

- If the fracture line runs in such a manner that the associated muscles tend to hold the fragments together, the fracture is described as *favourable*
- If the associated muscles tend to pull the fragments apart, the fracture is described as *unfavourable*.

Radiographic limitations

As mentioned earlier, the limitations of the radiographic image mean that these appearances can be influenced by:

- The position and severity of the fracture
- The degree of displacement or separation of the fragments
- The position of the film and X-ray tubehead in relation to the fracture line(s), as shown in Figure 30.7.

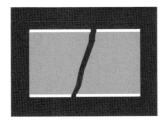

A One radiolucent fracture line with no displacement of the fragments

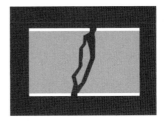

B Two radiolucent fracture lines with no displacement of the fragments

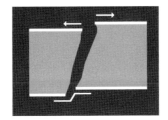

C Wide radiolucent fracture line and step deformity due to separation and displacement of the fragments

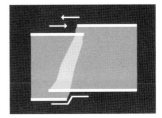

D Radiopaque line due to overlap of the fragments and step deformity also evident

Fig. 30.6 Diagrams illustrating the radiographic appearances of fractures depending on the bony displacement, separation or overlap that could be present.

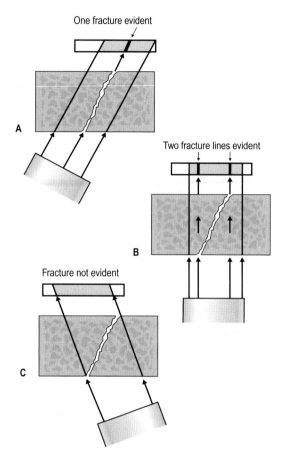

Fig. 30.7 Diagrams illustrating how the position of the film and X-ray tubehead in relation to a fracture can affect the final image.

Important points to note

- It is because of these limitations that at least two views, at different angles, are required.
- If displacement and separation are minimal, there may be **no radiographic evidence** of a fracture at all.

Interpretation of fractures

To emphasize, yet again, the importance of the principles outlined in Chapter 20, before any attempt is made to diagnose a fracture the *quality* of the radiographs should be assessed.

While doing the *overall* critical assessment, it is worth remembering that many patients who have recently been injured may be very difficult to radiograph because of pain, medication, overlying soft tissue wound dressings or other injuries which they may have sustained at the same time. In addition, blood in the antra, nose and pharynx may adversely affect film contrast.

Clinicians should not be too critical of the radiographer; the radiographs obtained are probably the best possible under the circumstances. However, due allowance should be made for these likely technique difficulties when interpreting the final radiographs.

Systematic approach

A suggested sequence for examining radiographs when attempting to diagnose mandibular fractures is shown in Figure 30.8.

Postoperative and follow-up appraisal

When using radiographs postoperatively or in the follow-up appraisal, a similar systematic approach is adopted, but particular attention should be paid to:

- The alignment and approximation of the bone fragments
- The position of intra-osseous wires, bone plates or other fixation
- Healing and bone union
- The condition of any teeth involved in the fracture line
- Evidence of infection or other complications.

Examine the lateral view of the mandible
(usually a panoramic radiograph)

1 Trace the outline of the mandible from one condyle to the other along the lower border

2 Note particularly:
              Any alteration in the outline shape
              Step deformities

3 Examine the ramus and body of the mandible, paying particular attention to the sites where fractures are most common — angle
                  condylar necks
                  body
                  canine region
                  ramus
                  coronoid process

4 Note particularly:
              The presence of radiolucent fracture line(s)
              The direction of the fracture lines
              The degree of separation of the bone fragments
              Any radiopaque line(s) indicating overlying
                  bone ends

Examine the second view of the mandible
(usually a PA jaws)

5 Repeat steps(1) – (4) for the relevant areas of the mandible shown on the second view

Examine the intra-oral views of the teeth

6 Note particularly:
              The relationship of the teeth to the fracture line
              The state of the teeth, including:
                  fractured crowns or roots
                  caries
                  size of restorations
                  periodontal condition
                  apical condition

Fig. 30.8 Suggested sequence to follow when examining radiographs for mandibular fractures.

Examples of mandibular fractures

Examples of fractures of different sites of the mandible, preoperatively and postoperatively, are shown in Figures 30.9–30.17.

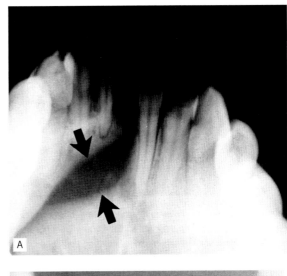

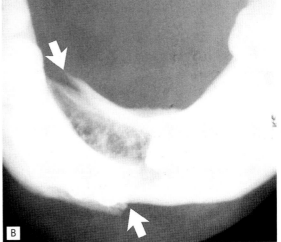

Fig. 30.9A Lower 45° occlusal and **B** Lower 90° occlusal showing a fracture in the symphyseal region (arrowed). Note the lower 45° occlusal shows the displacement in the vertical plane, while the lower 90° occlusal shows the displacement in the horizontal plane.

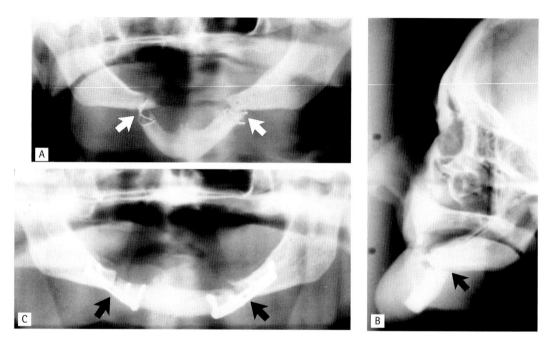

Fig. 30.10A Panoramic radiograph showing bilateral fractures of the canine region, so-called *bucket handle* fractures (arrowed), after the first attempted fixation with intra-osseous wires. **B** True lateral skull. Note the extensive displacement of the anterior segment of the mandible owing to the unopposed pull of the muscles attached to this fragment. This is described as an unfavourable fracture. The inadequate intra-osseous wires are again evident. **C** Panoramic radiograph after fixation with bone plates (arrowed).

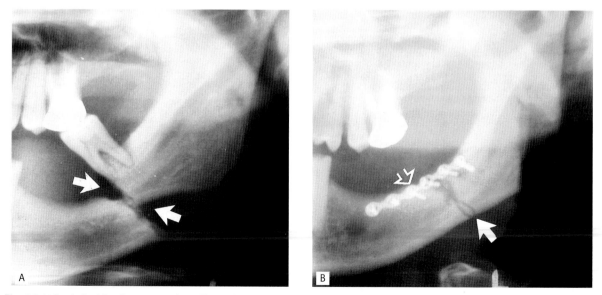

Fig. 30.11A Left side of a panoramic radiograph showing an unfavourable markedly displaced fracture of the body of the mandible (arrowed). **B** Left side of a panoramic radiograph taken postoperatively showing accurate reduction of the fragments (solid arrow) and fixation with a bone plate (open arrow). The lower molar has been extracted.

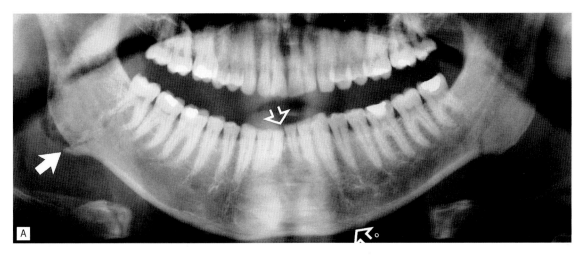

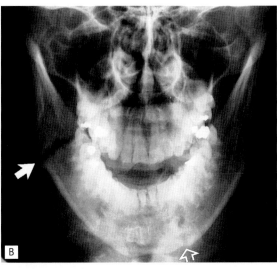

Fig. 30.12A Panoramic radiograph showing bilateral fracture of the mandible – through the right angle and symphyseal/left canine region. Note that the fracture through the angle appears radiopaque as the bony fragments are overlying one another (solid arrow) and that the symphyseal/canine region fracture (open arrow) is almost totally obscured by the overlying ghost shadow of the cervical spine. **B** PA jaws showing the fracture through the angle clearly as a radiolucent line (solid arrow) while the symphyseal/canine region fracture is still difficult to see (open arrow) as a result of superimposition of the cervical spine. **C** Postoperative panoramic radiograph showing reduction and fixation of the bone fragments (arrowed) using bone plates. Arch bars and islet wiring around the teeth are also evident.

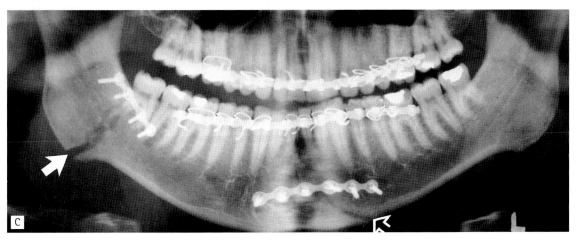

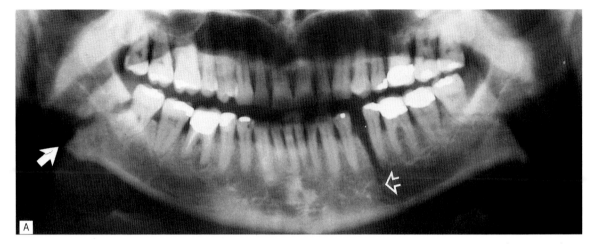

Fig. 30.13A Panoramic radiograph showing a bilateral fracture of the mandible through the right angle (solid arrow) and left body (open arrow) with minimal displacement.

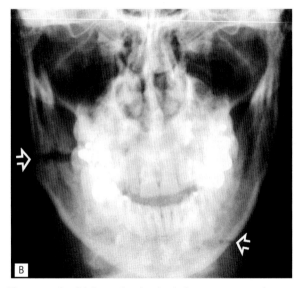

Fig. 30.13B PA jaws showing both fractures arrowed.

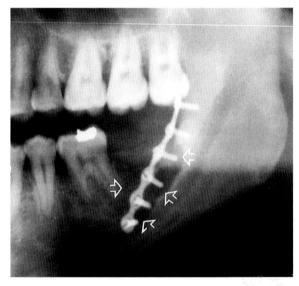

Fig. 30.14 Left side of a panoramic radiograph showing extensive bone resorption (arrowed) as a result of infection around a bone plate that had been used for fracture fixation.

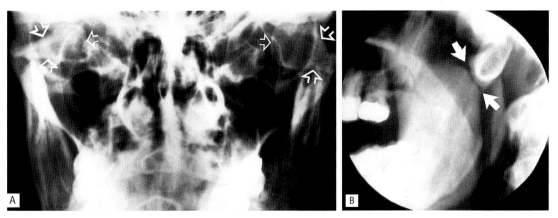

Fig. 30.15A   Central portion of a PA jaws showing bilateral fractures of the condylar necks with marked medial displacement of both condylar heads (arrowed). **B** An oblique lateral of the left side showing the fracture line (arrowed). Note that although the condylar shape is altered, it is not possible to deduce whether it has been displaced medially or laterally from the oblique lateral view alone.

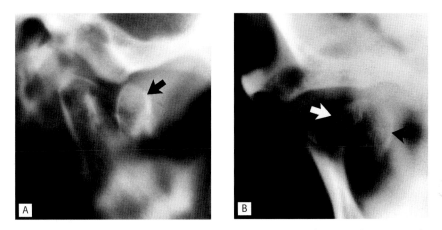

Fig. 30.16A   Sagittal and **B** coronal spiral tomographs showing an intracapsular fracture of the head of the right condyle. The anteromedially displaced fractured fragment of the head is arrowed.

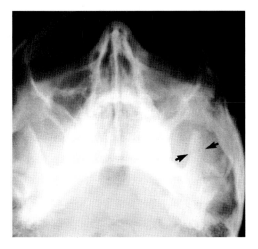

Fig. 30.17   Occipitomental showing a fracture of the left coronoid process (arrowed).

FRACTURES OF THE MIDDLE THIRD OF THE FACIAL SKELETON

This is probably one of the most difficult and confusing topics in dental radiology. The problem now concerns *multiple-bone* fractures instead of the relatively simple *one-bone* fractures encountered with the mandible. Owing to the complexity of the facial skeleton, there is a fundamental requirement of a sound knowledge of anatomy.

In addition, the knowledge required by the clinician can again be summarized as follows:

- **Where** the middle third of the face tends to fracture
- **Which** radiographic views are required to show each of the fracture sites
- **What** radiological features indicate the presence of fracture(s)
- **How** to assess the radiographs for fractures.

Classification and the main fracture sites

Most injuries to the middle third of the face are from the front, forcing part or parts of the facial skeleton downwards and backwards along the cranial base. The resulting lines of fracture follow the lines of weakness of the facial skeleton, as shown in Figure 30.18. This allows a broad classification based on site, as follows:

- *Dento-alveolar* fractures
- *Central middle third* fractures, including:

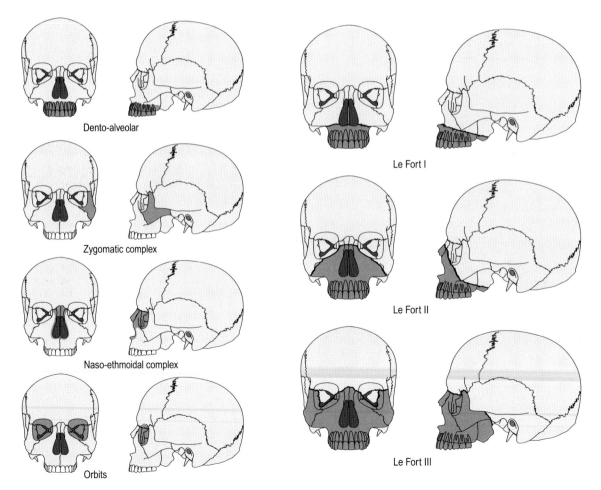

Dento-alveolar

Zygomatic complex

Naso-ethmoidal complex

Orbits

Le Fort I

Le Fort II

Le Fort III

Fig. 30.18   Diagrams of the skull from the front and side illustrating the main sites of middle third facial fractures.

- Le Fort's type I, bilateral detachment of the alveolar process and palate, or the low-level subzygomatic fracture of Guérin
  - Le Fort's type II, pyramidal, subzygomatic fracture of the maxilla
  - Le Fort's type III, high-level suprazygomatic fracture of the central and lateral parts of the face
- Fractures of the *zygomatic complex*, including:
  - Zygoma depressed with fractures at several sites
  - Fracture of the zygomatic arch
- Fractures of the *naso-ethmoidal complex*
- Fractures of the *orbit*, including:
  - Fractures of the orbital rim (usually as part of a complex fracture)
  - Orbital blow-out fracture.

Radiographic investigation

As mentioned earlier, radiographic investigation of facial fractures depends upon available facilities, the general state of the patient, associated injuries, particularly intracranial and spinal (odontoid peg), and the severity of the facial trauma.

Nevertheless, in **all cases** radiographic investigation should include a *true lateral skull* projection to exclude fractures of the cranial base, a characteristic feature of which is the presence of a fluid level in the sphenoidal air sinus.

Important points to note
- In a casualty department, the patient is usually X-rayed lying down as shown in Chapter 14. The true lateral projection should be taken with the patient supine (brow up), and with the X-ray beam horizontal, to show the possible fluid level. This projection is therefore sometimes referred to as a *brow-up lateral* or *shoot-through lateral* (see Fig. 14.1A).
- The projections that can be used for the different fracture sites are summarized in Table 30.2. Again the principle of requiring a minimum of two views at right angles applies but, as indicated, several views may be necessary.
- A useful tip to remember is that the occipito-mental radiographs should be viewed initially from a distance of about a metre to allow an

easy comparison of both sides and to detect any facial asymmetry.

Postoperative and follow-up appraisal
Again, systematic viewing sequences are adopted when using radiographs postoperatively or in the follow-up appraisal of fractures, but special attention should be paid to:

- The alignment and approximation of the bone fragments
- The position of bone plates and other fixation
- Healing and bone union
- The condition of the antra
- Evidence of infection or other complications.

Table 30.2 Summary of the common radiographic projections used to show the various middle third fracture sites

Fracture type/site	Commonly used investigations
Dento-alveolar	Periapicals Upper standard occlusal Upper oblique occlusal
Le Fort I	0° occipitomental (0° OM) 30° occipitomental (30° OM) True lateral skull (*brow-up*)
Le Fort II	0° occipitomental (0° OM) 30° occipitomental (30° OM) True lateral skull (*brow-up*)
Le Fort III	0° occipitomental (0° OM) 30° occipitomental (30° OM) True lateral skull (*brow-up*) CT or cone beam CT
Zygomatic complex	0° occipitomental (0° OM) 30° occipitomental (30° OM) CT or cone beam CT Submentovertex (SMV)
Naso-ethmoidal complex	True lateral skull (*brow-up*) 0° occipitomental (0° OM) 30° occipitomental (30° OM) Soft tissue lateral view of the nose Postero-anterior (25°) CT or cone beam CT
Orbit	0° occipitomental (0° OM) True lateral skull (*brow-up*) Posteroanterior (25°) CT or cone beam CT

Interpretation of middle third fractures

Systematic approach

In view of the numerous possible fracture sites, an ordered sequence to viewing is essential. One suggested approach can be summarized as follows:

- Examine the 0° OM using an approach based broadly on that suggested originally by McGrigor and Campbell (1950), often referred to as *Campbell's lines* (Fig. 30.19).
- Examine the 30° OM as shown in Figure 30.20.
- Examine the true lateral skull as shown in Figure 30.21.
- Examine any other films.

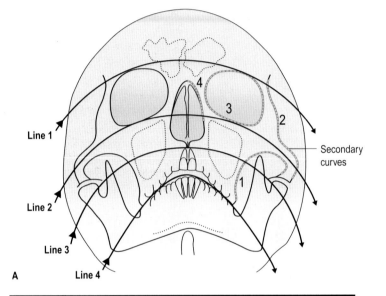

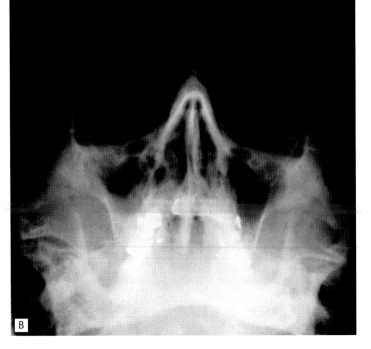

Fig. 30.19 Suggested systematic approach to interpretation of the 0° OM. **A** Diagram of a 0° OM showing Campbell's curvilinear lines and the secondary curves. **B** An example of a 0° occipitomental. **C** An explanation of Campbell's lines and the secondary curves.

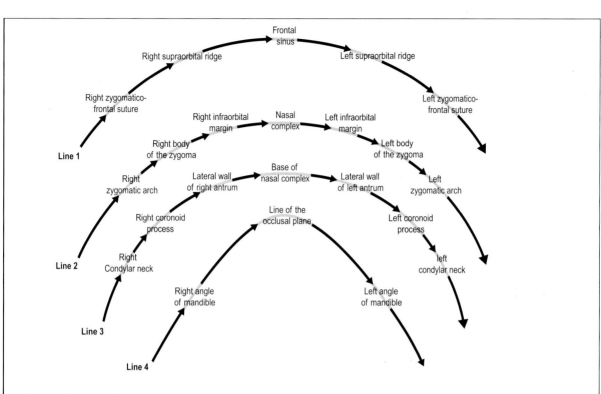

Step I :   Compare both sides by traversing across the radiograph following Campbell's lines
Step II :   Compare both sides of the radiograph tracing the *secondary curves,* indicated on one side of the diagram:

   Curve 1 - Lateral wall of the antrum and the inferior surface of the body of the zygoma and zygomatic arch
   Curve 2 - Superior margin of the zygomatic arch and the lateral aspect of the body of the zygoma and orbital margin
   Curve 3 - Inner aspect of the orbital rim
   Curve 4 - Outer curvature of the nasal complex

In both steps (I) and (II) the features to note include:
   • Any alteration or asymmetry in bony outline or shape
   • Step deformities
   • Widening of suture lines
   • The presence of radiolucent fracture line(s)
   • The direction of the fracture lines
   • The degree of separation of the bone fragments
   • Any radiopaque lines or shadows indicating overlying bone ends

Particular attention should be paid to the radiographic sites on a 0° OM where middle third facial fractures are usually identified including:
   • Zygomatico-frontal sutures
   • Frontonasal sutures
   • Zygomatico-temporal sutures (zygomatic arch)
   • The inferior margins of the orbits
   • The lateral margins of the antra
   • The nasal septum and complex

Note: All of these sites are automatically checked if the suggested systematic sequences for viewing the occipitomental radiograph are followed.

Step III :   Examine the antra — compare both sides and check for opacity and/or fluid levels suggesting haemorrhage into the antra

C

Fig. 30.19   *Continued.*

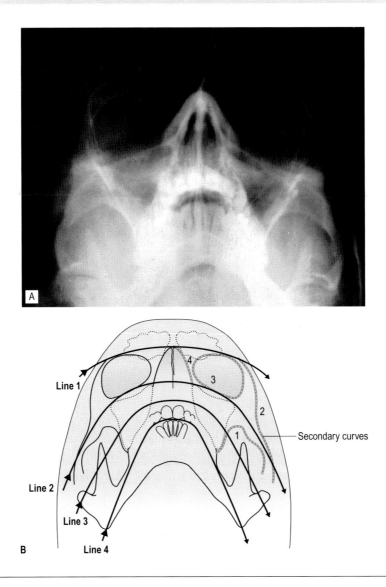

Fig. 30.20 Suggested systematic approach to interpretation of the 30° OM. **A** An example of a 30° occipitomental. **B** Diagram of a 30° OM showing Campbell's curvilinear lines and the secondary curves. **C** An explanation of the systematic approach.

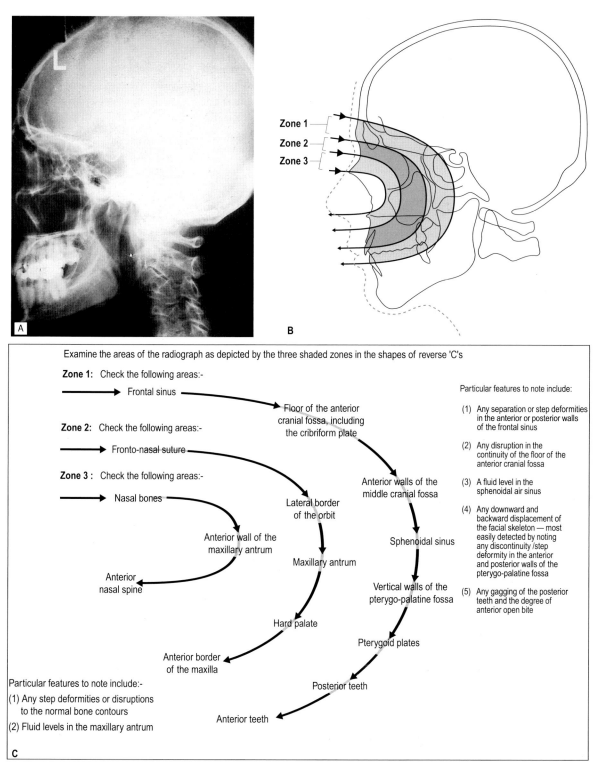

Examine the areas of the radiograph as depicted by the three shaded zones in the shapes of reverse 'C's

Zone 1: Check the following areas:-

→ Frontal sinus

Zone 2: Check the following areas:-

→ Fronto-nasal suture

Zone 3 : Check the following areas:-

→ Nasal bones

Floor of the anterior cranial fossa, including the cribriform plate

Anterior walls of the middle cranial fossa

Lateral border of the orbit

Anterior wall of the maxillary antrum

Sphenoidal sinus

Maxillary antrum

Anterior nasal spine

Vertical walls of the pterygo-palatine fossa

Hard palate

Anterior border of the maxilla

Pterygoid plates

Posterior teeth

Anterior teeth

Particular features to note include:

(1) Any separation or step deformities in the anterior or posterior walls of the frontal sinus

(2) Any disruption in the continuity of the floor of the anterior cranial fossa

(3) A fluid level in the sphenoidal air sinus

(4) Any downward and backward displacement of the facial skeleton — most easily detected by noting any discontinuity /step deformity in the anterior and posterior walls of the pterygo-palatine fossa

(5) Any gagging of the posterior teeth and the degree of anterior open bite

Particular features to note include:-

(1) Any step deformities or disruptions to the normal bone contours

(2) Fluid levels in the maxillary antrum

Fig. 30.21 Suggested systematic approach to interpretation of the true lateral skull. **A** An example of a true lateral skull. **B** Diagram of a lateral skull showing the three curved zones. **C** An explanation of the systematic approach to the zones.

Examples of middle third facial fractures

Examples of injuries to different parts of the facial skeleton are shown in Figures 30.22–30.29.

Orbital blow-out fracture

Following a direct blow to the globe of the eye, the orbital rim remains intact but the force of the blow is transmitted either downwards or medially. The very thin bones of the orbital floor can break and allow the contents of the globe to herniate downwards into the antrum. Superimposition on conventional radiographs makes this type of fracture difficult to detect, hence the need for CT (if available) or cone beam CT to determine the site and severity of the injury (see Fig. 30.30).

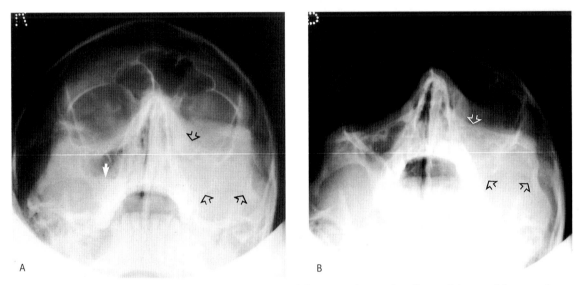

Fig. 30.22A 0° OM and **B** 30° OM showing a fracture of the left zygomatic complex. Three of the usual fracture sites are arrowed: the lower border of the orbit, the zygomatico-temporal suture (zygomatic arch) and the lateral wall of the antrum. There is a fluid level evident in the right antrum (white arrow).

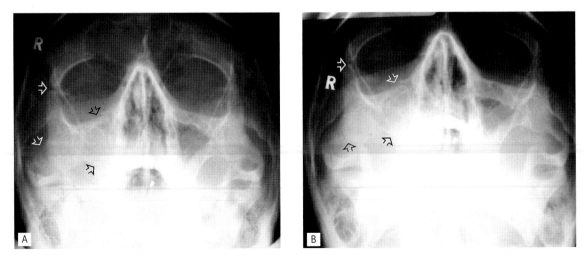

Fig. 30.23A 0° OM and **B** 30° OM showing a fracture of the right zygomatic complex. The main fracture sites are arrowed.

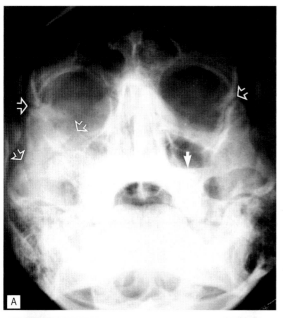

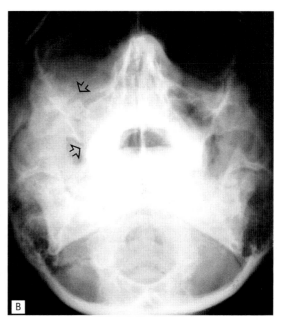

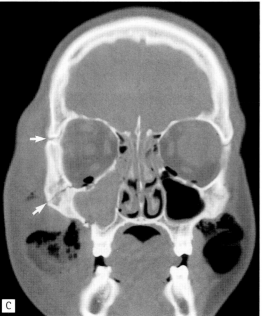

Fig. 30.24A 0° OM, **B** 30° OM and **C** Coronal section CT of different patients showing multiple middle third fracture sites, the more obvious of which are arrowed. In addition, the CT scan shows the right antrum to be totally opaque, the extensive soft tissue swelling and air in the orbits and soft tissues. (Kindly supplied by Dr J. Luker.)

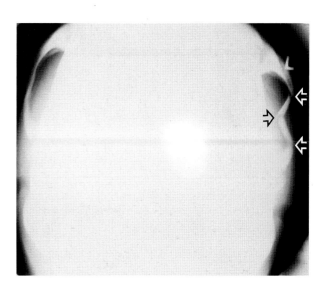

Fig. 30.25 Submentovertex (reduced exposure) showing a depressed fracture of the left zygomatic arch. Typically this type of injury results in three fracture sites which are arrowed.

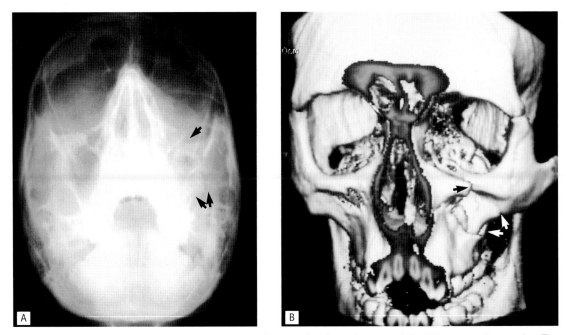

Fig. 30.26A   OM and **B** three-dimensional reconstructed CT scan showing a fracture of the left zygomatic complex. The more obvious fracture sites are arrowed. (Kindly supplied by Mr N. Drage.)

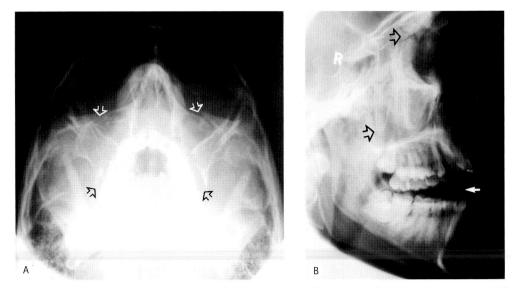

Fig. 30.27A   30° OM and **B** true lateral skull showing Le Fort II fracture. The more obvious fractures are arrowed including the pterygopalatine fossa walls. As a result of the backward displacement of the facial skeleton the posterior teeth are in occlusion and there is an anterior open bite (solid arrow).

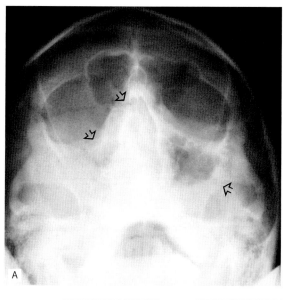

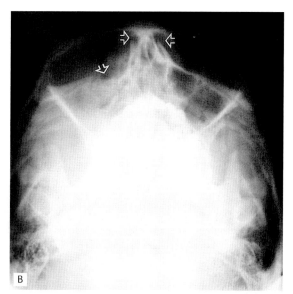

Fig. 30.28A   0° OM and **B** 30° OM and **C** true lateral skull showing multiple middle facial fractures including the nasal complex (arrowed). The facial skeleton has again been displaced backwards producing an anterior open bite.

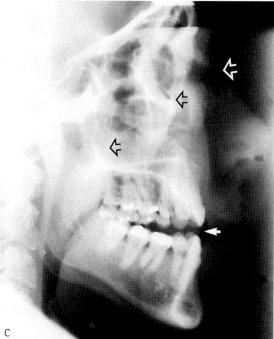

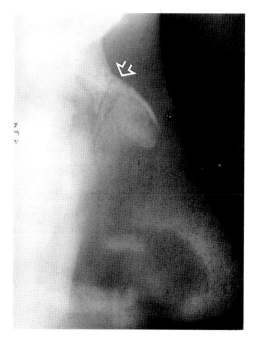

Fig. 30.29   Soft tissue lateral view of the nose showing fracture of the nasal bones (arrowed).

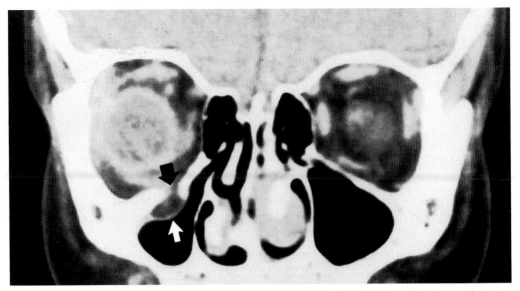

Fig. 30.30 Coronal section CT showing an orbital blow-out fracture of the right orbital floor (black arrow). The *hanging drop* appearance in the antrum is readily evident (white arrow). (Kindly supplied by Mrs J. E. Brown.)

OTHER FRACTURES AND INJURIES

Facial fractures are often associated with some other injury involving the head and neck. These can be divided broadly into:

- Fractures of the skull vault
- Fractures of the cranial base
- Fractures of the cervical spine
- Intracranial injuries.

It is beyond the scope of this book to discuss these injuries in detail, but the more commonly used radiographic investigations are summarized in Table 30.3.

Table 30.3 Summary of the commonly used radiographic investigations for fractures of the cranium, cervical spine and intracranial injuries

Fracture type/site	Commonly used investigations
Skull vault	Posteroanterior (PA skull) (for the frontal bones)
	True lateral skull (for the sides of the skull, including the parietal bones, frontal bones, squamous temporal bones, sphenoid bone — greater wings)
	Anteroposterior (AP skull) or Towne's view (for the occipital bone)
	Tangential views of trauma site to show depressed fractures
Cranial base	True lateral skull (*brow-up*)
	Submentovertex (SMV)
	CT
Cervical spine	True lateral of the neck
	Anteroposterior of the neck
	Anteroposterior with the mouth open (for the odontoid peg)
	CT
Intracranial injuries	CT
	MR

Chapter **31**

The temporomandibular joint

INTRODUCTION

The temporomandibular joint (TMJ) is one of the most difficult areas to investigate radiographically. This fact is underlined by the many types of investigations that have been developed over the years. Several plain radiographic projections and various modern imaging modalities are used for showing different parts of the complex joint anatomy. The clinical problems are complicated by the broad spectrum of conditions that can affect the joints, which can present with very similar signs and symptoms, and by prolonged searches for objective signs to explain TMJ pain dysfunction.

From the investigative point of view the knowledge required by clinicians includes:

- The normal anatomy of the TMJ
- What investigations are available, and in particular for each investigation:

- The clinical indications
- How the investigation is performed
- The clinical information provided
- The limitations and disadvantages
- The radiographic features of the more common pathological conditions that can affect the joints.

NORMAL ANATOMY

The basic components of the TMJ include:

- The mandibular component, i.e. the head of the condyle
- The disc
- The temporal component, i.e. the glenoid fossa and articular eminence
- The capsule surrounding the joint (see Figs 31.1 and 31.2).

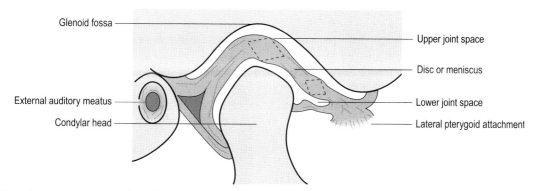

Fig. 31.1 Diagram of a sagittal section through the right TMJ showing the various components.

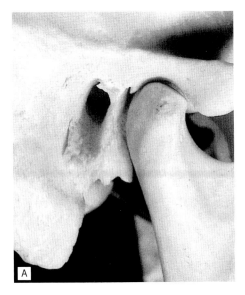

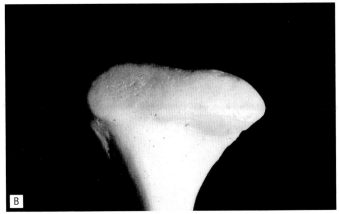

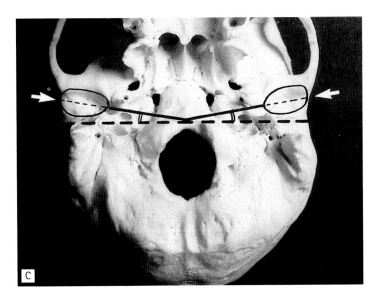

Fig. 31.2A   The bony components of the joint from the side. **B** The head of the condyle from the anterior aspect. **C** The base of the skull from below. The glenoid fossae (arrowed) and their angulation to the coronal plane have been drawn in.

In addition to this knowledge of the *static* anatomy, clinicians need to be aware of the types and range of joint movements which result in the condyles moving *downwards* and *forwards* when patients open their mouths. These include:

- Hinge or rotation of the condyle within the fossa
- Translation or excursive movement of the condyle down the articular eminence. The disc being attached to the condyle also moves forwards as shown in Figure 31.3.

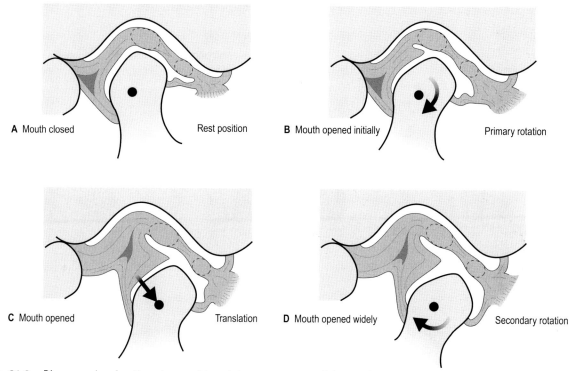

A Mouth closed   Rest position

B Mouth opened initially   Primary rotation

C Mouth opened   Translation

D Mouth opened widely   Secondary rotation

Fig. 31.3   Diagrams showing the rotary and translatory movements of the condyle during normal mouth opening.

INVESTIGATIONS

Modern imaging of the TMJ is dependent on the facilities available but could include:

- Conventional panoramic radiography
- Specific field limitation TMJ panoramic programmes
- Transpharyngeal radiography
- Multidirectional tomography
- Cone beam CT
- Magnetic resonance (MR)
- Computed tomography (CT)
- Arthrography
- Arthroscopy.

Previously described *transorbital* and *trancranial* views are now seldom used and are only of historical interest.

Dental panoramic radiography

Main indications

The main clinical indications include:

- TMJ pain dysfunction syndrome
- To investigate disease within the joint
- To investigate pathological conditions affecting the condylar heads
- Fractures of the condylar heads or necks
- Condylar hypo/hyperplasia.

Technique summary (see Ch. 17 for details)

Conventional panoramics usually image both condylar heads, although to guarantee this the technique can be modified by raising the X-ray tubehead and cassette carriage assembly to a slightly higher level in relation to the patient (so-called *high* panoramic as shown in Fig. 31.4).

Diagnostic information

The information provided includes:

- The shape of the condylar heads and the condition of the articular surfaces from the lateral aspect
- A direct comparison of both condylar heads.

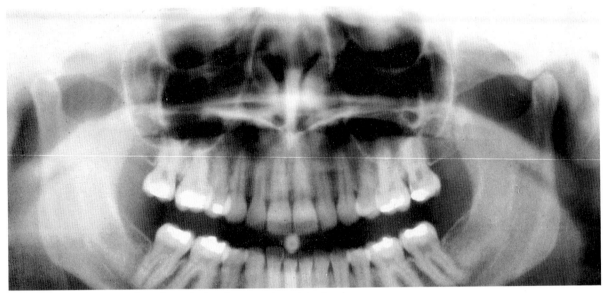

Fig. 31.4 A high panoramic radiograph showing normal condylar heads.

Panoramic TMJ programmes

Main indications

The main clinical indications are the same as for a conventional panoramic radiograph. If the equipment includes specific TMJ programmes these should be regarded as the views of choice as additional information can be provided when the mouth is opened.

Technique summary

The technique can be summarized as follows:

- The patient is positioned with their Frankfurt plane angled 5 degrees downwards within a panoramic unit with their mouth closed but using a special nose/chin support as shown in Figure 31.5A instead of the bite-peg
- The head is accurately positioned using the light beam markers and immobilized using the temple supports
- The distance from the external auditory meatus to the canine light is measured and the anteroposterior position of the chin support adjusted manually to ensure that the condyles appear in the middle of the image

- During the exposure, first the left and then the right condyle is imaged in the closed position
- The equipment automatically returns to the start position
- The patient is instructed to open the mouth, as shown in Figure 31.5B
- The left and right condyles are then exposed in the open position and the resultant image is shown in Figure 31.6.

Diagnostic information

The information provided includes:

- The shape of the condylar heads and the condition of the articular surfaces from the lateral aspect
- The range of movement of the condyles when the mouth is open
- A direct comparison of both condylar heads.

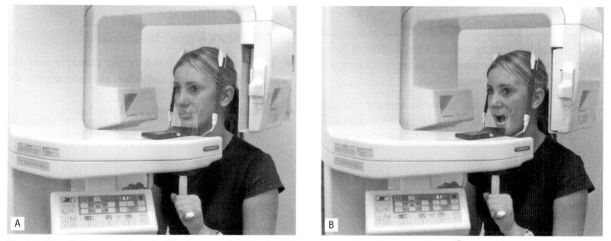

Fig. 31.5A Patient positioned with the mouth closed within a panoramic unit using the special nose/chin support and **B** positioned with the mouth open.

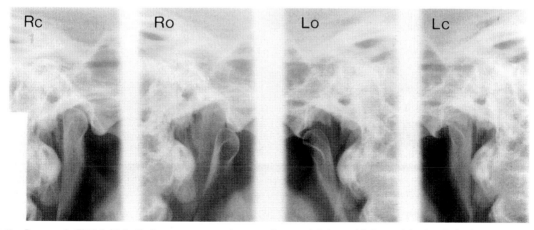

Fig. 31.6 Panoramic TMJ field limitation programme images of normal right and left condylar heads in the mouth closed (c) and open (o) positions.

Transpharyngeal radiography

Main indications

The main clinical indications include:

- TMJ pain dysfunction syndrome
- To investigate the presence of joint disease, particularly osteoarthritis and rheumatoid arthritis
- To investigate pathological conditions affecting the condylar head, including cysts or tumours
- Fractures of the neck and head of the condyle.

Technique and positioning

This projection can be taken with a dental X-ray set and an extraoral cassette. The technique can be summarized as follows:

1. The patient holds the cassette against the side of the face over the TMJ of interest. The film and the mid-sagittal plane of the head are parallel. The patient's mouth is open and a bite-block is inserted for stability.
2. The X-ray tubehead is positioned in front of the opposite condyle and beneath the zygomatic arch. It is aimed through the sigmoid notch, slightly posteriorly, across the pharynx at the condyle under investigation, as shown in Figure 31.7. Usually this view is taken of both condyles to allow comparison.

Diagnostic information

The information provided includes:

- The shape of the head of the condyle and the condition of the articular surface from the lateral aspect (Fig. 31.8)
- A comparison of both condylar heads.

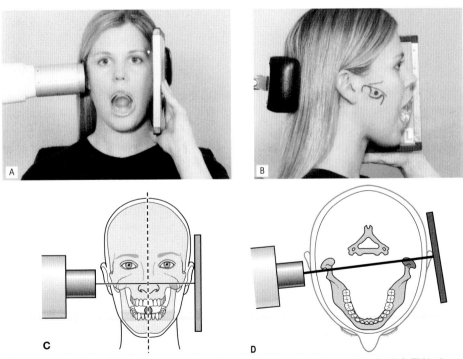

Fig. 31.7A Positioning for the left transpharyngeal — the patient is holding the film against the left TMJ, the mouth is open and the X-ray beam is aimed across the pharynx. **B** The side of the face with various anatomical structures — the zygomatic arch, condyle, sigmoid notch and coronoid process — drawn in to clarify the centring point of the X-ray beam which is marked. **C** Diagram of the positioning from the front showing the film parallel to the mid-sagittal plane and the X-ray beam aimed across the pharynx. **D** Diagram of the positioning from above, showing the X-ray beam aimed slightly posteriorly across the pharynx.

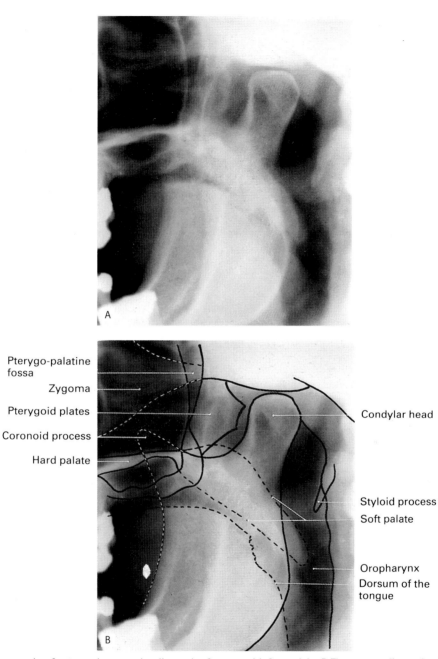

Fig. 31.8A   An example of a transpharyngeal radiograph of a normal left condyle. **B** The same radiograph with the major anatomical features drawn in.

Multidirectional tomography

Modern multidirectional tomographic equipment such as the Scanora® unit, described in Chapter 16 enables high resolution tomographic images of the bony elements of the TMJ to be obtained in both the near-sagittal and coronal planes.

Main indications

The main clinical indications include:

- Full assessment of the whole of the joint to determine the presence and site of any bone disease or abnormality
- To investigate the condyle and articular fossa when the patient is unable to open the mouth
- Assessment of fractures of the articular fossa and intracapsular fractures.

Technique summary

The procedure can be summarized as follows:

- An initial computer-controlled sagittal orientation programme is selected, which enables the correct angulation for ideal cross-sectional imaging to be assessed, by taking relatively thick (16 mm) tomographic views of the TMJ at four different angles (see Figs 31.9 and 31.10).
- The optimal angulation is chosen, fed into the unit and narrow (2 or 4 mm), detailed, computer-controlled, spiral tomographic cross-sectional slices of the joint are produced, as shown in Figure 31.11A.
- Similarly, coronal orientation and detailed tomographic programmes can be selected to produce narrow (6 mm) coronal tomographic slices, as shown in Figure 31.11B.

Diagnostic information

The information provided includes:

- The size of the joint space
- The position of the head of the condyle within the fossa
- The shape of the head of the condyle and condition of the articular surface including the medial and lateral aspects
- The shape and condition of the articular fossa and eminence
- Information on all aspects of the joints
- The position and orientation of fracture fragments.

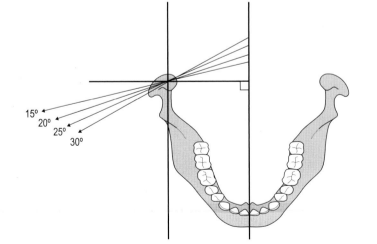

Fig. 31.9 Diagram showing the different angulations of the Scanora® TMJ orientation programme, enabling the correct angulation for detailed cross-sectional tomography to be determined.

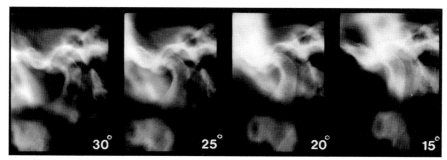

Fig. 31.10   Examples of the 16 mm thick tomographs taken at the four different angulations of the Scanora® orientation programme. The 25° angulation was considered the most satisfactory and used to produce the detailed tomographs shown in Figure 31.11A.

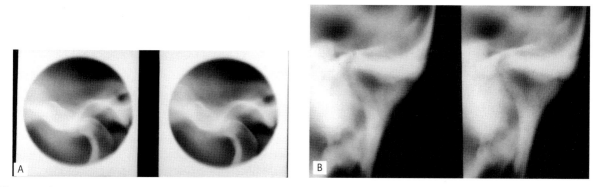

Fig. 31.11A   Two 4-mm thick, near-sagittal, detailed spiral tomographic slices of the left TMJ using the 25° orientation programme. Note the small round collimated beam that is used to restrict the radiation to the exact area of interest. B Two 6-mm thick coronal tomographs of the same left condylar head.

Cone beam CT

Cone beam CT (CBCT) described in Chapter 19 is increasingly being used to image the bony elements of the TMJ as shown in Figures 31.12 and 31.13. As with multidirectional tomography, sectional or slice images of all aspects of the joints are produced, but in addition, using appropriate software, 3-D images can be created.

Main indications

The main clinical indications are the same as for multidirectional tomography and include:

- Full assessment of the whole of the joint to determine the presence and site of any bone disease or abnormality
- To investigate the condyle and articular fossa when the patient is unable to open the mouth
- Assessment of fractures of the condylar head and articular fossa and intracapsular fractures.

Diagnostic information

The information provided includes:

- The shape of the condyles and the condition of the articular surfaces
- The condition of the glenoid fossae and eminences
- The nature of any disease affecting the condylar heads.

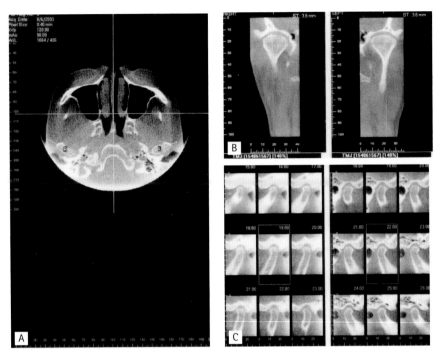

Fig. 31.12A   Axial, B coronal and C various near-sagittal images of normal right and left TMJs obtained using the I-CAT®
cone beam CT. (Reproduced with the kind permission of Imaging Sciences International, Inc.)

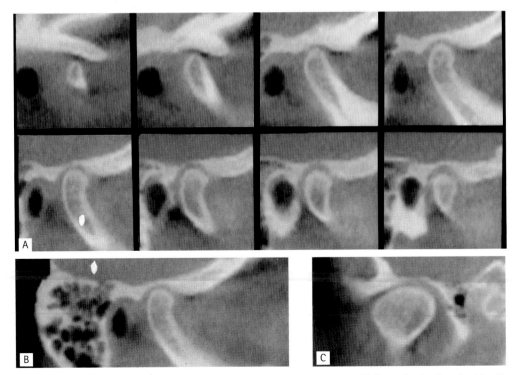

Fig. 31.13A   and B series of near-sagittal and C coronal images of a normal right TMJ obtained using the NewTom® cone
beam CT. (Kindly provided by Prof K. Tsiklakis.)

Magnetic resonance (MR)

Magnetic resonance imaging described in Chapter 19 is now established as one of the more useful investigations of the bony **and** soft tissue elements of the TMJ. It is particularly useful for determining the position and form of the disc when the mouth is both open and closed (see Fig. 31.14). As mentioned in Chapter 19, cineloop or pseudodynamic echo sequences are generally used for TMJ imaging:

- When diagnosis of internal derangements is in doubt
- As a preoperative assessment before disc surgery.

Computed tomography (CT)

Computed tomography described in Chapter 19, like ordinary tomography, provides sectional or slice images of the joint. The advantages of CT are that it can produce images of the hard and soft tissues in the joint, including the disc, in different planes.

Diagnostic information

This includes:

- The shape of the condyle and the condition of the articular surface
- The condition of the glenoid fossa and eminence
- The position and shape of the disc
- The integrity of the disc and its soft tissue attachments
- The nature of any condylar head disease.

Arthrography

Main indications

These include:

- Longstanding TMJ pain dysfunction unresponsive to simple treatments
- Persistent history of locking
- Limited opening of unknown aetiology.

Main contraindications

These include:

- Acute joint infection
- Allergy to iodine or the contrast medium.

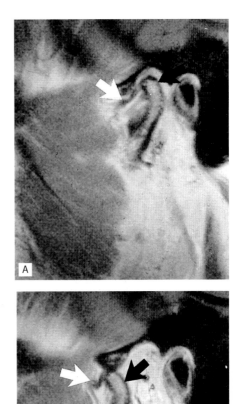

Fig. 31.14A Lateral MR scan of a left TMJ in the closed position and **B** in the open position. The condylar head (black arrow) and anteriorly positioned disc (white arrow) are indicated. (Kindly supplied by Mr B. O'Riordan.)

Technique (Fig. 31.15)

This can be summarized as follows:

1. Non-ionic aqueous contrast medium (e.g. iopamidol-Niopam® 370) is injected carefully into the lower joint space, using fluoroscopy to aid the accurate positioning of the needle

2. The primary record is obtained ideally using video-recorded fluorography or cinefluorography which allows imaging of the joint components as they move. Only the lateral aspects of the joints are seen
3. Thin-section, multidirectional (e.g. hypocycloidal) tomography of the joint can also be performed if required, to provide information on the medial and lateral aspects of the joint. Typically, five or six slices, 2–3 mm apart, are used with the patient's mouth open and closed
4. If further information is required, the contrast medium can be introduced into the upper joint space and the investigation repeated.

Diagnostic information

The information provided includes:

- Dynamic information on the position of the joint components and disc as they move in relation to one another
- Static images of the joint components with the mouth closed and with the mouth open. Any anterior or anteromedial displacement of the disc can be observed
- The integrity of the disc, i.e. the presence of any perforations.

Note: Outlining the **lower** joint space usually provides the more useful information on the disc.

Arthroscopy

Arthroscopy gives direct visualization of the TMJ and allows certain interventional procedures to be performed; these include:

- Washing out the joint with saline
- Introduction of steroids directly into the joint
- Division of adhesions
- Removal of loose bodies from within the joint.

Arthroscopy is usually considered as the last line of investigation before full surgical exploration of the joint is carried out.

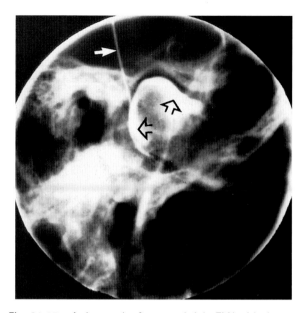

Fig. 31.15 Arthrograph of a normal right TMJ with the mouth closed. The needle (white arrow) and the contrast medium outlining the lower joint space (open black arrows) are indicated.

MAIN PATHOLOGICAL CONDITIONS AFFECTING THE TMJ

The main pathological conditions that can affect the TMJ include:

- TMJ pain dysfunction syndrome (myofascial pain dysfunction syndrome)
- Internal derangements
- Osteoarthritis (osteoarthrosis)
- Rheumatoid arthritis
- Juvenile rheumatoid arthritis (Still's disease)
- Ankylosis
- Tumours
- Fractures and trauma
- Developmental anomalies.

TMJ (myofascial) pain dysfunction syndrome

This is the most common clinical diagnosis applied to patients with pain in the muscles of mastication, often worst in the early morning and evening, with occasional clicking and stiffness. The aetiology is said to include anxiety or depression, malocclusion, or muscle spasm.

Main radiographic features

These include:

- Normal condylar head shape and articular surface
- Normal glenoid fossa shape
- Possible increase or reduction in the overall size of the *joint space* — an increase in the size of the joint space is only indicative of inflammation
- Possible displacement of the condylar head anteriorly or posteriorly in the glenoid fossa when the mouth is closed and the teeth are in occlusion
- Reduction in the range of condylar movement.

Note In their booklet *Making Best Use of a Department of Clinical Radiology* 5th edn, published in 2003 the Royal College of Radiologists in the UK state that in relation to TMJ dysfunction, radiographs 'do not often add information as the majority of temporomandibular joint problems are due to soft tissue dysfunction rather than bony changes, which appear late and are often absent in the acute phase'.

Internal derangements

Symptoms include clicking which may be painful, pain from the joint and/or musculature, trismus and hesitation of movement and locking usually with failure of opening. Conventional radiography may have revealed an alteration in the position of the head of the condyle, implying an abnormality in disc position. MRI is the investigation of choice to show:

- Disc position — it may dislocate anteriorly or anteromedially
- Disc movement relative to the condyle during opening and closing.

Osteoarthritis

This degenerative arthrosis increases in incidence with age and commonly causes pain in the stressbearing joints, such as the hips and spine. It is now thought to be a systemic disease, or a complication of internal derangement of a joint, and stress merely causes the affected joint to be painful. Radiographic signs of osteoarthritis of the TMJ are often seen in the elderly, but are frequently of no clinical significance. Symptoms, if they occur, can include painful crepitus and trismus and are usually persistent.

Main radiographic features
(see Figs 31.16–31.18)

These include:

- Osteophyte (bony spur) formation on the anterior aspect of the articular surface of the condylar head. The radiological appearance of small osteophyte formation is often referred to as *lipping*; extensive osteophyte formation is referred to as *beaking*
- Flattening of the head of the condyle on the anterosuperior margin
- Subchondral sclerosis of the condylar head which becomes dense and more radiopaque — a process sometimes referred to as *eburnation*
- A normal outline to the glenoid fossa though it may also become sclerotic
- Very rarely, there may be evidence of:
  - Osteophyte formation posteriorly
  - Subchondral cysts
  - Erosion of the articular surface of the condylar head.

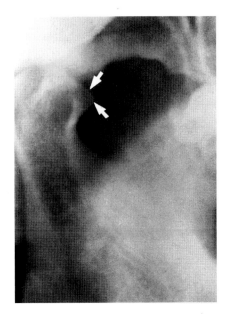

Fig. 31.16 Transpharyngeal of a right condyle showing advanced osteoarthritic change with pronounced anterior osteophyte formation (*beaking*) (arrowed).

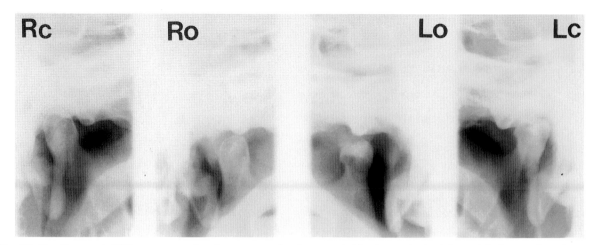

Fig. 31.17 Panoramic TMJ programme showing an example of osteoarthritic change in the left condyle (arrowed) — the shape of the head of the condyle is altered and there is evidence of early anterior osteophyte formation. The right condyle is normal. (Kindly provided by Dr J. Luker.)

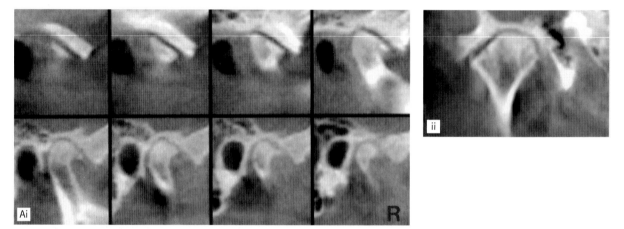

Fig. 31.18 Near sagittal and coronal NewTom® cone beam CT images showing **A** osteoarthritic flattening and anterior osteophyte formation affecting the right condyle.

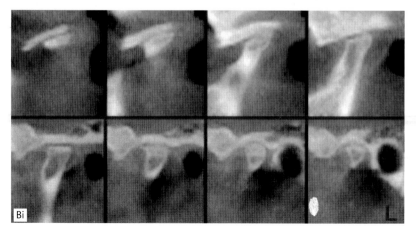
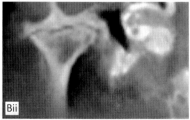

Fig. 31.18B Flattening and erosion of the articular surface affecting the left condyle. (Kindly provided by Prof K. Tsiklakis.)

Rheumatoid arthritis

Rheumatoid arthritis is a generalized, chronic inflammatory, connective tissue disease affecting many joints. TMJ involvement can be found, particularly in severe rheumatoid arthritis, but even then TMJ symptoms are usually minor.

Main radiographic features (see Figs 31.19–31.21)

These include:

- Flattening of the head of the condyle
- Erosion and destruction of the articular surface of the head of the condyle which may be extensive causing the outline to become irregular
- Occasional osteophyte formation on the condylar head
- Hollowing of the glenoid fossa
- Reduction in the range of movement
- Features are usually bilateral and fairly symmetrical.

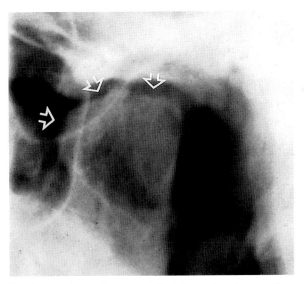

Fig. 31.19 Transpharyngeal of a left condyle showing the typical erosion and destruction of the articular surface (arrowed) caused by severe rheumatoid arthritis.

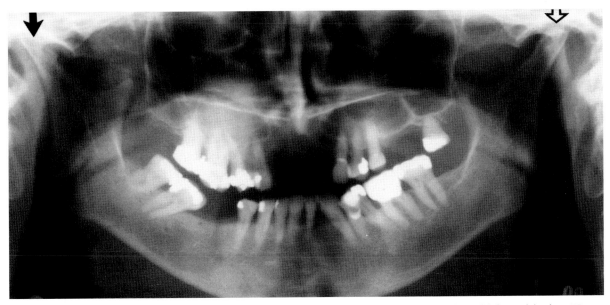

Fig. 31.20 Panoramic radiograph showing advanced rheumatoid arthritic change in both right and left condyles in a 75-year-old woman with widespread joint involvement. The right (solid arrow) shows marked flattening while the left (open arrow) shows erosion of the articular surface. Despite these pronounced changes the patient was symptom-free.

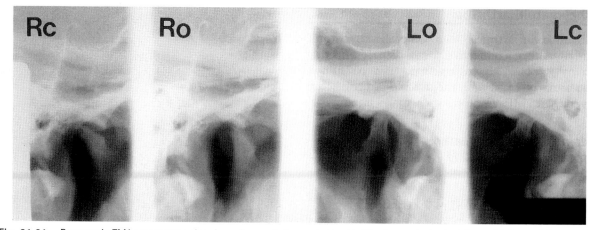

Fig. 31.21   Panoramic TMJ programme showing advanced rheumatoid arthritic change in both right and left condyles. (Kindly provided by Mr N. Drage.)

Juvenile rheumatoid arthritis (Still's disease)

The radiographic features of juvenile rheumatoid arthritis are similar to the adult disease. In severe cases, the disease may cause interference with normal condylar growth producing micrognathia, or it may result in TMJ ankylosis.

Ankylosis

True ankylosis, i.e. fusion of the bony elements of the joint (see Fig. 31.22), is uncommon but is usually the result of:

- Trauma, particularly condylar head fractures and birth injury, and bleeding into the joint
- Infection
- Severe juvenile rheumatoid arthritis.

Tomography, cone beam CT or CT are the investigations of choice because of the obvious problems of opening the mouth.

Main radiographic features

These include:

- Little or no evidence of a joint space
- Bony fusion between the head of the condyle and the glenoid fossa with total loss of the normal anatomical outlines
- Associated evidence of condylar neck hypoplasia and mandibular underdevelopment on the

affected side producing asymmetry, if the ankylosis precedes completion of mandibular growth. A prominent antegonial notch on the affected side is often evident.

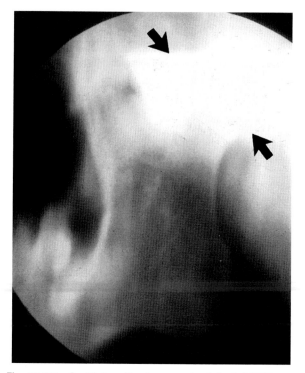

Fig. 31.22   Sagittal section tomograph of the left TMJ showing complete ankylosis and bony fusion of the condyle and glenoid fossa (arrowed).

Tumours

Benign or malignant tumours develop occasionally in the head of the condyle. The radiographic features depend on the type and nature of the tumour involved, but there is usually an alteration in the shape of the condylar head. Typical examples include osteoma, chondroma (see Fig. 31.23) and chondrosarcoma.

Fractures and trauma

Fractures of the condylar necks are common after a blow to the chin (see Ch. 30). Very occasionally with this type of injury the condylar neck does not fracture but the head of the condyle either fractures, a so-called intra-capsular fracture (see Fig. 31.24) or is forced upwards, through the glenoid fossa into the middle cranial fossa (see (Fig. 31.25). Tomography, cone beam CT or CT will demonstrate the extent of any injury. Trauma can also result in unilateral or bilateral dislocation (see Fig. 31.26).

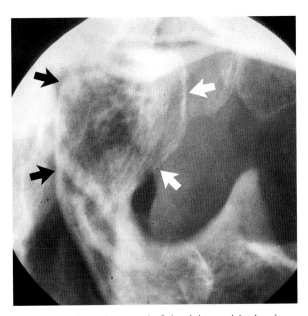

Fig. 31.23 Transpharyngeal of the right condyle showing gross, expansive enlargement of the head (arrowed). The lesion is round, well defined and with a moderately well-corticated outline — these features all indicate a slow-growing, benign lesion which proved to be a chondroma.

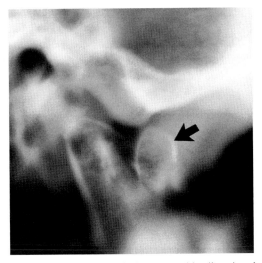

Fig. 31.24 Near-sagittal spiral tomographic slice showing an intracapsular fracture of the head of a right condyle. The anteriorly displaced fractured fragment of the head is arrowed.

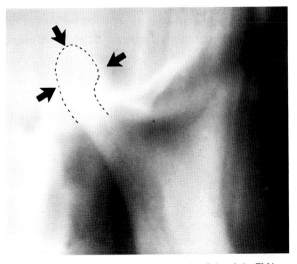

Fig. 31.25 Sagittal section tomograph of the right TMJ showing the condylar head (drawn in and arrowed), fractured through the glenoid fossa into the middle cranial fossa.

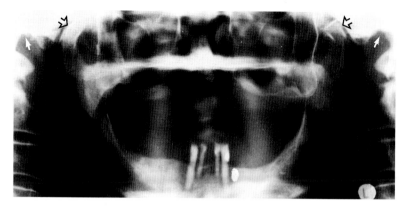

Fig. 31.26 Panoramic radiograph showing bilateral dislocation of the condyles (open arrows) out of the glenoid fossae (white arrows). (Kindly provided by Mr N. Drage.)

Developmental anomalies

Developmental defects affecting the TMJ are usually investigated using conventional radiography. They can be divided into:

- Condylar hypoplasia (unilateral or bilateral) (see Fig. 31.27)
- Condylar hyperplasia (unilateral or bilateral) (see Fig. 31.28)
- Bifid condyle (see Fig. 25.30)
- Post-radiotherapy
- Defects associated with specific disease or syndromes, for example:
  - First arch syndrome
  - Mandibular facial dysostosis (Treacher Collins syndrome).

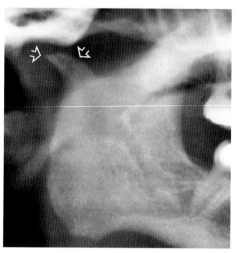

Fig. 31.27 Part of a panoramic showing marked condylar hypoplasia of the right condyle (arrowed).

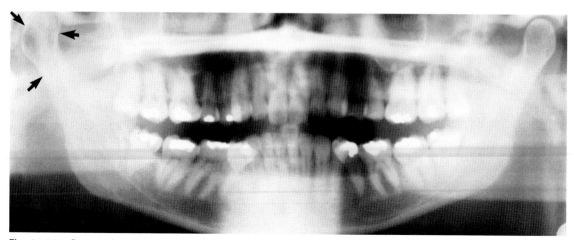

Fig. 31.28 Panoramic radiograph showing condylar hyperplasia particularly of the right condyle and elongation of the condylar neck (arrowed). The head of the condyle on the left is also slightly enlarged.

FOOTNOTE

The bony abnormalities illustrated are often detected as incidental findings on panoramic radiographs taken for some other clinical condition. For those patients with specific signs and symptoms relating to the TMJ the type of investigation chosen will depend on the history, the clinical presentation and the facilities available. Knowledge of the respective merits and limitations of the different investigations allows the clinician to use the most appropriate for each patient.

Chapter 32

Bone diseases of radiological importance

INTRODUCTION

There are many diseases and abnormalities of bone. Some are localized to the jaws while others can affect the whole skeleton. It is beyond the scope of this book to consider them all. This chapter summarizes a somewhat diverse, but important group of bone conditions which can affect the facial skeleton and which are of radiological importance.

Unfortunately, several of the bone diseases described, although totally different in nature, can present very similar appearances radiographically. To differentiate them, clinicians need to consider all relevant factors including — the age of the patient, the distribution of the disease (whether it is generalized or localized) and which bones are involved, as well as noting the specific radiographic features.

Using the *atlas* approach adopted in Chapter 25, an example of each of the conditions is shown together with a summary of the main radiographic features seen in the skull and facial skeleton. It is worth remembering that bone is a constantly changing, dynamic tissue. Thus diseases of bone can present a spectrum of radiographic appearances depending on the behaviour and maturity or stage of the disease and/or lesion(s). The examples shown represent only a small part of that spectrum.

The diseases of bone described include:

- **Developmental or genetic disorders**
  - Cleidocranial dysplasia
  - Osteopetrosis

- **Infective or inflammatory conditions**
  - Osteoradionecrosis
  - Osteomyelitis

- **Hormone-related disorders**
  - Hyperparathyroidism
  - Acromegaly

- **Blood dyscrasias**
  - Sickle cell anaemia
  - Thalassaemia

- **Diseases of unknown cause**
  - Fibrous dysplasia
  - Paget's disease of bone.

DEVELOPMENTAL OR GENETIC DISORDERS

Cleidocranial dysplasia

This is a rare developmental disturbance affecting the skull and clavicles. The abnormalities of dentition can be gross but usually affect only the permanent teeth. Examples are delayed eruption and multiple supernumeraries (see Fig. 32.1).

Main radiographic features

These can include:

- Aplasia or hypoplasia of the clavicles

- Evidence in the skull vault of:
  - A widened cranium
  - Delayed ossification of the fontanelles
  - A large number of wormian bones
  - Frontal and occipital bossing
  - Basilar invagination
- Evidence in the jaws of:
  - Small, underdeveloped maxillae
  - Delayed eruption of many permanent teeth, sometimes with associated cyst formation
  - Multiple supernumerary teeth.

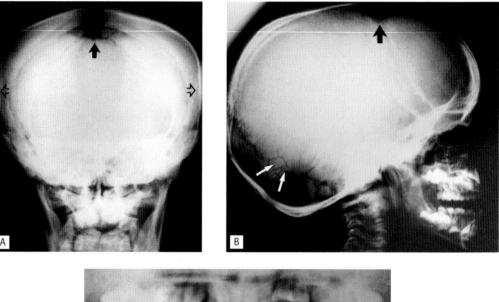

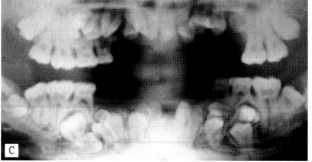

Fig. 32.1 Cleidocranial dysplasia. **A** PA skull showing the cranial features of widened cranium (open arrows) and open fontanelle (solid arrow). **B** True lateral skull of another patient also showing the open fontanelle (black arrow) and also small wormian bones (white arrows). The enlargement of the occiput is also obvious. **C** Panoramic radiograph showing the dental anomalies of delayed eruption and multiple supernumerary teeth.

Osteopetrosis (Albers–Schönberg disease)

This hereditary disease is characterized by sclerosis of the skeleton (so called *marble bones*), fragile bones and secondary anaemia. Bone formation is normal but bone resorption is reduced, resulting in the presence of excessive calcified tissue and lack of marrow space (see Fig. 32.2). Cranial base changes may produce compression of the cranial nerves.

Main radiographic features

These can include:

- Evidence in the skull of:
  - A uniformly dense and radiopaque skull vault
  - Loss of the normal skull markings and structure
  - Gross thickening and increased opacity of the cranial base with narrowing of the foramina
- Occasional involvement of the jaws. This involvement is always bilateral and includes:
  - Thickening of the lamina dura around the teeth in the early stages (an almost pathognomonic finding in adults)
  - Gradual thickening of the trabeculae and a reduction in the size of the marrow spaces producing an overall increase in bone density
  - Usually normal teeth, but they may be deformed.

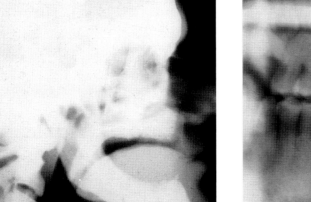
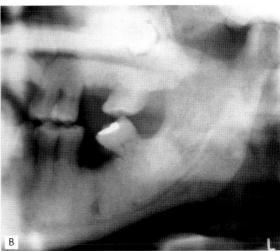

Fig. 32.2   Osteopetrosis. **A** True lateral skull showing the cranial features of radiopaque, dense vault and thickened base. **B** Left side of a panoramic radiograph showing loss of the normal trabecular pattern and replacement with dense thickened bone.

INFECTIVE OR INFLAMMATORY CONDITIONS

Osteomyelitis

This spreading, progressive inflammation of bone and bone marrow, more frequently affects the mandible than the maxilla. It is caused usually by local factors such as periapical infection, pericoronitis, acute periodontal lesions, extractions or trauma. The inflammatory response may be acute or chronic depending on the virulence of the infecting organism and the resistance of the patient. It results ultimately in the destruction of the infected bone (see Fig. 32.3). The reaction of the surrounding bone and periosteum is very variable and often age-related. There may be surrounding sclerosis of the bone forming poorly-defined patchy opacity. Sequestra (small pieces of necrotic bone) can be exfoliated over a period of several weeks. The periosteum around the affected area can lay down new bone (the so-

called periosteal reaction). In children this can be pronounced and is described as *proliferative periostitis*. This typically affects the mandible in young girls, following apical or pericoronal infection associated with the lower first molar producing a non-tender, bony hard swelling of the lower border. Radiographically the proliferative periostitis results in a laminated, so called *onion-skin*, appearance (see Fig. 32.3D)

Main radiographic features of acute osteomyelitis

These can include:

- Ragged, patchy or *moth-eaten* areas of radiolucency — the outline of the area of destruction is irregular and poorly defined
- Evidence of small radiopaque sequestra of dead bone occasionally within the radiolucency

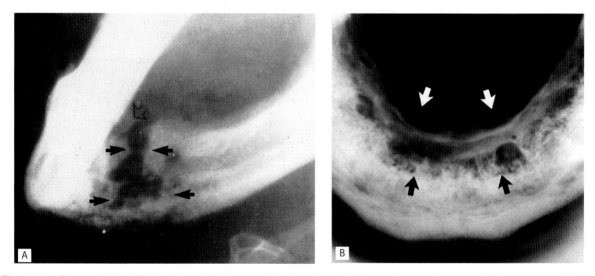

Fig. 32.3 Osteomyelitis. **A** Oblique lateral of the mandible showing typical ragged or *moth-eaten* radiolucent areas of bone destruction (solid arrows) and a sequestrum of dead bone (open arrow). **B** Lower 90° occlusal showing irregular bone destruction (black arrows) and lingual involucrum formation (white arrows).

- Evidence of new subperiosteal bone formation, usually beyond the area of necrosis, particularly along the lower border of the mandible.

Main radiographic features of chronic osteomyelitis

These can include:

- Localized patchy or *moth-eaten* areas of bone destruction
- Sclerosis of the surrounding bone

- Evidence of small radiopaque sequestra of dead bone sometimes within the area of bone destruction
- Evidence of an involucrum surrounding the area of destruction following extensive subperiosteal bone formation.

Note: The radiographic appearance of osteomyelitis varies considerably depending on the type of underlying inflammatory response and the age of the patient.

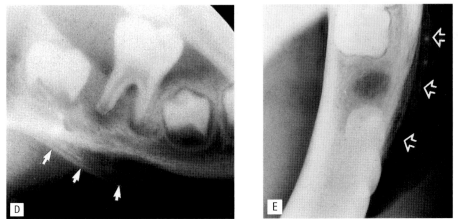

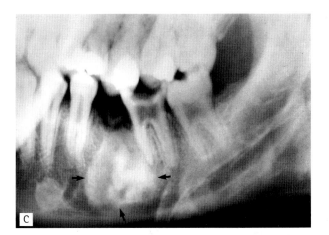

Fig. 32.3C   Oblique lateral showing chronic dense sclerosing osteomyelitis (arrowed). **D** Proliferative periostitis-oblique lateral of a 9-year-old girl showing bone destruction around the first molar and the *onion-skin* layering periosteal reaction affecting the lower border (arrowed). **E** Part of a lower occlusal showing another example of *onion-skin* layering periosteal new bone formation.

Osteoradionecrosis

The high doses of radiation used in radiotherapy reduce drastically the vascularity and reparative powers of bone. The mandible is particularly susceptible. Subsequent trauma (e.g. tooth extraction) or infection may produce osteomyelitis with rapid destruction of the irradiated bone, sequestra formation and poor healing. Radiographically osteoradionecrosis resembles other types of osteomyelitis, although the border between necrotic and normal bone may be more sharply defined and subperiosteal new bone formation is not usually evident (see Fig. 32.4). A history of radiotherapy enables the differential diagnosis to be made.

Main radiographic features

These can include:

- Ragged, patchy or *moth-eaten* radiolucent areas of bone destruction
- Occasional evidence of radiopaque sequestra of dead bone
- Little evidence of healing.

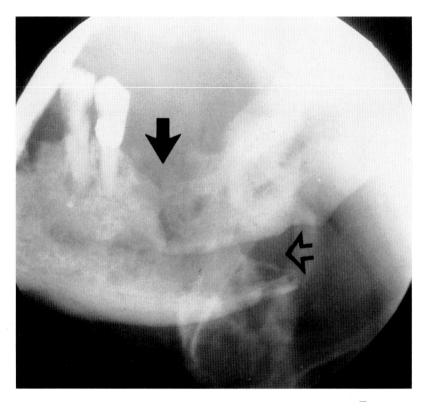

Fig. 32.4 Osteoradionecrosis — oblique lateral of the mandible following the extraction of $\overline{6|}$, showing the typical destructive appearance (solid arrow), which has resulted in a pathological fracture (open arrow). Radiotherapy had been given several years previously.

HORMONE–RELATED DISEASES

Hyperparathyroidism

Primary hyperparathyroidism, caused by either hyperplasia or an adenoma of the parathyroids, or secondary hyperparathyroidism caused by kidney disease, results in increased secretion of parathormone. This causes generalized skeletal bone resorption leading to osteopenia (generalized decrease in bone density), bone pain or even pathological fracture and raises the plasma calcium levels (see Fig. 32.5). Localized cyst-like central giant cell lesions (brown tumours) can also develop in the jaws and long bones. The term *osteitis fibroa cystica* is used to describe severe chronic skeletal hyperparathyroidism following brown tumour degeneration and fibrosis.

Main radiographic features

These can include:

- Evidence in the skull vault of osteopenia producing a fine overall stippled pattern to the bone — hence the description *pepper-pot* skull
- Evidence in the jaws of:
  - Osteopenia (in mandible and maxilla) producing a very fine trabecular pattern, often described as *ground glass*
  - Loss of the lamina dura surrounding all the teeth and thinning or loss of the normal thick cortical bone of the lower border of the mandible
  - Occasional localized radiolucent cyst-like central giant cell lesions (brown tumours, see Ch. 27)
  - Usually normal teeth.

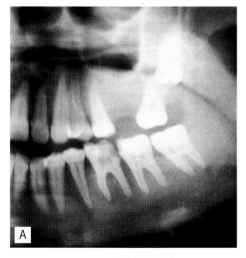

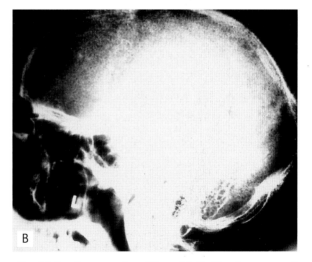

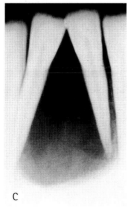

Fig. 32.5 Hyperparathyroidism. **A** Left side of a panoramic radiograph showing the typical bone changes including loss of the lamina dura, fine *ground glass* trabecular pattern, and thinning of the cortical bone of the lower border and inferior dental canal. **B** True lateral skull showing the *pepper-pot* appearance in the skull vault. **C** Periapical showing a radiolucent central giant cell lesion (brown tumour) between the lower incisors which have been displaced but not apparently resorbed.

Acromegaly

This is a disturbance of bone growth caused by hypersecretion of growth hormone (GH) usually as the result of a pituitary adenoma developing after puberty. Characteristic features include renewed growth of certain bones, particularly the jaws, hands and feet, and overgrowth of some soft tissues (see Fig. 32.6).

Main radiographic features

These can include:

- Evidence in the skull of:
  - Thickening of the bones of the skull vault which become enlarged and deformed
  - Enlargement and distortion of the pituitary fossa

- Evidence in the jaws of:
  - Enlargement of the mandible; the length of the horizontal and ascending rami are both increased causing it to become prognathic with an increased obliquity of the angle and with loss of the antegonial notch
  - The body of the mandible may also be bent or bowed downwards anterior to the angle
  - Enlargement of the inferior dental canal
  - Thickening and enlargement of the alveolar bone with spacing and fanning out of the teeth, particularly anteriorly, resulting in an open bite.

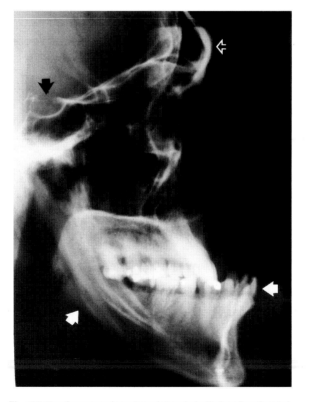

Fig. 32.6 Acromegaly — true lateral skull showing frontal bossing (open white arrow), enlarged pituitary fossa (black arrow), grossly enlarged and prognathic mandible with increased obliquity of the angle (solid white arrows).

BLOOD DYSCRASIAS

Sickle cell anaemia

This hereditary, chronic, haemolytic blood disorder affects principally black populations. It is characterized by abnormal haemoglobin which results in fragile erythrocytes which become sickle-shaped under conditions of hypoxia. These abnormal red blood cells have a decreased capacity to carry oxygen and are destroyed rapidly producing anaemia.

In homozygotes, the radiographic changes reflect the haemopoietic system's response to the anaemia including:

- Increased production of red blood cells and hyperplasia of the bone marrow at the expense of the cancellous bone
- Bone infarcts (see Fig. 32.7).

Main radiographic features

These can include:

- Evidence in the skull vault of:
  - Thickening of the frontal and parietal bones
  - Widening of the diploic space
  - Thinning of the inner and outer tables
  - Generalized osteoporosis
  - The *hair-on-end* appearance (rare)
- Evidence in the jaws of:
  - A generalized coarse trabecular pattern, fewer trabeculae are evident and the spaces between them appear larger
  - The remaining trabeculae between the roots of the teeth can become aligned horizontally to produce a *step ladder* appearance
  - Enlargement of the maxillae, with protrusion and separation of the upper anterior teeth
  - Osteosclerotic areas resulting from the infarcts
  - Usually normal teeth with normal lamina dura.

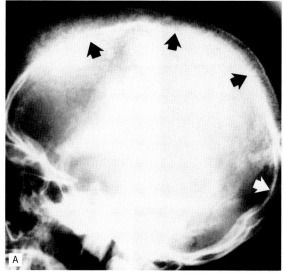
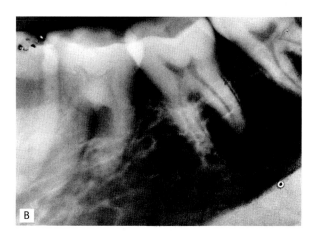

Fig. 32.7 Sickle cell anaemia. **A** True lateral skull showing widening of the diploic space and thinning of the inner and outer tables and early *hair-on-end* appearance anteriorly (arrowed). **B** Periapical showing the generalized coarse trabecular pattern in the mandible.

Thalassaemia (Cooley's anaemia)

This hereditary haemoglobinopathy is characterized by chronic haemolytic anaemia and mainly affects people from the Mediterranean area. The defect lies in an inability to make enough normal globin chains thus creating abnormal red blood cells which have a shortened life expectancy. Again the radiographic features result from the bone marrow proliferation required to produce more red blood cells with subsequent remodelling of all affected bones (see Fig. 32.8).

Main radiographic features

These can include:

- Evidence in the skull vault of:
  - Widening of the diploic space
  - Thinning of the inner and outer tables
  - Remodelling of the trabeculae to give sparse lines which may radiate outwards from the inner table producing the *hair-on-end* appearance
- Evidence in the jaws of:
  - Generalized coarse trabecular pattern with very large marrow spaces
  - Expansion, which may lead to encroachment on, and subsequent obliteration of the maxillary antra
  - Thinning of all cortical structures, most noticeably the lower border of the mandible
  - Apparent spike-shaped or shortened tooth roots
  - No evidence of bone infarcts.

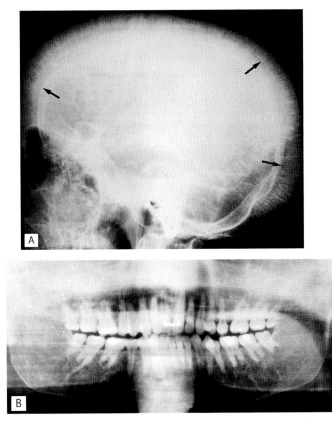

Fig. 32.8 Thalassaemia. **A** True lateral skull showing pronounced *hair-on-end* appearance (black arrows) and involvement of the maxilla with obliteration of the antra. **B** Panoramic radiograph showing the altered trabecular pattern throughout the mandible and maxilla with very large marrow spaces, obliteration of the antra and thinning of the lower border cortex. (Kindly supplied by Mrs J.E. Brown.)

DISEASES OF UNKNOWN CAUSE

Fibrous dysplasia

As mentioned in Chapter 28, fibrous dysplasia is categorized as a *bone-related lesion* in the WHO 2005 Classification. It is described by the WHO as a genetically-based sporadic disease of bone affecting single or multiple bones. It usually develops in childhood and is manifest before the age of 10. It is characterized by the proliferation of fibrous tissue and resorption of normal bone in one or more localized areas, and subsequent replacement with poorly formed, haphazardly arranged new bony trabeculae. Clinical varieties include:

- *Monostotic fibrous dysplasia*, characterized by a lesion affecting a single bone, including the jaws, particularly the posterior part of the maxilla (see Fig. 32.9).
- *Polyostotic fibrous dysplasia*, characterized by multiple bone lesions and subdivided into:
  - *Jaffe type*, without endocrine disturbances
  - *McCune–Albright syndrome*, with endocrine disturbances and skin pigmentation.

Main radiographic features of monostotic fibrous dysplasia affecting the jaws

- A localized rounded zone of relative radiolucency containing a variety of fine trabecular patterns, described as *ground glass, fingerprint* and *orange peel*. The more mature the lesion the more radiopaque it appears.
- Poor definition of the edge of the lesion which merges imperceptibly with the surrounding normal bone (see Fig. 28.18).
- Loss of the lamina dura with thinning of the periodontal ligament shadow.
- Enlargement of the affected bone.
- In the maxilla encroachment on, or obliteration of, the antrum and spread into particularly the zygoma and sphenoid bones of the cranial base.
- Associated teeth occasionally displaced, but rarely resorbed.

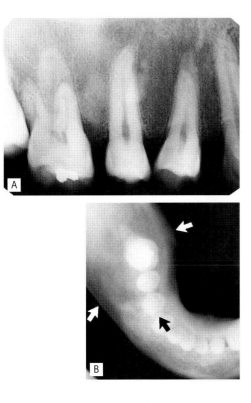

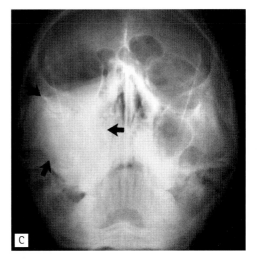

Fig. 32.9 Fibrous dysplasia. **A** Periapical showing the overall fine stippled trabecular pattern (*orange peel*), and loss of the lamina dura around the 6/. **B** Lower 90° occlusal centred on the right side again showing the *ground glass* appearance and expansion but involving the mandible in the premolar and molar regions (arrowed). The anterior part of the mandible is unaffected. **C** 0° OM showing expansion of the right posterior maxilla spread into the zygoma and total obliteration of the right antrum (arrowed).

Paget's disease of bone (osteitis deformans)

In this disease of the elderly, the normal processes of bone deposition and resorption are disturbed severely, but only in certain bones and usually symmetrically. The main features are an enlarged head and thickening of the affected long bones which bend under stress. Typically the early stages of the disease are characterized by bone resorption and the later stages by bone deposition, although there is no clear-cut distinction between the two stages (see Fig. 32.10).

Main radiographic features of early-stage Paget's disease

- In the skull vault scalloped, circumscribed zones of osteoporosis spreading gradually across the calvarium, described as *osteoporosis circumscripta*
- Involvement of the maxilla and/or the mandible. If either is involved, the whole of the bone concerned shows radiographic changes which include:
  - Generalized osteoporosis of the affected bones producing a fine trabecular pattern, described as *ground glass*
  - Enlargement of the affected bone
  - Loss of the lamina dura surrounding all the teeth.

Main radiographic features of late-stage Paget's disease

- Evidence in the skull vault of:
  - Haphazard deposition of sclerotic bone in the earlier zones of osteoporosis producing an appearance resembling *cottonwool* patches
  - Enlargement and distortion of the shape of the skull including basilar invagination
- Evidence in the jaws of:
  - Haphazard deposition of sclerotic bone also resembling *cottonwool* patches
  - Enlargement and distortion of the shape of the affected jaw, particularly the alveolus
  - Encroachment of bone on the sinuses
  - Separation and displacement of the teeth often with extensive hypercementosis
  - Loss of the lamina dura and periodontal ligament shadows.

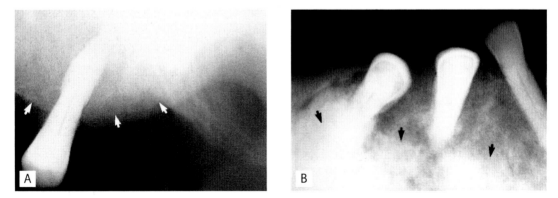

Fig. 32.10 Paget's disease of bone. **A** Periapical showing the early porotic stage in the maxilla; note the overall fine trabecular pattern (*ground glass*), loss of the lamina dura and enlargement of the maxilla (arrowed). **B** Periapical showing the typical late stage in the mandible. Note the *cottonwool* patches of sclerotic bone (arrowed), loss of the lamina dura, enlargement of the bone, malposition of the teeth and the associated hypercementosis.

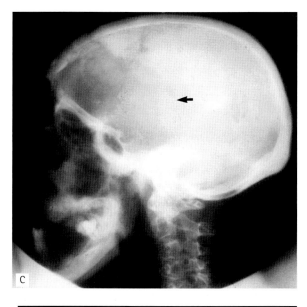

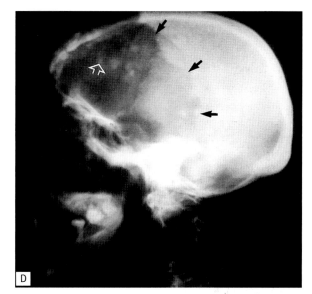

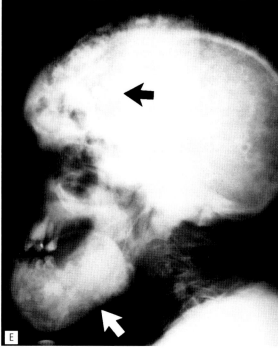

Fig. 32.10C True lateral skull showing early cranial vault involvement — the frontal region appears radiolucent and the scalloped line of *osteoporosis circumscripta* is arrowed. D Same patient 12 months later — the scalloped line of *osteoporosis circumscripta* has progressed posteriorly (black arrows) and there is early haphazard deposition of bone in the frontal region (open white arrow). E True lateral skull of a different patient showing the typical late stage appearance of *cottonwool* patches affecting the frontal region of the skull vault (black arrows) and the mandible (white arrow). The occipital region is still in the early stages.

Chapter 33

The salivary glands

SALIVARY GLAND DISORDERS

Disorders of the major salivary glands are relatively common, with a large spectrum of underlying diseases. This has led to a variety of classifications. However, the presenting symptoms and complaints allow a broad division into six main categories:

- Acute intermittent generalized swelling of a gland, often related to meals
- Acute generalized swelling of one or more glands
- Chronic generalized swelling, often involving more than one gland
- Discrete swelling within or adjacent to a gland
- Dry mouth
- Excess salivation.

The important causes of these complaints are summarized in Table 33.1.

INVESTIGATIONS

Several investigations can be used on the salivary glands, the most appropriate often being decided by the patient's presenting symptoms. The main investigations include:

- Plain radiography
- Sialography
- Ultrasound
- Magnetic resonance (MR)
- Radioisotope imaging
- Flow rate studies
- Computed tomography (CT)
- Biopsy.

Table 33.1 A summary of the main salivary gland complaints and their causes

Salivary gland complaint	Cause
Acute intermittent generalized swelling	Obstructive disorders including: Sialolithiasis—salivary stones Stricture or stenosis of the duct, usually secondary to surgery, stones or infection Recurrent parotitis of childhood
Acute generalized swelling	Infection, either: Viral, e.g. mumps Bacterial-ascending sialadenitis
Chronic generalized swelling	Sjögren's syndrome, either primary or secondary Sialosis Chronic infection HIV disease Cystic fibrosis Sarcoidosis
Discrete swelling	Intrinsic tumour, benign or malignant Extrinsic tumour Cysts Overlying lymph nodes
Dry mouth	Sjögren's syndrome Post-radiation damage Mouth breathing Dehydration Functional disorders, including: Drugs, such as tricyclic antidepressants Neuroses, particularly chronic anxiety states
Excess salivation	Psychological (false ptyalism) Reflex, e.g. due to local stimulation Heavy metal poisoning

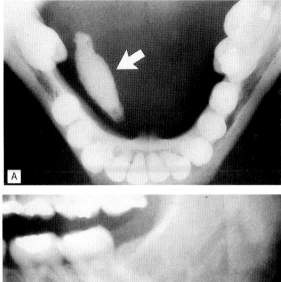

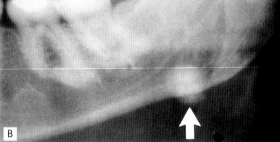

Fig. 33.1A Lower 90° occlusal showing a large radiopaque calculus (arrowed) in the right submandibular duct. **B** Part of a panoramic radiograph showing another calculus (arrowed) in the left submandibular gland.

Plain radiography

The most common disorder of the major salivary glands is obstruction caused either by salivary stones (calculi) or stricture of the ducts. A large proportion of salivary calculi are radiopaque (approximately 40–60% in the parotid and 80% in the submandibular glands) so patients presenting with obstructive symptoms of acute intermittent swelling require routine radiographs to determine the presence and position of the stone(s), as shown in Figure 33.1.

The radiographic projections used commonly for the parotid and submandibular glands are summarized in Table 33.2.

Sialography

Sialography can be defined as the radiographic demonstration of the major salivary glands by introducing a radiopaque contrast medium into their ductal system. It is also very effective for the diagnosis of obstruction whether caused by stones or strictures. It is widely used and is probably still the most common specialized salivary gland investigation.

The procedure is divided into three phases.

- The preoperative phase
- The filling phase
- The emptying phase.

Preoperative phase
This involves taking preoperative (scout) radiographs, if not already taken, before the introduction of the contrast medium, for the following reasons:

- To note the position and/or presence of any radiopaque obstruction
- To assess the position of shadows cast by normal anatomical structures that may overlie the gland, such as the hyoid bone
- To assess the exposure factors.

Filling phase
The relevant duct orifice needs to be found clinically, probed and dilated, and then cannulated. This is shown in Figure 33.2. together with a diagram of the normal anatomy of the major

Salivary gland	Radiographic projections used
Parotid	Panoramic radiograph
	Oblique lateral
	Rotated PA or AP
	Intra-oral view of the cheek
Submandibular	Panoramic radiograph
	Oblique lateral
	Lower 90° occlusal (to show the duct)
	Lower oblique occlusal (to show the gland)
	True lateral skull with the tongue depressed
	Rotated AP (below mandible)

Table 33.2 A summary of the commonly used radiographic projections for the parotid and submandibular glands

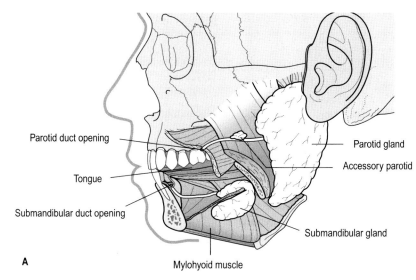

Parotid duct opening

Tongue

Submandibular duct opening

Parotid gland

Accessory parotid

Submandibular gland

A   Mylohyoid muscle

Parotid   Submandibular

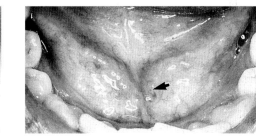

Clinical observation of the duct orifices

Dilatation of the duct orifices

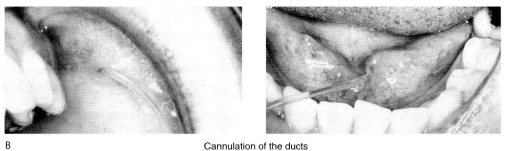

B   Cannulation of the ducts

Fig. 33.2A   Diagram showing the normal anatomy of the parotid and submandibular salivary glands, ducts and duct orifices. **B** Clinical photographs showing these duct orifices (arrowed), being dilated and cannulated.

salivary glands and ducts. The contrast medium can then be introduced.

Three main techniques are available for introducing the contrast medium, as described later. When this is complete, the filling phase radiographs are taken, ideally at least two different views at right angles to one another.

Emptying phase

The cannula is removed and the patient allowed to rinse out. The use of lemon juice at this stage to aid excretion of the contrast medium is often advocated but is seldom necessary. After one and five minutes, the emptying phase radiographs are taken, usually oblique laterals. These films can be used as a crude assessment of function.

Contrast media used

The types of contrast media (see Ch. 19) suitable for sialography are all iodine-based, and include:

- *Ionic aqueous solutions*, including:
  - Diatrizoate (Urografin®)
  - Metrizoate (Triosil®)
- *Non-ionic aqueous solutions*, including:
  - Iohexol (Omnipaque®)
- *Oil-based solutions*, including:
  - Iodized oil, e.g. Lipiodol® (iodized poppy seed oil)
  - Water-insoluble organic iodine compounds, e.g. Pantopaque®.

Most radiology departments use aqueous solutions. Their relative advantages and disadvantages are summarized in Table 33.3.

Note: Since the contrast medium is not being introduced into the bloodstream, there is no need to use the safer, but more expensive, non-ionic contrast media discussed in Chapter 19.

Main indications

The main clinical indications for sialography include:

- To determine the presence and/or position of calculi or other blockages, whatever their radiodensity

Table 33.3 A summary of the advantages and disadvantages of oil-based and aqueous contrast media

Contrast medium	Advantages	Disadvantages
Oil-based	Densely radiopaque, thus shows good contrast High viscosity, thus slows excretion from the gland	Extravasated contrast may remain in the soft tissues for many months, and may produce a foreign body reaction High viscosity means considerable pressure needed to introduce the contrast, calculi may be forced down the main duct
Aqueous	Low viscosity, thus easily introduced Easily and rapidly removed from the gland Easily absorbed and excreted if extravasated	Less radiopaque, less easy to see in line ducts Excretion from the gland is very rapid unless used in a closed system

- To assess the extent of ductal and glandular destruction secondary to an obstruction
- To determine the extent of glandular breakdown and as a crude assessment of function in cases of dry mouth.

Contraindications

The main contraindications include:

- Allergy to compounds containing iodine although gadolinium may be used as an alternative
- Periods of acute infection/inflammation, when there is discharge of pus from the duct opening
- When clinical examination or routine radiographs have shown a calculus close to the duct opening, as injection of the contrast medium may push the calculus back down the main duct where it may be inaccessible.

Sialographic techniques

The control of infection measures detailed in Chapter 9 are of particular importance, and should be adhered to during sialography. In addition, the wearing of eye protection glasses and a mask by operators is recommended.

The three main techniques available for introducing the contrast medium into the ductal system, having cannulated the relevant duct orifice, include:

- Simple injection
- Hydrostatic
- Continuous infusion pressure-monitored.

These techniques can be summarized as follows:

Simple injection technique
Oil-based or aqueous contrast medium is introduced using gentle hand pressure until the patient experiences tightness or discomfort in the gland, (about 1.0 ml for the parotid gland, 0.8 ml for the submandibular gland).

Advantages
- Simple
- Inexpensive.

Disadvantages
- The arbitrary pressure which is applied may cause damage to the gland
- Reliance on patient's responses may lead to underfilling or overfilling of the gland.

Hydrostatic technique
Aqueous contrast media is allowed to flow freely from an overhead resevoir into the gland under the force of gravity until the patient experiences discomfort.

Advantages
- The controlled introduction of contrast medium is less likely to cause damage or give an artefactual picture
- Simple
- Inexpensive.

Disadvantages
- Reliant on the patient's responses
- Patients have to lie down during the procedure, so they need to be positioned in advance for the filling-phase radiographs.

Continuous infusion pressure-monitored technique
Using aqueous contrast medium, a constant flow rate is adopted and the ductal pressure monitored throughout the procedure.

Advantages
- The controlled introduction of contrast media at known pressures is not likely to cause damage
- Does not cause overfilling of the gland
- Does not rely on the patient's responses
- May give information on the presence of obstruction.

Disadvantages
- Complex equipment is required
- Time consuming.

Each of these techniques has its advocates, and with experience, each produces satisfactory results. The technique employed is therefore dependent on the operator and the facilities available.

In addition, sialography may also be performed using advanced imaging modalities, e.g. CT sialography and MR sialography (see Fig. 33.20).

Sialographic interpretation

Once again, the essential requirements include:

- A systematic approach
- A detailed knowledge of the radiographic appearances of normal salivary glands
- A detailed knowledge of the pathological conditions affecting the salivary glands.

Systematic approach
A suggested systematic approach for viewing sialographs is shown in Figure 33.3.

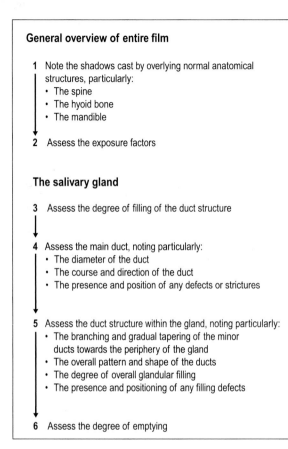

General overview of entire film

1 Note the shadows cast by overlying normal anatomical
   structures, particularly:
   • The spine
   • The hyoid bone
   • The mandible

2 Assess the exposure factors

The salivary gland

3 Assess the degree of filling of the duct structure

4 Assess the main duct, noting particularly:
   • The diameter of the duct
   • The course and direction of the duct
   • The presence and position of any defects or strictures

5 Assess the duct structure within the gland, noting particularly:
   • The branching and gradual tapering of the minor
     ducts towards the periphery of the gland
   • The overall pattern and shape of the ducts
   • The degree of overall glandular filling
   • The presence and positioning of any filling defects

6 Assess the degree of emptying

Fig. 33.3 A systematic approach for viewing sialographs.

Normal sialographic appearances of the parotid gland

These include:

- The main duct is of even diameter (1–2 mm wide) and should be filled completely and uniformly.
- The duct structure within the gland branches regularly and tapers gradually towards the periphery of the gland, the so-called *tree in winter* appearance (see Fig. 33.4).

Normal sialographic appearances of the submandibular gland

These include:

- The main duct is of even diameter (3–4 mm wide) and should be filled completely and uniformly
- This gland is smaller than the parotid, but the overall appearance is similar with the branching duct structure tapering gradually towards the periphery — the so-called *bush in winter* appearance (see Fig. 33.5).

Pathological appearances

Based on the suggested systematic approach to sialographic assessment, the main pathological changes can be divided into:

- Ductal changes associated with:
  - Calculi
  - Sialodochitis (ductal inflammation/infection)

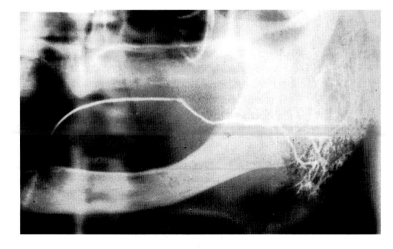

Fig. 33.4 Sialograph showing a normal left parotid gland, the *tree in winter* appearance.

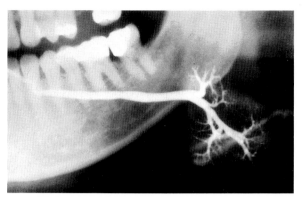

Fig. 33.5   Sialograph showing a normal left submandibular gland, the *bush in winter* appearance.

- *Glandular changes* associated with:
  - Sialadenitis (glandular inflammation/infection)
  - Sjögren's syndrome
  - Intrinsic tumours.

Sialographic appearances of calculi include:

- Filling defect(s) in the main duct
- Ductal dilatation proximal to the calculus
- The emptying film usually shows contrast medium retained behind the s0tone.

See Figures 33.6–33.8.

Sialographic appearances of sialodochitis include:

- Segmented sacculation or dilatation and stricture of the main duct, the so-called *sausage link* appearance
- Associated calculi or ductal stenosis.

See Figures 33.7 and 33.8.

Sialographic appearances of sialadenitis include:

- Dots or blobs of contrast medium within the gland, an appearance known as *sialectasis* (see Fig. 33.9) caused by the inflammation of the glandular tissue producing saccular dilatation of the acini
- The main duct is usually normal.

Sialographic appearances in Sjögren's syndrome include:

- Widespread dots or blobs of contrast medium within the gland, an appearance known as

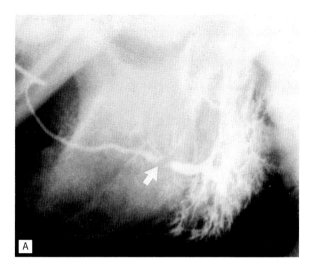

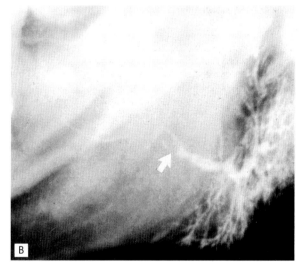

Fig. 33.6A   Sialograph of a left parotid gland showing a filling defect at the posterior end of the main duct (arrowed), caused by a stone in the duct. Ductal dilatation is evident beyond the stone. **B** Emptying film of the same gland showing the contrast medium retained behind the filling defect (arrowed), confirming the diagnosis of salivary calculus in the main duct.

punctate sialectasis or *snowstorm* (see Fig. 33.10). This is caused by a weakening of the epithelium lining the intercalated ducts, allowing the escape of the contrast medium out of the ducts
- Considerable retention of the contrast medium during the emptying phase
- The main duct is usually normal.

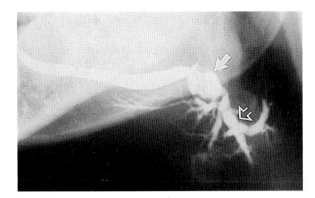

Fig. 33.7 Sialograph of a left submandibular gland, showing a normal main duct, a large calculus (solid arrow) at the posterior end of the main duct and associated segmental sacculation or dilatation and stricture of the ducts beyond the stone. Within the gland (open arrow) the *sausage-link* appearance is caused by sialodochitis.

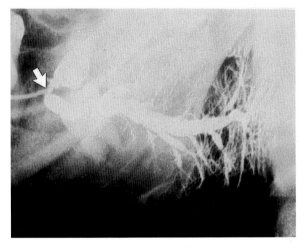

Fig. 33.8 Sialograph of a left parotid showing gross dilatation of the main duct caused by sialodochitis secondary to stenosis at the orifice (arrowed).

An understanding of the underlying disease processes explains why the sialographic appearances of sialadenitis and Sjögren's syndrome (two totally different conditions) are so similar. This is shown diagrammatically in Figure 33.11.

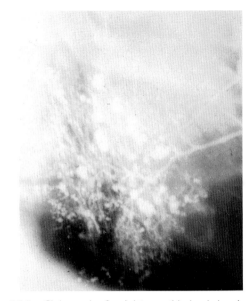

Fig. 33.9 Sialograph of a right parotid gland showing the dots or blobs of contrast medium within the gland — the appearance known as *sialectasis*, caused by sialadenitis. Note the main duct is normal.

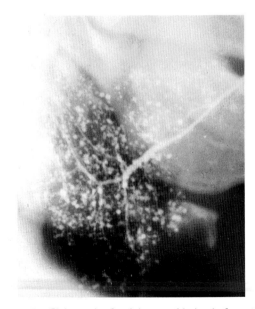

Fig. 33.10 Sialograph of a right parotid gland of a patient with Sjögren's syndrome. The main duct is normal and there are widespread dots or blobs of contrast medium throughout the gland, the *snowstorm* appearance of *punctate sialectasis*.

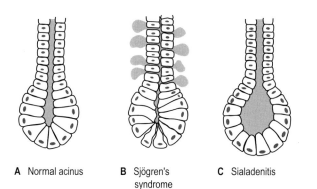

A Normal acinus   **B** Sjögren's syndrome   **C** Sialadenitis

Fig. 33.11   Diagrams showing an intercalated ductule and acinus. **A** In a normal gland. **B** In Sjögren's syndrome, the epithelium lining the intercalated ductule becomes weakened allowing escape of the contrast medium out of the duct so producing the dots or blobs. **C** In sialadenitis, the acinus becomes dilated allowing the collection of contrast into a dot or blob.

Sialographic appearances of intrinsic tumours include:

- An area of underfilling within the gland, owing to ductal compression by the tumour
- Ductal displacement — the ducts adjacent to the tumour are usually stretched around it, an appearance known as *ball in hand* (see Figs 33.12 and 33.13)
- Retention of contrast medium in the displaced ducts during the emptying phase.

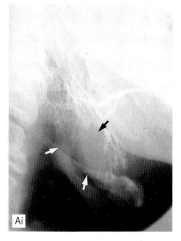

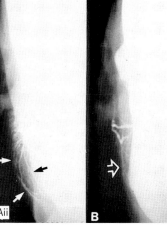

Fig. 33.12A(i)   Sialograph of a right parotid showing a large area of underfilling in the lower lobe (arrowed) caused by an intrinsic tumour (biopsy confirmed a pleomorphic adenoma). A(ii) Rotated AP view showing the lateral bowing and displacement of the ducts (arrowed) around the tumour. **B** Rotated AP view of a normal parotid gland for comparison.

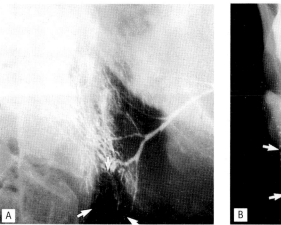

Fig. 33.13A   Sialograph of a right parotid gland showing a large area of underfilling in the lower lobe (arrowed) caused by an intrinsic tumour (pleomorphic adenoma). **B** Rotated AP view showing extensive ductal displacement, the appearance described as *ball in hand* (arrowed).

Interventional sialography

Conventional sialographic techniques can be supplemented and expanded into minimally invasive interventional procedures by using *balloon catheters* and small *Dormia baskets* under fluoroscopic guidance. The *balloon catheter*, as the name implies, can be inflated once positioned within a duct to produce dilatation of ductal strictures. The *Dormia basket* may be used to retrieve mobile ductal salivary stones (see Fig. 33.14). Both these procedures are now being used successfully to relieve salivary gland obstruction without the need for surgery.

Ultrasound

Ultrasound imaging of the salivary glands as shown in Figure 33.15 is becoming increasingly common. Modern high resolution scanners produce excellent images and that coupled with the numerous advantages shown below has elevated ultrasound to the imaging modality of choice for many patients with salivary gland disorders as shown in Figures 33.16–33.18.

Indications

- Discrete and generalized swellings both intrinsic and extrinsic to the salivary glands
- Salivary obstruction.

Advantages

- Ionizing radiation is not used
- Provides good imaging of superficial masses
- Useful for differentiating between solid and cystic masses and for identifying the nature and location of the margins of a lesion
- Different echo signals from different tumours
- Assessment of blood flow using colour Doppler
- Identification of radiolucent stones
- Lithotripsy of salivary stones
- Ultrasound-guided fine-needle aspiration (FNA) biopsy possible
- Intra-oral ultrasound possible with small probes.

Disadvantages

- The sound waves used are blocked by bone, so limiting the areas available for investigation
- Provides no information on fine ductal architecture.

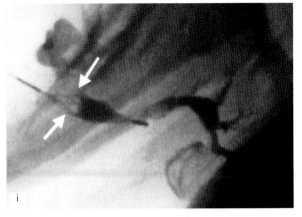

i

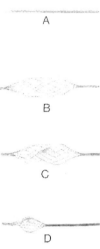

A

B

C

ii   D

Fig. 33.14 (i) Fluoroscopic sialograph showing an open Dormia basket in the left submandbular duct. The stone has been captured and is inside the basket (white arrows). Contract media is evident in the dilated main duct within the gland. (Kindly provided by Mrs J.E.Brown.) (ii) The Meditech (Boston Scientific) Dormia basket – **A** closed for insertion beyond the stone; **B** open ready to draw back; **C** open with the stone inside and **D** closed around the stone ready for withdrawal.

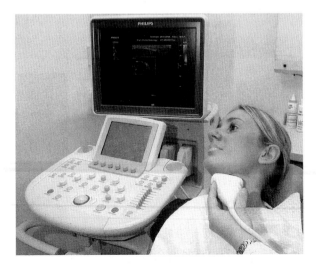

Fig. 33.15 Patient undergoing ultrasound investigation of the left submandibular gland.

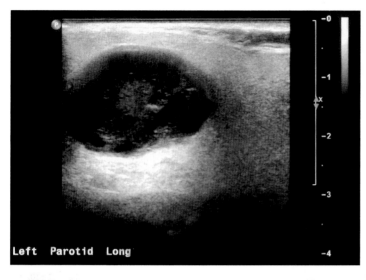

Fig. 33.16 Ultrasound image of a pleomorphic adenoma in the parotid gland. The benign tumour shows well defined margins and is generally hypoechoic (dark) with *through transmission* suggesting low density and a high water content. (Kindly provided by Mrs J.E. Brown.)

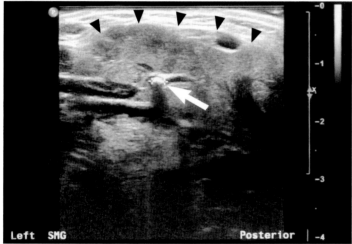

Fig. 33.17 Ultrasound image of a submandibular gland (the margin of the gland is marked by the black arrow heads) containing a small calculus (white arrow) within the hilum of the main duct. The stone measured 2.2 mm in diameter and was radiolucent on plain radiography. The dilated duct to the right of the stone is also evident. (Kindly provided by Mrs J.E. Brown.)

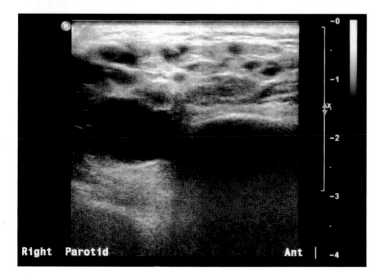

Fig. 33.18 Ultrasound image showing the changes typically seen within the parotid gland in Sjögren's syndrome. The multiple small hypoechoic (dark) areas represent lymphoepithelial infiltration of the gland parenchyma. (Kindly provided by Mrs J.E. Brown.)

Magnetic resonance (MR)

Indications

- Discrete swelling or lump both intrinsic and extrinsic to the salivary glands
- Generalized swelling, e.g. Sjögren's syndrome.

Advantages

- Ionizing radiation is not used
- Provides excellent soft tissue detail, readily enables differentiation between normal and abnormal
- Provides accurate localization of masses (see Fig. 33.19) and may be able to distinguish benign from malignant tumours
- The facial nerve may be identifiable
- Images in all planes are available
- *Co-localization* possible with PET scans
- MR sialography may be performed (see Fig. 33.20) together with MR spectroscopy
- Water in the ducts and glands can be visualized to create MR sialographs without the use of contrast agents (see Fig. 33.20)
- MR spectroscopy can be performed to differentiate different tissues by their chemical constituents.

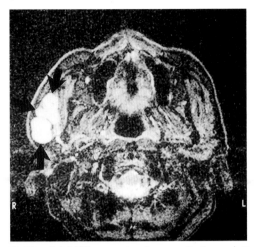

Fig. 33.19 Axial MR scan, showing a well-circumscribed benign mass in the right parotid gland (arrowed). Histopathology revealed a pleomorphic adenoma.

Disadvantages

- Provides no information on salivary gland function
- Limited information on surrounding hard tissues
- May not distinguish benign lesions with high water content from cysts.

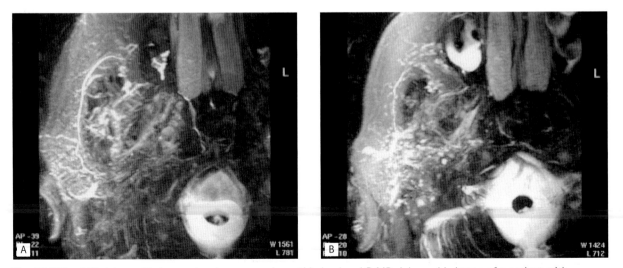

Fig. 33.20A MR sialographic image showing a normal parotid gland and **B** MR sialographic image of a patient with Sjögren's syndrome. (Kindly provided by Dr V. Rushton.)

Radioisotope imaging

Indications

- Dry mouth as a result of salivary gland diseases such as Sjögren's syndrome
- To assess salivary gland function
- PET for salivary gland tumours.

Advantages

- Provides an indication of salivary gland function (see Fig. 33.21)
- Allows bilateral comparison and images all four major salivary glands at the same time
- Computer analysis of results is possible
- Can be performed in cases of acute infection
- *Co-localization* of PET with CT or MR scans (see Ch. 19).

Disadvantages

- Provides no indication of salivary gland anatomy or ductal architecture
- Relatively high radiation dose to the whole body
- The final images are not disease-specific.

Flow–rate studies

These are used to investigate salivary gland function. Comparative flow rates of saliva from the major salivary glands are measured over a time period.

Indications

- Dry mouth
- Poor salivary flow
- Excess salivation.

Advantages

- Ionizing radiation is not used
- Simple to perform
- Provides information on salivary gland function.

Disadvantages

- Provides only limited information — no indication of the nature of underlying disease
- Time consuming.

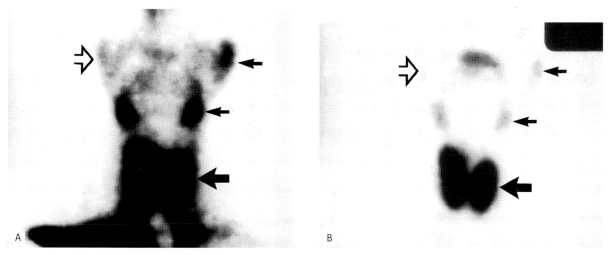

Fig. 33.21 Two radioisotope scans showing the thyroid (large arrow) and salivary glands (small arrows). **A** 2 minutes after the injection of technetium. **B** 15 minutes after the injection of technetium. In the 2-minute image, note the large amount of background activity owing to the technetium still in the bloodstream and in both scans the lack of uptake by the non-functioning RIGHT parotid (open arrow).

Computed tomography (CT)

Indication

- Discrete swellings both intrinsic and extrinsic to the salivary glands.

Advantages

- Provides accurate localization of masses, especially in the deep lobe of the parotid
- The nature of the lesion can often be determined
- Images can be enhanced by using contrast media, either in the ductal system (CT sialography) or more commonly intravenously
- *Co-localization* possible with PET scans.

Disadvantages

- Provides no indication of salivary gland function
- Risks associated with intravenous contrast media if used (see Ch. 19)
- Fine duct detail is not well imaged
- High radiation dose
- May be difficult to distinguish tumours in the submandibular gland from normal gland tissue (due to similar density).

Bibliography and suggested reading

Part 1
Introduction (Ch. 1)

Coren S, Porac C, Ward LM 1979 Sensation and perception. Academic Press, New York

Cornsweet TN 1970 Visual perception. Academic Press, New York

Lindsay PH, Norman DA 1977 Human information and processing. 2nd edn. Academic Press, New York

Part 2
Radiation physics and equipment (Chs 2–7)

Armstrong SJ 1990 Lecture notes on the physics of radiology. Clinical Press, Bristol

Berkhout WE, Beuger DA, Sanderink GC, Stelt van der PF 2004 The dynamic range of digital radiographic systems: dose reduction or risk of overexposure? Dentomaxillofacial Radiology 33:1–5

Curry TS, Dowdey JE, Murry RC 1990 Christensen's physics of diagnostic radiology. 4th edn. Lea and Febiger, Philadelphia

Graham DT 1996 Principles of radiological physics. 3rd edn. Churchill Livingstone, Edinburgh

HSE 1992 Fitness of equipment used for medical exposure to ionising radiation. Health and Safety Guidance Note PM77

IPEM 2005 Recommended standards for the routine performance testing of diagnostic X-ray imaging systems. IPEM Report No. 91

Mason RA, Bourne S 1998 A guide to dental radiography. 4th edn. Oxford University Press, Oxford

Meredith WJ, Massey JB 1977 Fundamental physics of radiology. 3rd edn. John Wright, Bristol

NRPB 1994 Guidelines on radiology standards in primary dental care. National Radiological Protection Board, Vol. 5, No. 3 1994

NRPB/DH 2001 Guidance notes for dental practitioners on the safe use of X-ray equipment.

Smith NJD 1989 Dental radiography. 2nd edn. Blackwell Scientific, Oxford

Strather JW, Muirhead CR, Edwards AA et al 1988 Health effects models developed from the UNSCEAR report. National Radiological Protection Board, Chilton, NRPB-R226. HMSO, London

Sumner D, Wheldon T, Watson W 1991 Radiation risks: an evaluation. 3rd edn. The Tarragon Press, Glasgow

Tanner RJ, Wall BF, Shrimpton PC, Hart D, Bungay DR 2000 Frequency of medical and dental X-ray examinations in the UK –1997/98. NRPB-R320 (2000), Chilton

Wilks R 1987 Principles of radiological physics. 2nd edn. Churchill Livingstone, Edinburgh

Part 3
Radiation protection (Ch. 8)

Approved code of practice: the protection of persons against ionising radiation arising from any work activity. The ionising radiations regulations 1985. HMSO, London

Bury B, Hufton A, Adams J 1995 Radiation and women of childbearing potential. British Medical Journal 310:1022–23

EC 2004 European guidelines on radiation protection in dental radiology - the safe use of radiographs in dental practice. European Commission, Radiation Protection 136

FGDP (UK) 2004 Selection criteria for dental radiography. 2nd edn. Faculty of General Dental Practice (UK) of the Royal College of Surgeons of England

Frederiksen NL, Benson BW, Sokolowski TW 1994 Effective dose and risk assessment from film tomography used for dental implant diagnostics. Dentomaxillofacial Radiology 23:123–127

Guidance notes for dental practitioners on the safe use of X-ray equipment 2001. NRPB/DoH, London

Health and Safety at Work, etc. Act 1974. HMSO, London

ICRP publication 34 1982 Protection of the patient in diagnostic radiology. Pergamon, Oxford

ICRP publication 60 1990 Recommendations of the International Commission on Radiological Protection. Annals ICPR 21. Nos 1–3. Pergamon, Oxford

Lecomber AR, Downes SL, Mokhtari M, Faulkner K 2000 Optimisation of patient doses in programmable dental panoramic radiography. Dentomaxillofacial Radiology 29:107–112

Napier I D. 1999 Reference doses for dental radiography. British Dental Journal 186:8 392–396

NCRP 2003 Radiation protection in dentistry. National Council on Radiation Protection and Measurements, Report No. 145

NRPB 1994 Guidelines on radiology standards in primary dental care. National Radiological Protection Board, Vol. 5, No. 3 1994

NRPB 1999 Guidelines on patient dose to promote the optimisation of protection for diagnostic medical exposures. National Radiological Protection Board, Vol. 10, No. 1 1999

Russel JGB 1989 Diagnostic radiation, pregnancy and termination. British Journal of Radiology 62:92–94

Shrimpton PC, Wall BF, Jones DG et al 1986 A national survey of doses to patients undergoing a selection of routine X-ray examinations in English hospitals. National Radiological Protection Board, Chilton, NRPB-R200

Ionising Radiations Regulations 1999. SI 1999 No 3232. HMSO, London

Ionising Radiation (Medical Exposure) Regulations 2000. SI 2000 No 1059. HMSO, London

Sharp C, Shrimpton JA, Berry RF 1998 Diagnostic medical exposures – advice on exposure to ionising radiation during pregnancy. Joint guidance from National Radiological Protection Board

Sherer MAS, Visconti PJ, Ritenour ER 2002 Radiation protection in medical radiography. 4th edn. Mosby, London

White SC 1992 Assessment of radiation risk from dental radiography. Dentomaxillofacial Radiology 21:118–126

Part 4
Radiography (Chs 9–19)

Ahuja A, Evans R 2000 Practical head and neck ultrasound. Greenwich Medical Media, London

Armstrong P, Wastie ML 1998 Diagnostic imaging. 4th edn. Blackwell Scientific, Oxford

Barnes L, Eveson JW, Reichart P, Sidransky D 2005 World Health Organization classification of tumours – pathology and genetics of head and neck tumours. IARC, Lyon 2005

Bergeron RT, Osborn AG, Som PM 1990 Head and neck imaging. 2nd edn. CV Mosby, St Louis

British Orthodontic Society 2000 Guidelines for the use of radiographs in clinical orthodontics. 2nd edn. London

Chapman S, Nakielny R 1993 A guide to radiological procedures. WB Saunders, London

Delbalso AM 1990 Maxillofacial imaging. WB Saunders, Philadelphia

Hedrick WR, Hykes DL, Starchman DE 1995 Ultrasound physics and instrumentation. 3rd edn. CV Mosby, St Louis

Horner K 1992 Quality assurance: 1 Reject analysis, operator technique and the X-ray set. Dental Update 19:75–80

Horner K 1992 Quality assurance: 2 The image receptor, the darkroom and processing. Dental Update 19:120–122

IPEM 1991 Quality assurance in dental radiology. IPEM report No.67

Jacobson A 1995 Radiographic cephalometry. Quintessence, Chicago

Jones ML, Oliver RG 1994 Walther and Houston's orthodontic notes. 5th edn. Butterworth-Heinemann, Oxford

Kidd EAM 2005 Essentials of dental caries. 3rd edn. Oxford University Press, Oxford

Langland OE, Langlais RP 1997 Principles of dental imaging. Williams and Wilkins, Baltimore

Langland OE, Langlais RP, McDavid WD, Delbalso AM 1989 Panoramic radiology. Lea and Febiger, Philadelphia

Manson-Hing LR 1990 Fundamentals of dental radiography. 3rd edn. Lea and Febiger, Philadelphia

Mason RA, Bourne S 1998 A guide to dental radiography. 4th edn. Oxford University Press, Oxford

Maisey M, Jeffrey P 1991 Clinical applications of positron emission tomography. British Journal of Clinical Practice 45:265–272

McDonald F, Ireland AJ 1998 Diagnosis of the orthodontic patient. Oxford University Press, Oxford

NRPB/DH 2001 Guidance notes for dental practitioners on the safe use of X-ray equipment

Proceedings of the second symposium on digital imaging in dental radiology, Amsterdam 1992. Dentomaxillofacial Radiology 21:179–221

Proceedings of the third symposium on digital imaging in dental radiology, Noorwijkerhout, The Netherlands 1995. Dentomaxillofacial Radiology 24:67–106

Razmus TF, Williamson GF 1996 Current oral and maxillofacial imaging. WB Saunders, Philadelphia

Schild HH 1990 MRI made easy (…well almost). Schering AG, Berlin

Sharp PF, Gemmell HG, Smith FW 1998 Practical nuclear medicine. 2nd edn. Oxford University Press, Oxford

Smith NJD 1989 Dental radiography. 2nd edn. Blackwell Scientific Publications, Oxford

Sutton D, Young JWR 1990 A short textbook of clinical imaging. Springer-Verlag, London

The British standards glossary of dental terms BS 4492: 1983

White SC, Pharoah MJ 2004 Oral radiology principles and interpretation. 5th edn. CV Mosby, St Louis

World Health Organization Quality assurance in diagnostic radiology. WHO, Geneva

Yuh WTC, Tali ET, Afifi AK et al 1994 MRI of head and neck anatomy. Churchill Livingstone, New York

Part 5
Radiology (Chs 20–33)

Albrektson T, Zarb GA 1989 The Branemark osseointegrated implant. Quintessence, Chicago

Andreasen JO, Andreasen FM 2001 Textbook of traumatic injuries to the teeth. 4th edn. Munksgard, Copenhagen

Armstrong P, Wastie ML 1998 Diagnostic imaging. 4th edn. Blackwell Scientific, Oxford

Blair GS 1973 Hydrostatic sialography, an analysis of a technique. Oral Surgery 36:116–130

Brocklebank L 1996 Dental radiology (understanding the X-ray image). Oxford University Press, Oxford

Browne RM, Edmondson HD, Rout PGJ 1995 Atlas of dental and maxillofacial radiology. Mosby-Wolfe, London

Cawson RA, Odell EW 2002 Essentials of oral pathology and oral medicine. 7th edn. Churchill Livingstone, Edinburgh

Cawson RA, Binnie WH, Eveson JW 1993 A colour atlas of oral disease – clinical and pathologic correlations. 2nd edn. Wolfe Medical, London

Cawson RA, Eveson JW 1987 Oral pathology and diagnosis. William Heinemann Medical, London

Cawson RA, Langdon JD, Eveson JW 1996 Surgical pathology of the mouth and jaws. Wright, Oxford

Coleman GC, Nelson JF 1993 Principles of oral diagnosis. Mosby Year Book, St Louis

Ferguson MM, Evans A Mason WN 1977 Continuous infusion pressure-monitored sialography. International Journal of Oral Surgery 6:94–98

FGDP (UK) 2004 Selection criteria for dental radiography. 2nd edn. Faculty of General Dental Practice (UK) of the Royal College of Surgeons of England

Gibilisco JA 1985 Stafne's oral radiographic diagnosis. 5th edn. WB Saunders, Philadelphia

Harnsberger HR 1995 Handbook of head and neck imaging. 2nd edn. CV Mosby, St. Louis

Heffez LB, Mafee MF, Rosenberg H 1995 Imaging atlas of the temporomandibular joint. Williams and Wilkins, Baltimore

Horner K, Rout J, Rushton V 2002 Interpreting dental radiographs. Quintessence, London

Howe GL 1985 Minor oral surgery. 3rd edn. John Wright, Bristol

Hutchinson IL, Hopper C, Conar HS 1990 Neoplasia masquerading as periapical infection. British Dental Journal 168:228–294

Keller JD 1990 Basics of head and neck film interpretation. Little, Brown, Boston

Kidd EAM 2005 Essentials of dental caries. 3rd edn. Oxford University Press, Oxford

Langlais RP, Langland OE, Nortge CJ 1995 Diagnostic imaging of the jaws. Williams and Wilkins, Baltimore

Langland OE, Sippy FH, Langlais RP 1984 Textbook of dental radiology. 2nd edn. Charles C Thomas, Illinois

Logan BM, Reynolds PA, Hutchings RT 2004 McMinn's colour atlas of the head and neck anatomy. 3rd edn. Mosby, Edinburgh

Ludlow JB, Davies-Ludlow LE, Brooks SL 2003 Dosimetry of two extra-oral direct digital imaging devices:–NewTom cone beam CT and Orthophos Plus DS panoramic unit. Dentomaxillofacial Radiology 32:229–234

McGowan DA, Baxter PW, James J 1993 The maxillary sinus and its dental implications. Butterworth-Heineman, Oxford

Miles DA, Van Dis ML 1994 The clinical approach to radiologic diagnosis. The dental clinics of North America. WB Saunders, Philadelphia, Vol. 38

Miles DA, Van Dis ML, Kaugars GE, Lovas JGL 1991 Oral and maxillofacial radiology – radiologic/pathologic correlations. WB Saunders, Philadelphia

Neville BW, Damn DD, Allen CM, Bouquot JE 2002 Oral and maxillofacial pathology. 2nd edn. WB Saunders, Philadelphia

Norman J de B, Bramley P 1990 A textbook and colour atlas of the temporomandibular joint. Wolfe Medical, London

Palmer RM 2000 A clinical guide to implants in dentistry. British Dental Association, London

Poyton HG, Pharoah MJ 1989 Oral radiology. 2nd edn. BC Decker, Toronto

RCR 2003 Making the best use of a department of clinical radiology. 5th edn. The Royal College of Radiologists, London

Roberts G, Longhurst P 1996 Oral and dental trauma in children and adolescents. Oxford University Press, Oxford

Robinson PD 2000 Tooth extraction – a practical guide. Wright, Oxford

Rout PGJ, Browne RM 1997 Self-assessment picture tests. Oral radiology. Mosby-Wolfe, London

Rudolphy MP, van Amerongen JP, ten Cate JM 1994 Radiopacities in dentine under amalgam restorations. Caries research 28:240–245

Sailer HF, Pajorola GF 1999 Oral surgery for the general dentist. Thieme, Stuttgart

Tyndall AA, Brooks SL 2000 Selection criteria for dental implant site imaging: a position of the American academy of Oral and Maxillofacial Radiology. Oral Surg Oral Med Oral Path Oral Radiol Endod 89(5):630–637

Van der Waal I 1991 Diseases of the jaws diagnosis and treatment. Munksgaard, Copenhagen

White SC. Pharaoh MJ 2004 Oral radiology – principles and interpretation. 5th edn. CV Mosby, St Louis

White SC, Heslop EW, Hollander LG, Mosier KM, Ruprecht A, Shrout MK 2001 An official report of the American Academy of Oral and Maxillofacial Radiology. Oral Surg Oral Med Oral Path Oral Radiol Endod 91(5):498–511

Wood NK 1999 Review of diagnosis, oral medicine, radiology, and treatment planning. 4th edn. CV Mosby, St Louis

Wood NK, Goaz PW 1991 Differential diagnosis of oral lesions. 4th edn. CV Mosby, St Louis

Wood RE 1988 Handbook of signs in dental and maxillofacial radiology. Warthog, Toronto

Worth HM 1963 Principles and practice of oral radiographic interpretation. Year Book Medical, Chicago

Worthington P, Beirne OR 1991 Implants. Oral and maxillofacial surgery clinics of North America. WB Saunders, Philadelphia, Vol. 3

Wright EF 2005 Manual of temporomandibular disorders. Blackwell Munsgaard, Iowa

Index

Page numbers in **BOLD** indicate illustrations/images.

A

Abscess, of the periodontium
  gingival, 285
  pericoronal, 285
  periodontal, 279, 285, **286**
Abscess, periapical, 270, **271, 272**
Absorption, 21, 46
Absorption efficiency, of intensifying
     screens, 46
Absorption unsharpness, 208
  see also Cervical *burn-out*
Accuitomo, 235, **235, 236**
Acne scars, calcified, 356, 371
Acquired defects of teeth, 300
Acquired immune deficiency syndrome
    (AIDS), 87
Acromegaly, 301, 431, 438, **438**
Acute apical periodontitis, 270, **271-272**
Acute effects of whole body radiation,
    29
Acute inflammation, signs of, 270
Acute sinusitis, 375, **376**
  see also Maxillary antra
Additional teeth, 299, **302**
  see also Hyperdontia
Adenomatoid odontogenic tumour
    (AOT), 331, 341, 354, 356, 361,
    361, 372
Adequate training in radiation
    protection, 75
Adhesive restorations, 256, **256**
Aggressive periodontitis, 279, 285, **286**
ALARP principle, 33
Albers-Schönberg disease, 370, 433,
    433
Alpha particles, 227
Aluminium filter, in X-ray tubehead 36,
    36
Aluminium wedge filter, in
    cephalostat, **171,** 172, **174**

Alveolar bone fractures, 388
Ameloblastic fibroma, 331, 340, **340,**
    354
Ameloblastic fibro-odontoma, 331, 341,
    361, **361**
Ameloblastoma, 331, 338, **338–339,** 354,
    384
  Unicystic, 338
Amelogenesis imperfecta, 299, **302**
ANB, cephalometric angle, **175,** 176
Aneurysmal bone cyst, 331, 337, 351,
    351, 354
Angiography, 223, **224,** 225
Ankylosis,TMJ, 422, 426, **426**
Annihilation radiation, 228
Annual radiation dose limits, 76–80
Anode, in X-ray tube, 17, **17**
Anodontia, 299
  see also Hypodontia
Anterior nasal spine (ANS)
    cephalometric point, 174, **175**
    normal radiographic anatomy, **136,**
    336
Anti-scatter grid, 150, **151,** 171, **171**
Antra *see* Maxillary antra
Antral disease, 375–385
Antral halo appearance, **273,** 377
Antrolith, 381
Apert's syndrome, 301, **308**
Apical periodontitis
  acute, 271, **272**
  chronic, 271, **272-273**
Aprons *see* Lead protection
Approximal caries, 252, **252-253,** 255
Arthritis *see* Osteoartritis, Rheumatoid
    arthritis
Arthrography, TMJ 223, 413, 421–422,
    422
Arthroscopy, TMJ, 413, 422
Articular eminence (TMJ), anatomy of,
    411-413

Articulare (Ar),cephalometric point,
    175, **175**
Atomic physics 15-18, 21-23
Atomic mass number (A), 16
Atomic number (Z), 16
Atomic particles 15-16
Atomic structure, **15,** 15–16
Attenuation, 21
Audits, 220
Authorization, 70
Automatic processing, 57–58, **58**
Average gradient, 45, **45**
Avulsion, 387

B

Back scatter, 23, **23**
Background fog density, **43,** 44
Background radiation 27
Ball in hand appearance, 453, **453**
Balloon catheter, 454
  see also Interventional sialography
Barium meal, 223, **224**
Barrier envelopes, **41,** 49, **52,** 88, **88-89**
Beaking, TMJ,423, **423-424**
Beam-indicating device (BID), 36, **36, 37**
  see also Spacer cone
Bending of film packet, effect of, 210,
    211, 213
Benign tumours *see* Tumours and
    tumour-like lesions
Beta particles, 227
Bifid condyle, 301, **307,** 428
Bifid root, 300, **304**
Bimolar technique, 146, **147**
  see also Oblique lateral radiography
Biofilm of plaque, 251
Biological effects of radiation, 29–33
Bisected angle technique, 106–115
  see Periapical radiography

Bite blocks, 93, **93-96**
Bitewing radiography, 125-133
    assessment of quality, 132-133
    ideal technique requirements, 125–126, 126
    image receptor holders for, 127
    main indications, 125
    positioning techniques, 127–130, **127-130**
    resultant radiographs, 130–133
    suggested guidelines for interpreting, 263
Blood dyscrasias, 431, 439–440, **439-440**
    see also Sickle cell anaemia; Thalassaemia
Blooming, 65, **66**
Blow-out fracture see Orbital blow-out fracture
Blurring, 210, **210**, 213
    see also Penumbra effect; Image unsharpness
Bone conditions of variable radiopacity, 356, 359–370, **359-370**
Bone cysts, 331, 337, **337**, 351, **351**
Bone diseases 431-440
    blood dyscrasias, 4a9–440, **439-440**
    developmental or genetic disorders, 432–433, **432-433**
    diseases of unknown cause, 441–443, **441-443**
    hormone-related diseases, 437–438, **437-438**
    infective or inflammatory conditions, 434–436, **434-436**
Bone loss, periodontal assessment, 277, **282-283**
Bone-related lesions, 331, 349–354, **349-354**, 356, 368–369, **368-369**
    aneurysmal bone cyst, 331, 337, 351, **351**, 354
    brown tumour in hyperparathyoidism, 331,350, 354,437, **437**
    central giant cell lesion (granuloma), 331, 349, **349**, 354
    cherubism, 331, 350, **350**, 354
    familial gigantiform cementoma, 331, 356, 367, 372
    fibrous dysplasia, 331, 356, 368, **368** 372, 431, 441, **441**
    florid osseous dysplasia, 331, 353, **353**, 356, 367, **367**, 372
    focal osseous dysplasia, 331, 356, 366, **366**, 372
    ossifying fibroma, 331, 356, 369, **369**, 372
    periapical osseous dysplasia, 331, 352, **352**, 356, 366, **366**, 372
    simple bone cyst, 331, 337, **337**, 354

Stafne's bone cavity, 331, 354, **354**
Bone tumours, 274, 343–348, **343-348**
    see also Tumours and tumour-like lesions
Braking radiation, 19
Brånemark implant system, 289, **290**
Bremsstrahlung radiation, 19
Brightness, image, 63, **63**
British Standards Glossary of Dental Terms, 135, 151, 176
Brow-up lateral projection, 401
Brown tumour in hyperparathyroidism, 331, 350, 354, 437, **437**
Broad-beam linear tomography, **181**, 181–185, **184-185**, 188, **188**
Buccal bifurcation cyst, 332
Bucket handle fracture, **396**
Burkitt's lymphoma, 331, 347, **347**
Burn-out, 256–258, **257**, 262, 288
    see also Cervical *burn-out*
Bush in winter appearance, 450, **451**

C

Calcifications, superimposed soft tissue, 356, 370-371
    calcified acne scars, 356, 371
    calcified lymph nodes, 356, 370, **370**
    calcified tonsils, 356, 371, **371**
    phleboliths, 356, 371, **371**
    salivary calculi, 356, 370, **370**, 445, **446**, 450, **451-452**, 454, **454**
Calcifying cystic odontogenic tumour, (calcifying odontogenic cyst), 331, 341, 354, 362, **362**, 372
Calcifying epithelial odontogenic tumour (CEOT), 331, 341, 354, 360, **360**, 372
Calcium tungstate intensifying screens, 46, **46**, 47
Calculi, salivary, 356, 370, **370**, 445, **446**, 450, **451-452**, 454, **454**
    sialographic appearances of, 451, **451-452**
    see also Interventional sialography
Campbell's lines, 402, **402**, 404
Cancer induction, estimating the risk of, 31–32
Canines
    mandibular
        bisected angle technique, **111**
        paralleling technique, 96, **102**
    maxillary
        bisected angle technique, **109**
        paralleling technique, 96, **98**

radiographic assessment of unerupted, 316–321, **316-321**
Carcinomas, metastatic, 346, **346**
Caries, 251-264
    classification of, 251–252
    diagnosis and detection of, 252–255
    limitations of radiographic detection of, 258–262, **259-262**
    other important radiographic appearances, 256–258
    radiographic appearance of, **253**, **255**
    risk, 253–254
    suggested guidelines for interpretation, 263–264
Cassettes, 47–48, **47-48**
    quality assurance checks, 218, **219**
Cathode, in X-ray tube, 17, **17**
Cementoblastoma, 356, 363, **363**, 372
Cemento-enamel junction, 278, **278**
Central giant cell lesion (granuloma), 331, 349, **349**, 354
Central haemangioma, 331, 343, **343**, 354
Cephalometric planes and angles, **175**, 175–176
Cephalometric points, 174–175, **175**
Cephalometric radiography, cephalometric posteroanterior of the jaws, **176**, 176–177
    equipment, 169–171, **170-172**
    main indications, 169
    main projections, 173–176
Cephalometric tracing, 174–176, **175**
Cephalostat units, 170-171, **173**
Cervical *burn-out*, 256–258, **257**, 262
Cervical spine
    ghost shadow on panoramic radiographs, 196, **199**, 288
    normal radiographic appearance, **158-159**, 140-143
    radiography of, 410
Characteristic curve, 43, **43-44**
Characteristic spectrum, **19**, 19–20
Charge-coupled device (CCD), 50-51, **50-51**
    see also Solid-state sensors
Chemical processing of images, **55**, 55–58
    quality assurance programme, 218–219
Chemical solutions, 57
Cherubism, 331, 350, **350**, 354
Children's radiography
    Bitewing, 129-131, **129-131**
    oblique lateral, 145, **147**
    periapical, 120, **121**
    specific requirements, 86-87
    under GA, **86**
Chondroma, 331, 356, 372, 427, **427**

Chondrosarcoma, 331, 344, 427
Chronic periodontitis, 279, 281-282, **282-285**
Chronic inflammation, hallmarks of, 271
Chronic sinusitis
   see also Maxillary antra
Circuitry of X-ray machines, **39**, 39–40
Cleft lip, 301
Cleft palate, 301, **307-308**
Cleidocranial dysplasia, 301, 431, 432, **432**
Coin test, 217–218, **218**
Collective effective dose, 26
Collimators
   in cephalometry, **170**, 171, 173, **173**
   in X-ray tubehead, 36, **36-37**
   incorporated in image receptor holder, **94**
   rectangular types, **36-37**
   secondary, 173, **173**
Collisions, electron, 17–18, **18**
Co-localization, 228, 456, 458
Combined spectra, 20, **20**
Complex odontome, 356, 358, **358**
Complimentary metal oxide detectors (CMOS), 50
Compound odontome, 356, 358, **358**
Compton effect, 21, **22**, 22–23
Computed tomography (CT), 223, 228–236, **228, 229, 231**
   facial fractures, 401, **407, 408, 410**
   implant assessment, 292, 293, **294**
   maxillary antra, 376, **377, 385, 386**
   salivary glands, 458
   temporomandibular joint, 421
Computer digital processing, 59–66
Concresence, 300, **303**
Condylar hyperplasia, 428, **428**
Condylar hypoplasia, 307, 428, **428**
Cone beam computed tomography (CBCT), 59, 232–235, **232-235**
   implant assessment, 291–293, **292-293**
   maxillary antra, 376, **376**
   temporomandibular joint, 419, **420, 424**
Condylar head
   normal anatomy, **412-413**
   normal radiographic appearances, **161, 167, 417, 420**
   see also Temporomandibular joint
Condylar neck
   fracture of, 392, **399**
   hyperplasia, 428, **428**
   hypoplasia, **307, 428, 428**
   normal radiographic appearances, **158-163**
Condyle *see* Temporomandibular joint
Cone cutting see Coning off

Congenital syphilis, 300, **304**
Coning off, 113, **123**, 129, **133**, 214, **214**
Continuous infusion pressure monitored sialography, 449
Continuous spectrum, 19, **19**
Contrast, 10, 44, **44**
   effect of, 11, **12, 64**
   image processing, 63–64
   image quality, 9, 207–208
   inadequate, **209**, 210, 212
   variation in, **10**
   visual perception 11, **12**, 258, **258**
Contrast media/studies, 223–226
   angiography, 223, **224**, 225
   arthography, 223, 413, 421-422, **422**
   barium studies, 223, **224**
   harmful effects/complications of, 225
   sialography, 223, **224**, 446-453, **450-453**
   types of, 223 - 225
Control of infection, 87-90, **88-90**
   in sialography, 449
   main infections of concern, 87
Controlled areas for radiation exposure, 71, **71**
Control panels, 37, **38**, 191, **193**
Conversion efficiency, intensifying screens, 46
Cooley's anaemia, 440, **440**
   see also Thalassaemia
Copper-beaten appearance, **308**
   see also Craniosynostosis
Copper block, in X-ray tube, 17, **17**
Coronoid process
   fracture of, 392, **399**
   normal radiographic appearances, **152-159, 417**
Cosmic radiation, 27
Cottonwool patches, 326, **442**
Cranial base foraminae, normal radiographic appearances, **167**
Cranial fossa floor, normal radiographic appearances, **156-157, 164-167**
Craniofacial dysostosis *see* Crouzon's syndrome
Craniostat *see* Cephalostat
Craniosynostosis, **308**
Craniotome, 149–150, **150**, 182, **182**
Cretinism, 300
Crista galli, normal radiographic appearance, **156-157**
Critical examination report of equipment, 71–72
Critical voltage (Vc), 20
Crouzon's syndrome, 301, **308**
Cysts, 331–337
   antral, 375, 381–382, **382-383**
   bone, 331, 337, **337**, 351, **351**
   buccal bifurcation, 332

classification of, 331
dentigerous (follicular), 331, 334, **334**, 381, **383**
eruption, 334
Gorlin's *see* Calcifying cystic odontogenic tumour
lateral periodontal, 331, 333, **333**
nasopalatine duct/incisive canal, 331, 336, **336**
non-odontogenic, 331, 336-337
odontogenic, 331, 332-335
odontogenic keratocyst, 331, 335, **335**
periapical radicular, 270, **271-274**, 331, 332, **332**
residual radicular, 331, 333, **333**

D

D-speed film, 32, 44
Dark film, 209, **209**, 212
Darkroom, quality assurance programme, 217–218
DC X-ray generating equipment, 39-40
Deciduous teeth, periapical tissues of, 266, **267**
Delayed eruption, causes of, 300
DentOptix, 52, 60, **60**
Demineralization, 251
Dens-in-dente (invaginated odontome), 300, **304**
Dense bone island, 355
Dental caries *see* Caries
Dental panoramic tomography *see* Panoramic radiography
Dental X-ray generating equipment, 35-40
Dentigerous cyst, 331, 334, **334**, 381, **383**
Dentinogenesis imperfecta, 299, **302**
Dento-alveolar fractures, 400
Description of radiographic lesions, 323–327, **324-326**
Developer solution, 57
Developing teeth, periapical tissues of, 268, **268**
Developmental abnormalities, classification of, 299–301
   tooth number, 299, **301-302**
   tooth position, 300, **306**
   radiographic assessment of mandibular third molars, 309–315, **309–315**
   radiographic assessment of unerupted maxillary canines, 316–321, **316–321**
   tooth shape, 300, **303-304**
   tooth size, 300, **302-303**
   tooth structure, 299-300, **301-303**

Developmental abnormalities, *cont'd*
  skeletal – mandible and maxilla, 300-
      301, **306-308**
  rare diseases and syndromes, 301,
      308, 335, 432, **432**
Differential diagnosis
  describing lesions, 323–327
  lesions of variable radiopacity in the
      jaw, 355–372, **357-372**
  radiolucent lesions of the jaws,
      329–54, **332-354**
  step-by-step guide to lesions of
      variable opacity,355-356, **355**
  step-by-step guide to radiolucent
      lesions, 329–330, **330**
Digital imaging, 48-53, 59–66
  advantages, 65
  disadvantages, 65
  image processing, 59–66, **59-66**
      see also Computer digital processing
  image receptors, 48-53, **49-52**
      see also Digital sensors
Digital sensor holders
  bisected angle technique, **107**,
      107–108
  bitewing, 127, **127**
  paralleling technique, 92–95, **93–95**
Digital sensors, 48-53, **49-52**
Digital volume tomography *see* Cone
      beam computed tomography
      (CBCT)
Digora Optime, 52, 60, **60**
Digora PCT, 52, 60
Dilaceration, 300, **305, 321**
Diphtheria, 87
Direct action/damage on cells, **30**,
      30–31
Direct-action (non-screen) film, **41**,
      41–42
Disabled patients, radiography of,
      86–87
Disposable bite blocks, 90, **90**
Dormia basket, 454, **454**
      see also Interventional sialography
DNA damage, **30**, 30–31
Docking station, 49, **49**
Doppler effect, 237, **238**
Dose limitation, 76-80
Dose limits, 76-80
  general public, 79-80
  patients, 76-77
  radiation workers, 77, 79
Dose monitoring, 80-81
Dose rate, 27
Dose reference level (DRL), 73
Dose-response curves, **31**, 32
Dose units, 25–28
Doses encountered in diagnostic
      radiology, 26

Dosimetry, 25–28
Down's syndrome, 279, 299
Driven snow appearance, 341, 360, **360**
Dry mouth, causes of, 445

E

E-speed film, 32, 44
Eagle's syndrome, 301, **308**
Eburnation, TMJ, 423
Ectodermal dysplasia, 299, **304**
Edentulous patients radiography of,
      120, **120**
Education and training
      recommendations, 75
Eezee-grip film holder, 118, **118**
Effective dose (E), 26
Effects of X-rays, biological, 29–33
Ehlers-Danlos syndrome, 300
Electromagnetic spectrum, 15
Electrons, 15-16
  interactions, 17–20
  shells,16
Electron volt (eV), 16
Emmenix film holder, **107, 116**
Emissions, intensifying screens
      spectral, 47, **47**
Employee's duties, radiation
      protection, 73
Employer's duties, radiation
      protection, 73–74
Emulsion, film, 39-43, **39-43**
Enamel-dentine junction (EDJ), **253**
Enamel pearl, 300, **305**
Enameloma, 300, **305**
Endodontics, 118–119, **118-119**, 273
Endoray, image receptor holder, **118**
Endosteal implants, 289
Eosinophilic granuloma, 331, 348, **348**
      see also Langerhans cell disease
Equivalent dose (H), 25–26
Eruption cyst, 334
Ethmoidal sinuses, 386, **386**
*European Guidelines on Radiation
      Protection in Dental Radiology,*
      27, 32
Ewing's tumour, 331, 347
Excess cancer incidence, 31
Excess salivation, causes of, 445
Excitation, 16–17
Exostoses, 359, **359**
Exposure factors, 247, **248**
  in caries detection, 259, **259**
  in periodontal assessment, 288
      see also Over-exposure; Under-
      exposure
Exposure time selector, on control
      panel, 37, 38

Extra cusps, 300
Extraoral digital sensors, 51, **51-52**
External auditory meatus
  in cephalometric radiography, 171
  normal radiographic appearances,
      164-167
External root resorption
acute apical periodontitis, 270
trauma, 388, **390**
tumours, 274, **274, 338, 342, 344**
Extrinsic primary malignant tumours
      involving bone, 331, 345, **345**
Eye protection, in infection control, 88,
      88

F

Facial fractures *see* Middle third
      fractures
Familial gigantiform cementoma, 331,
      356, 367, 372
Fetus, effects of X-rays on, 30
Fibroma, 331
Fibrosarcoma, 331, 344
Fibrous dysplasia, 331, 356, 368, **368**,
      372, 431, 441, **441**
Field limitation techniques in
      panoramic radiography, 195,
      196
Filament, in X-ray tube, 17, **17**
Film *see* Radiographic film
Film badges, 80, **80**
Film emulsion, 42, **42**
Film faults
  bitewing technique, 132-133, **133**, 214
  examples of, 209–211, **209-211**
  panoramic technique, 202, **203-206,**
      214, **214**
  periapical technique, 122, **123,** 214
  summary of, 212-213
Film packet contents, 41-42, **42**
Film packet holders *see* Image receptor
      holders
Film packets, **41**, 41–42, **42**, 129, **129**
Film reject analysis, 215-216
Film/screen contact, 48,
  quality control test for, 218, **219**
Film speed, 44, **44**
Film storage, 48
Filtration, 19
      see also Aluminium filter
Finger print appearance, 368, 441, **441**
Fixer solution, 57
Floating teeth, 345, 348, **348**
Florid osseous dysplasia, 331, 353, **353**,
      356, 367, **367**, 372
Flow-rate studies, 445, 457
Fluorescent phosphors, 45, 46

Focal corridor, 190
Focal osseous dysplasia, 331, 356, 366, **366**, 372
Focal plane,tomography, 179-182, **181, 182**
  see also Focal trough
Focal spot size, 37, **38**
Focal spot to skin distance (fsd), 36, **37, 38**, 92, **92**
Focal trough, 179, 187-190, **187-190**, 194-195, **195**
Focusing device, in X-ray tube, 17, **17**
Fog, 207-208
  background fog density, **43**, 43-44
Fogging effect, 217, **218**
Forbidden zone, 16
Forehead-nose position, 156-161, **156-161**, **176**, 176-177
Foreign bodies, 371, **372**
  antral, 381
  inhaled, radiography of, 388
  localization of, **7-8**
  swallowed, radiography of, 388
Forward scatter, 23, **23**
Fourth-generation CT scanners, 228-289, **229**
Fractures
  affecting the maxillary antra, 380, **380-381**
  alveolar bone, 388
  cervical spine, 410
  cranial base, 410
  mandibular, **392**, 392-399, **393, 395-399**
  middle third of facial skeleton, **400**, 400-409, **402-409**
  teeth, 387-388, **389, 391**
  temporomandibular joint, 427, **427**
Frankfort plane, 175, 194
Free radicals, 30-31
Frontal sinus
  normal radiographic appearances, **152-157, 164-167**
  radiography of, 386, **386**
Full mouth survey, 96
Furcation involvement, 280-281, **281, 284**
Fusion, 300, **303**

G

Gadolinium
  Intensifying screens, 46
  MR contrast media, 241
Gagging, problems with, 117
Galileos (CBCT), **232, 235**
Gallium, 226

Gamma, film, 45, **45**
Gamma camera, 226
Gamma rays, 15, 227
Gardner's syndrome, 364
Gemination, 300, **303**
General public radiation dose limitation, 79-80
Genetic defects of teeth, 299
Genetic stochastic effects of radiation, 30
Geometric unsharpness, 208
  see also Penumbra effect
Ghost shadows, on panoramic radiographs 196, **198-199**
Giant cell lesions, 331, 349-351
  aneurysmal bone cyst, 331, 337, 351, **351**, 354
  brown tumour in hyperparathyroidism, 331, 350, 354, 437, **437**
  central giant cell lesion (granuloma), 331, 349, **349**, 354
  cherubism, 331, 350, **350**, 354
Gingival abscess, 285
Gingival diseases, 279, 280
Glenoid fossa (TMJ), anatomy of, **411-413**
Gnathion (Gn), cephalometric point, 175, **175**
Gonion (Go), cephalometric point, 175, **175**
Gorlin's cyst *see* Calcifying cystic odontogenic tumour
Granuloma *see* Central giant cell lesion; Periapical granuloma
Gray(Gy), 25-26
Ground glass appearance, 326
  fibrous dysplasia, 368, **368**, 441, **441**
  hyperparathyroidism, 437, **437**
  Paget's disease, 442, **442**
Guidance Notes for Dental Practitioners on the Safe Use of X-ray Equipment, 70-76
Guided tissue regeneration (GTR), 287, **287**
Guidelines on Radiological Standards in Primary Dental Care, 69

H

Hair-on-end appearance, 439, **439**, 440, **440**
Hand-Schuller-Christian disease, 331, 348
Hawe-Neos Kwikbite image receptor holders, **127-128**
Hawe-Neos Superbite image receptor holders, **94**

Hanging drop appearance, 380, **381, 410**
Hard copy printed digital images, 65-66
Hard palate, normal radiographic appearances, **136, 164-167, 197, 417**
Health and Safety at Work Act 1974, 69
Health and Safety Executive (HSE), 70
Health care workers (HCW), 87
Health Protection Agency (HPA), 27, 70
Heat, in X-ray production, 17-18
  removal, 18
Heat-producing collisions, 17-18, **18**
Hepatitis B, 87
Hepatitis C, 87
Herpes simplex virus, 87
High energy photons, 19, 23
  see also Compton effect
Histiocytosis X see Langerhans cell disease
Honeycomb appearance, 326
  ameloblastoma 338
  central giant cell lesion 349
  central haemangioma, 343, **343**,
  odontogenic myxoma 342,
Hormone-related diseases, 437-438
Human immunodeficiency virus (HIV), 87
Hutchinson's incisors, 300, **304**
Hydrostatic sialography,
Hyoid, normal radiographic appearance, **146, 197**
Hypercementosis, 356, 359, **359**
  in Paget's disease, 442, **442**
Hyperdontia, 299, **302**
Hyperparathyroidism, 350, 431, 437, **437**
Hypodontia, 299, **301**

I

Idiopathic lesions see Stafne's bone cavity
Image geometry, 208
Image processing, 55-66
chemical, 55-59
computer digital, 59-66
Image receptors, 41-53
  cassettes, 47-48, **47-48**
  digital, 48-53
  photostimulable phosphor plates, **52**, 52-53
  radiographic film, 41-47, **41-47**
  solid state sensors, 49-51, **49-51**
Image quality, 9-10, 207-209
  assessment of, 215-216, 246-248
  bitewing radiographs, 132-133

Image quality, *cont'd*
    panoramic radiographs, 201–202
    periapical radiographs, 121–122,
        123
    subjective rating of, 122, 132, 202,
        216
Image receptor holders,
    bisected angle technique, **107**,
        107–108
    bitewing technique, 127-128, **127-128**
    endodontics, 118, 118
    paralleling technique, 92–95, **93–95**
Implant assessment, 289-297
    main indications, 290
    postoperative evaluation and follow-
        up, 295–297
    radiographic examination, 291–294,
        291-295
    treatment planning considerations,
        290
Incisive canal cyst, 331, 336, **336**
Incisors, radiography of,
    mandibular
        bisected angle technique, **111**
        paralleling technique, 96, **101**
    maxillary
        bisected angle technique, **109**
        paralleling technique, 96, **97**
Indirect action/damage on cells, 31
Indirect-action film, 42–43, **43-44**
Infection control, 87–90
Infective conditions
    generalised affecting bone, 434–436,
        434-436
    maxillary antra, 376–379, **376–379**
    periapical tissues, 270–273, **271–273**
    periodontal tissues, 279-286, **279-286**
Infective hepatitis, 87
Inferior dental canal, relationship with
        lower third molars, 309-310,
        311
Inflammatory conditions
    generalised affecting bone, 434–436,
        434-436
    maxillary antra, 376–379, **376–379**
    periapical tissues, 270–273, **271–273**
    periodontal tissues, 279-286, **279-286**
Influenza, 87
Infradentale (Id), cephalometric point,
        175, **175**
Infraocclusal, 300, **306**
    see also Submersion
Injuries to teeth and supporting
        structures, 387-391, **389-390**
Innominate line, normal radiographic
        appearance, **154-155**
Intensifying screens, 45–48, **45**, **47-48**
Internal derangements,TMJ, 422, 423
Internal root resorption, 388, **390**

International Commission on
        Radiological Protection
        (ICRP), 69
Interventional sialography, 454, **454**
Intraoral radiography
    bitewing radiography, 125-133
    infection control measures,87-90, **88-90**
    occlusal radiography, 135-140
    periapical radiography, 97-124
Intraoral digital sensors, 49-50, **49-50**
Intrinsic primary malignant bone
        tumours, 331, 343-344, **343-344**
Inverse square law, 79, **79**
Involucrum, 435
    see also Osteomyelitis
Iodine
    contrast media, 225
    radioisotope, 226
Ionising Radiation (Medical Exposure)
        Regulations 2000, 69, 73-76
Ionising Radiations Regulations 1999,
        69, 70-73
Ionization, 16-17, 20-21, 31, **31**
Ionization chambers, 81, **81**
Isocentric skull unit, 149, **149**, **151**
Isotopes, 16

Jaffe type fibrous dysplasia, 441
Justification, in radiation protection, 69,
        74
Juvenile rheumatoid arthritis (Still's
        disease),TMJ, 426

K lines, 19-20, **19**
Keractocyst see Odontogenic
        keratocyst
Kilovoltage (kV), 17, 20, 22, 36-39
Krypton, 226
Kwikbite bitewing image receptor
        holder, **127-128**

L

L lines, 19-20, **19**
Lamina dura,
    effects of inflammation on, 270, **271-273**
    effects of superimposed shadows on,
        268, **269**
    importance in periapical
        interpretation, 266
Langerhans cell disease, 274, 331, 348,
        348
Lanthanum see Rare earth screens
Large cell lymphoma, 331, 347
Lateral periodontal cyst, 331, 333, **333**

Latitude, film, 44, **44**
Lead protection, 75–76, **76**
Le Fort fracture lines, **400**, 401
    see also Middle third fractures
Legislation, on radiation protection,
        69–81
Letter-Siwe disease, 331, 348
    see also Langerhans cell disease
Limitation,in radiation protection, 69
Lipping, TMJ, 423
Linear tomography, **181**, 181–185,
        184–185, **188**, **189**
Lithotripsy, 239, 454
Localization, 7-9, **7-9**, 317-321, **317-321**
    see also Parallax
Local Rules, 71
Long cone *see* Spacer cone
Low energy photons, 19-20
    see also Photoelectric effect
Lower 45° occlusal radiography, 135,
        139, **139**
Lower 90° occlusal radiography, 135,
        138, **138**
Lower oblique occlusal radiography,
        135, 140, **140**
Luxation injuries of the teeth, 387
Lymph nodes, calcified, 356, 370, **370**
Lymphography, 223
Lymphoreticular tumours of bone, 274,
        331, 347, **347**

M

Macrodontia, 300, **303**
Macrognathia, 301, **307**, 438, **438**
Magnetic resonance (MR), **239**,
        239–241, **240**
    implant assessment, 292, **295**
    maxillary antra, **378**, 383
    middle third fracture, **380**
    salivary glands, 456, **456**
    temporomandibular joint, 421, **421**
Maintenance of equipment, 70
Mandible
    fractures, 392, 392–399, **393**, **395–399**
    normal anatomy, **6**, 266
Mandibular facial dysostosis,
Mandibular incisal inclination,
        cephalometric angle, 175, 176
Mandibular occlusal projections, 135,
        138-140, **138-140**
Mandibular plane, cephalometric
        plane, **175**, 175–176
Mandibular third molars
    favourable/unfavourable root
        morphology, 310, **310**
    problems in periapical radiography,
        115-117, **116-117**

radiographic assessment, 309-315, **313-315**
relationship with ID canal, 310, **311**
Winter's lines, 310, 312, **312**
Mandibular torus, 301, 359, **359**
Manual processing, **56**, 56–57
Marble bone disease see Osteopetrosis
Marked film, 210, **211**, 213
Maxillary antra, 373-386
  antral disease, summary, 375
  investigation and appearance of disease, 376–385, **376-385**
  normal anatomy, 373
  normal appearance on conventional radiographs, **373–374**
Maxillary fractures *see* Middle third fractures
Maxillary incisal inclination, cephalometric angle, **175**, 176
Maxillary occlusal projections, 135-137, **136-137**
Maxillary plane, cephalometric plane, **175**, 176
Maxillofacial radiography
  equipment, 149–150, **149-151**
  main indications, 149
  main projections, 151–167, **151-167**
McCune-Albright syndrome, 441
Measles, 300
Median maxillary suture, normal radiographic appearance, **97**
Medical research, radiographic examinations for, 77
Menton (Me), cephalometric point, **175**, 175
Mesiodens, **302, 319, 320**
Microdontia, 300, **302**
Micrognathia, 301, **306**
Microsievert, 25
Missing teeth *see* Anodontia; Hypodontia
Molars, radiography of
  mandibular
    bisected angle technique, **112**
    oblique lateral radiography, **144, 145**, 146
    paralleling technique, 96, **104**
    positioning problems, 115, 115–117, **116, 117**
  maxillary
    bisected angle technique, **110**
    oblique lateral radiography, **144, 145**
    paralleling technique, 96, **100**
Milliamperage (mA), 17, 20, 37, 191, **193**
Milligray (mGy), 25
Millisievert (mSv), 25
Monitoring radiation, 80-81

dose rate, 27
methods, **80**, 80-81
Moon's/mulberry molars, 300, **304**
Moth-eaten appearance, 325
  infective conditions, 434–436, **434-436**
  tumours, 344–346, **344-346**, 365
Motion unsharpness, 208
Mucosal retention cyst, 381, **382**
Multidirectional tomography, 418, **418–19**
Multilocular lesions, summary of, 354
Multiple myeloma, 313, 347, **347**
Mumps, 87
Myofascial pain dysfunction syndrome, TMJ, 422-423
Myxoma, odontogenic, 313, 342, **342**, 354

N

Narrow-beam linear tomography, 188–189, **189**
Narrow-beam rotational tomography, **189**, 189–90
Nasal cartilages, radiographic shadows of, 196, 197
Nasal fossa, normal radiographic appearance, **136-137**
Nasal septum, normal radiographic appearances, **136**, 197
Nasion(N),cephalometric point, 174, **175**
Naso-ethmoidal complex fractures, 400-401, **409**
Nasolabial fold, radiographic appearance, 196, **197**
Nasolacrimal canal, normal radiographic appearance, **136**
Nasopalatine duct/incisive canal cyst, 331, 336, **336**
Nasopalatine foramen, 268
  normal radiographic appearance, **136**
  differentiation from nasopalatine duct cyst, 336
National Radiological Protection Board (NRPB) *see* Health Protection Agency (HPA)
Natural background radiation *see* Background radiation
Necrotizing periodontal diseases, 279
Neurofibroma, 331
Neutron number (N), 16
Neutrons, 15, 16
Nevoid basal cell carcinoma syndrome (Gorlin's syndrome), 335
Non-odontogenic cysts, 331, 336–337, **336-337**
  see also Cysts

Non-odontogenic tumours, 331, 343–348, **343-348**, 356
  see also Tumours and tumour-like lesions
Nose-chin position, 152-155, **152-155**
Nucleons, 16
Nucleus, 15, *15*

O

Oblique lateral radiography, 141-147
  basic technique principles, 142–143, **143**
  bimolar technique, 146, **147**
  equipment required for, 142, **142**
  main indications, 142
  positioning examples, 144–145, **144-145**
  terminology, **141**, 141–142
Occipital condyle, normal radiographic appearance, **167**
Occipitomental (0^0OM) projection, 151, 152, **153**
Occipitomental (30^0OM) projection, 151, 154, **155**
Occlusal caries, **253**
Occlusal radiography, 135-140
  mandibular, 138-140, **138-140**
  maxillary, 136-137, **136-137**
Odontogenic cysts, 331, 332–335, **332-335**
  see also Cysts
Odontogenic fibroma, 331, 342, **342**, 354
Odontogenic keratocyst, 331, 335, **335**
Odontogenic myxoma, 331, 342, **342**, 354
Odontogenic tumours, 331, 338–342, 356
  see also Tumours and tumour-like lesions
Odontoid peg, normal radiographic appearance, **156-157, 164-167**
Odontomes, 300, **304-306, 319-320**, 356, 358, **358**
Oil, in X-ray tubehead, 17
Onion skin appearance, 434, **434, 435**
Operator duties, 74
Optical density (OD), 43
Optimization, in radiation protection, 74
Optimum viewing conditions, 245–246, **246**
Orange peel appearance, 326
  fibrous dysplasia, 368, **368**, 441, **441**
  hyperparathyroidism, 437, **437**
  Paget's disease, 442, **442**
  fracture, 380, 401, 405
Orbital blow-out fracture, 380, **381**, 406, **410**

Orbitale (Or), cephalometric point, 174, **175**

Orbitomeatal line, 150, **151**

Orbits
normal radiographic appearance, **152-157, 164-167**

Orbix, 149, **149, 151**

Oro-antral communication, 380, **380**

Oropharynx, air shadow of, **164-165,** 196, **197, 417**

Orthodontics, radiography in, 169

Orthognathic surgery, 169

Osseointegration, 289, 291, **296**

Osseous dysplasias, 274, 331, 352–354, 356, 366–367,
florid osseous dysplasia, 331, 353, **353,** 356, 367, **367**
focal osseous dysplasia, 331, 366, **366**
periapical osseous dysplasia, 331, 352, **352,** 356, 366, **366**

Ossifying fibroma, 353, 356, 369, **369,** 372

Osteitis, sclerosing, **271**

Osteitis deformans, 370, 442, **442–443**
see also Paget's disease

Osteitis fibrosa cystica see
Hyperparathyroidism

Osteoarthritis, TMJ, 423, **423–424**

Osteoma, 356, 364, **364,** 372, 383, **386,** 427

Osteomyelitis, 431, 434–435, **434–435**

Osteopenia, 437

Osteopetrosis, 370, 431, 433, **433**

Osteoporosis circumscripta, 442, **443**
see also Paget's disease

Osteoradionecrosis, 431, 436, **436**

Osteosarcoma, 331, 344, **344,** 356, 358, 365, **365,** 372, 384, **385**

P

Packing density, intensifying screens, 46

Paget's disease of bone, 370, 431, 442, **442–443**

Pain dysfunction syndrome, TMJ, 422-423

Pair production, 21

Palatal torus, 301, 356, 359

Pale film, 209, **209,** 212

Panoramic radiography (dental panoramic tomography), 190-206
assessment of quality, 201-202
equipment, 40, 169, **170,** 171, 191, **192**
field limitation techniques, 195, **196**
ghost or artefactual shadows, 196, **198-199**
normal anatomy, 196, **197**

real or actual shadows, 196, **197**
selection criteria, 187–188
systematic sequence for viewing, **249**
technique and positioning, 194-195, **194-195**
technique and positioning errors, 202-206, **203-206**
temporomandibular joint programmes, 413–415, **414**
theory, 188–190, **188-190**

Papilloma, 383

Parallax, 317–20, **317–320**

Paralleling technique *see* Periapical radiography

Paranasal air sinuses, 386, **386**

Parotid salivary gland,
disorders, 445
duct cannulation, **447**
investigation of, 446, 451-458
normal anatomy, **447, 450, 450**
see also Sialography

Patient care, during radiography, 85–87

Patients radiation dose limitation, 76–77

Penumbra effect, 10, 37, **38,** 208

Pepper-pot skull, 437, **437**

Perception, of the radiographic image, 11-12, **11-12**

Periapical abscess, 270, **271, 272**

Periapical granuloma, 270, **271-273**

Periapical osseous dysplasia, 331, 352, **352,** 356, 366, **366**

Periapical radiography, 91-123
assessment of quality, 121-122, **123**
bisected angle technique,106-112, **106-112**
comparison of techniques, 113, **114-115**
ideal positioning requirements, 91
main indications, 91
paralleling technique, 92-105, **92-105**
positioning difficulties encountered, 115–124, **115-124**

Periapical tissues
effects of normal superimposed shadows, 268, **269-270**
guidelines for interpreting periapical images, 275
inflammatory changes, appearance of, 270–273, **270-273**
normal radiographic appearances of, 265–269, **265-269**

Pericoronal abscess, 285

Periodontal diseases
classification of, 279–280
evaluation of treatment measures, 287, **287**
limitations of radiographic diagnosis, 288, **288**

radiographic features of, 280–286, **280-286**

Periodontal ligament space
effects of superimposed shadows on, 268, **269-270**
importance in periapical interpretation, 266
inflammatory widening, 270, **271-272**
normal anatomy, **6, 266**
normal radiographic appearances, **97-104**

Periodontal tissues
limitations of radiographic diagnosis, 288, **288**
normal radiographic features, 278–279, **278-279**
see also Periodontal diseases

Periodontitis
acute apical, 270, **271, 272**
aggressive, 279, 285, **286**
chronic, 279, 281–284, **282-283**

Periosteal reaction *see* Osteomyelitis

Phleboliths, 356, 371, **371**

Phoenix abscess, 270

Phosphor storage plates, **52,** 52–53, 60, **60**
bitewing radiography, use in, **129**
control of infection measures, 88, **89**
cephalometric radiography, use in, 172
periapical radiography, use in, 92, **94**
skull and maxillofacial radiography, use in, 150

Planmeca digital sensor holders, **105, 118, 127**

Pleomorphic adenoma, **453, 455, 456**

Photoelectric effect, 21–22, **22,** 45

Photons, 15, 20

Photostimulable phosphor storage plates *see* Phosphor storage plates

Pindborg tumour *see* Calcifying epithelial odontogenic tumour

Pixels, 59, **59,** 61, **61, 64, 65**

Pneumatization, 373

Pogonion (Pog), cephalometric point, 175, **175**

Porion (Po), cephalometric point, 175, **175**

Positioning errors
bitewing radiography, 132–133, **133**
panoramic radiography, 194, **194-195,** 202, **204-205**
periapical radiography, 122, **123**

Positron emission tomography (PET), 227–228

Posterior nasal spine (PNS), cephalometric point, **175,** 175

Postero-anterior (PA) of the jaws, 158, **158–159**
Postero-anterior (PA) of the skull, 156, **156–157**
Postoperative evaluation, implants, 295–297, **296-297**
Practitioner duties, 74
Pregnancy, radiography in, 76
Premolars, radiography of,
mandibular
bisected angle technique, **112**
paralleling technique, 96, **103**
maxillary
bisected angle technique, **110**
paralleling technique, 96, **99**
Preparation of patient errors
bitewing radiography, 132–133, **133**
panoramic radiography, 202, **203**
periapical radiography, 122, **123**
summary, 214
Principle of line focus, 37, **38**
Processing of images, 55–66, 247-248
chemical, 55–58, **55-58**
computer digital, 59–66, **59-66**
equipment, 220, **220**
quality assurance programme, 218–219
Prosthion (Pr), cephalometric point, 175, **175**
Protons, 15-16
in magnetic resonance(MR), 239-241
Pseudocysts, 337, **337**
Pseudolocular lesions, summary of, 354
Pterygoid plates
involvement in middle third fractures, **400, 405**
normal radiographic appearances, **161-162, 164-167, 417**
Pterygo-palatine fossa
importance in middle third fractures, **400, 405**
normal radiographic appearances, **164-167, 365, 385**
tumour involvement, **385**
Pulpal necrosis, 270
Pulp canal anomalies, 300
Pulpstones, 300, **305**
Punctate sialectasis appearance, 451, **452**

Q

Quality assurance, 215–220
see also Image quality
Quality control
digital radiography, 220–221
film-based radiography, 215–220
Quality rating, subjective assessment, 122, 132, 202, 216

R

Rad, 25
Radiation
background, 27
damaging effects of, 29-30
estimated annual doses, 27
methods of causing cell damage, 30-31, **30-31**
occupational exposure, 27
risk of cancer induction, 31-32
Radiation-absorbed dose (D), 25
Radiation dose, 25–28
limitation, 76–80
monitoring and measuring, **80**, 80–81
Radiation protection and legislation, 69-81
Radiation Protection Adviser (RPA), 70–71
Radiation protection file, 74
Radiation Protection Supervisor (RPS), 71
Radiation weighting factor, 25, 26
Radicular periapical (dental) cyst, 270, **271-274**, 331, 332, **332**
Radiobiological effectiveness (RBE), 25
Radiodensity of lesions, importance of, 325–326
Radiographic baseline, 150, **151**
Radiographic film, 41–47
basic components, 42, **42**
characteristics, 43–45, **43-45**
faults with, **209–211**, 209–213
orientation, 42
types
direct-action (non-screen) film, **41**, 41–42
indirect-action film, 42–43, **43-44**
self-developing, 58, **59**
see also Film packets
Radioisotope imaging, **226**, 226–228
salivary glands, 457, **457**
Radioisotopes, 16
Radiological interpretation, introduction to, 245–250
Radiolucent lesions *see* Differential diagnosis
Radiolucent/opaque (variable opacity) *see* Differential diagnosis
Radon, 27
Rare earth intensifying screens, **46**, 46–47
Rayleigh scattering, 21
Rectified circuits, 39, **39**
Recurrent caries, 252
Referrer duties, 74
Rem, 25
Reject film analysis/assessment, 215–116

bitewing radiography, 132-133, **133**
panoramic radiography, 201-202, **203-206**
periapical radiography, 121-122, **123**
Remineralization, 251
Reparative secondary dentine, 258, **259**
Residual caries, 256, **256**
Residual radicular cyst, 331, 333, **333**
Resolution, image, 45, 208
Restorations, radiographic assessment of, 261-264, **261-262**
Reverse Towne's projection, **151**, 160, **160–161**
Rheumatoid arthritis, TMJ, 425, **425–426**
Rickets, 300
Rinn bitewing image receptor holders, **127**
Rinn Endoray holder, **118**
Rinn Green Stabe bite blocks, **107**
Rinn periapical image receptor holders, **93-95, 107**
Risk assessment, 70
Risks associated with X-rays, 29–33, 70
Root
abnormalities, 300
fractures, 388, **389–390**, 391
remnants, 356, 358, **358**
Root canal treatment *see* Endodontics
Rotated postero-anterior projection, 151, 162, **162–163**
Royal College of Radiologists (RCR), guidelines, 69, 376, 423
Rubella, 87

S

Salivary calculi, 356, 370, **370**, 445, **446**, 450, **451-452**, 454, **456**
sialographic appearances of, 451, **451-452**
Salivary glands, **447**
disorders of the, 445
investigations, 445–458
Sausage link appearance, 451, **452**
Scanora, spiral tomography unit, 183, **183**, 183–184, **184**
antral imaging, 376, **378**
implant imaging, 291, **291, 296**
TMJ imaging, **399, 418, 418-419**
Scattering, 21, **23**
Scattered radiation, 75, 150, 171, 208
Sclerosing osteitis, **271, 273**
Screens *see* Intensifying screens
Secondary caries, 251, **253**
Secondary (metastatic) bone tumours, 331, 346, **346**, 354
Selection criteria

caries, 253, **254**
implants, 291
overview, **78**
panoramic radiography, 187–188
periodontal tissues, 277–278
Selection Criteria for Dental Radiography,
        69–70, 74, **78**, 253, **254**
Self-developing films, 58, **59**
Sella (S), cephalometric point, 174, **175**
Sella turcica, normal radiographic
        appearance, **164-165**
Sequestra, **434**, 434, 435, 436
Shadowgraph, 3, 246
Shape of lesions, description of, 324,
        324-325
Shell teeth, 299, **302**
Short cone *see* Spacer cone
Sialadenitis, 451–452, **452**
Sialectasis appearance, 451, **452**
Sialodochitis, 451, **452**
Sialography, 223, **224**, 446–454
        contraindications, 448
        contrast media, 448
        examples of sialographs, **224, 450-454**
        interventional, 454, **454**
        main indications, 446–448, **447**
        techniques, 446–449
Sickle cell anaemia, 431, 439, **439**
Sievert (Sv), 25-26
Simple bone cyst, 331, 337, **337**
Simple injection sialography, 449
Single photon emission computed
        tomography (SPECT), 227
Sinusitis see Maxillary antra
Site of lesions, description of, 323–324
Size of lesions, description of, 324, **324**
Sjögren's syndrome, 451–452, **452, 453**
Skeletal developmental anomalies,
        300–301, **306-308**
Skull radiography, 149–167
        equipment, 149–150, **149-151**
        main indications, 149
        main projections, 151–167, **151-167**
        patient positioning, 150
        see also Cephalometric radiography
Skull units *see* Craniotome, Orbix
SLOB rule, 317
SN plane, cephalometric plane, **175**
SNA, cephalometric angle, **175**, 176
SNB, cephalometric angle, **175**, 176
Snowflakes appearance, 341, 361
Snowstorm appearance, 451, **452**
Soap-bubble appearance, 338, 342, 351
Soft palate, normal radiographic
        appearance, **164-165, 197, 417**
Soft tissue calcifications, 356, 370–371,
        370–371
Solid-state sensors, 49-51, **49–51**, 59
        bitewing radiography, **127**

cephalometric radiography, 172–173,
        172-173
endodontic radiography, **118**
paralleling technique, **94**, 96, **105**
Somatic deterministic effects, 29
Somatic stochastic effects, 29–30
Spacer cone, 36, **36, 37,**
Sphenoidal air sinus
        importance in middle third fractures,
        401, **405**
        normal radiographic appearances,
        152-153, 164-167
        radiographic investigation, 386
Spiking resorption, 344, 365
Spiral CT, 229, **229**
Squamous cell carcinoma, 331, 345, **345**,
        383, 384, **384, 385**
Squamous odontogenic tumour, 331
Staff training, quality control, 220
Stafne's idiopathic bone cavity, 331,
        353, 354, **354**
Standard reference film, 219, **219**
Step ladder appearance, 439
Step-up transformer, 36, **36, 150, 150**
Still's disease, TMJ, 426
Storage, film, 48
Strings of a tennis racket appearance, 342
Styloid process, normal radiographic
        appearance, **197**
        see also Eagle's syndrome
Subjective rating of image quality, 216
        bitewing radiography, 132
        panoramic radiography, 202
        periapical radiography, 122
Submandibular salivary gland
        disorders, 445
        duct cannulation, **447**
        investigation of, 446, **454-456**
        normal anatomy, **447, 450, 451**
        see also Sialography
Submentovertex projection, 151, 166,
        166–167
Submersion *see* Infraocclusal
Subperiosteal implants, 289
Subspinale (point A), cephalometric
        point, 175, **175**
Sunburst appearance, 343, 344, **365**
Sunray appearance, 343, 344, **365**
Superimposition, limitations imposed
        by, 7–8, **9**
Supernumerary teeth, 299, **302**, 356, **357**
Supplemental teeth, 299, **302**
Supramentale (point B), cephalometric
        point, 175, **175**
Swallowed foreign body, radiography
        of, 388
Syphilis, 87, 300, **304**
Systematic viewing

bitewing radiographs, 263–264
panoramic radiographs, 349, **349**
periapical images, 275

T

Target appearance, 371, **371**
Target, in X-ray tube, 17, **17, 36**
Taurodontism, 300, **305**
Technetium, 226, **226, 457**
Teeth
        developmental abnormalities,
        299–300, **301-306**, 356
        injuries to, 387–391, **389–391**
        unerupted/misplaced, 309-321, **309-321**, 356, 357, **357**
Temporomandibular joint, 411-429
        investigations, 413–422, **413-422**
        main pathological conditions
        affecting, 422–429, **422-429**
        normal anatomy, 411–413, **411-413**
Terbium, 46-47
Thalassaemia, 431, 440, **440**
Thermoluminescent dosemeters
        (TLDs), 80, **80**
Three-dimensional image
reconstruction, **233**
        see also Computed tomogtaphy (CT);
        Cone beam computed
tomography (CBCT)
Thulium, 46
Timer, of control panel, 37, **38**
Tissue weighting factor, 26
Tomography, 179-185, 188-190
        broad-beam linear tomography, **181**,
        181–185, **184–185**, 188, **188**
        equipment, 40, 182, **182-183**
        multidirectional, 181-182, **182**
        narrow-beam linear tomography,
        188–189, **189**
        narrow-beam rotational tomography,
        189, **189–190**
        original indications, 179–180
        theory, 180–181
        see also Computed tomography (CT);
        Cone beam computed
        tomography (CBCT);
        Panoramic radiography
Tongue, normal radiographic
        appearances, **138, 140, 197, 417**
Tonsils, calcified, 356, 371, **371**
Torus mandibularis *see* Mandibular
        torus
Torus palatinus *see* Palatal torus
Trabecullar bone, normal anatomy, **6**,
        266
Trabecullar pattern, **6, 97-104**
Training and education guidelines, 75

Tramlines, of ID canal, 310, **311**
Transmissible spongiform encephalopathies (TSEs), 87
Transpharyngeal radiography, 416–417, **416–417**
Transposition, 300, **306**
Trauma, 287-410
    antral, 380–381, **380–381**
    mandibular fractures, 390–399, **390-399**
    middle third of facial skeleton fractures, 400–409, **400-409**
    other fractures and injuries, 410
    teeth and supporting structures, 387–391, **389–391**
    temporomandibular joint, **399** 427, **427, 428**
Treacher Collins syndrome, 301
Tree in winter appearance, 450, **450**
True cephalometric lateral skull, 173, **174**
True lateral skull projection, 151, 164, **164–165**
Tubehead components, **36**, 36–37
Tuberculosis, 87
Tumours and tumour-like lesions, 331, 338–348, **338–348**, 356, 360–365, **360–365**
    adenomatoid odontogenic tumour (AOT), 331, 341, 354, 356, 361, **361**, 372
    ameloblastic fibroma, 331, 340, **340**, 354
    ameloblastic fibro-odontoma, 331, 341, 361, **361**
    ameloblastoma, 331, 338, **338–339**, 354, 384
    antral, 383–385, **384–385**
    bone, 274, 343–348, **343–348**
    Burkitt's lymphoma, 331, 347, **347**
    calcifying cystic odontogenic tumour (calcifying odontogenic cyst), 331, 341, 354, 362, **362**, 372
    calcifying epithelial odontogenic tumour (CEOT), 331, 341, 354, 360, **360**, 372
    central haemangioma, 331, 343, **343**, 354
    chondroma, 331, 356, 372, 427, **427**
    chondrosarcoma, 331, 344, 427
    classification of, 331
    eosionophilic granuloma, 331, 348, **348**
    Ewing's tumour, 331, 347
    extrinsic primary malignant tumours involving bone see Squamous cell carcinoma
    fibroma, 331
    fibrosarcoma, 331, 344
    keratocystic odontogenic tumour (odontogenic keratocyst), 331, 335, **335**
    Langerhans cell disease, 274, 331, 348, **348**
    large cell lymphoma, 331, 347
    multiple myeloma, 313, 347, **347**
    neurofibroma, 331
    odontogenic fibroma, 331, 342, **342**, 354
    odontogenic myxoma, 331, 342, **342**, 354
    osteoma, 356, 364, **364**, 372, 383, **386**, 427
    osteosarcoma, 331, 344, **344**, 356, 358, 365, **365**, 372, 384, **385**
    salivary gland, **238**, 445, 453, **453**, **455, 456**
    secondary metastatic, 331, 346, **346**, 354
    squamous cell carinoma, 331, 345, **345**, 383, 384, **384, 385**
    squamous odontogenic tumour, 331
    temporomandibular joint, 427, **427**
Turner tooth, 300, **303**

U

Ultrasound, **237**, 237–239, **238**
    salivary glands, **238**, 454, **454–455**
Ultraviolet intensifying screens, 46, **46**
Unborn child, effects of X-rays on, 30
Unerupted teeth, **302**, 356, 357, **357**
Unicystic ameloblastoma, 338
Unilocular lesions, summary of, 354
Unmodified scattering, 21
Upper oblique occlusal radiography, 135, 137, **137**
Upper standard occlusal radiography, 135–136, **136,** vertical parallax, 320, **320**
Urography, 223

V

Viewing conditions, optimum, 245–246, **246**
Voxel, 230, **230**, 232-235, **233-234, 236**

W

Wandering teeth, 300, **306**
Warning lights, of control panel, 37
Wave packets, 15, 20
Window level, CT, 230
Window width, CT, 230
Winter's lines, 310–312, **312**
Working procedures, quality control of, 220
World Health Organisation (WHO), 331
Wormian bones, 432, **432**
Worth film holder, **116**
Written procedures, 73-74

X

X-ray beam, 15
    characteristics, 10, 208
X-ray generating equipment
    cephalometric, 169-173, **170-173**
    dental, 35-40, **35-39**
    panoramic, 191-193, **192-193**
    quality control, 216–17
    regulations for, 72, 73
    skull, 149-151, **149-151**
X-ray producing collisions, 18, **18**
X-rays, 15
    attenuation, absorption, scattering, 21
    biological effects and risks of, 29–33
    interactions with matter, **21**, 21–23
    production of, 16–20
    properties and characteristics,20
    spectra, **19**, 19–20
X-ray tube, 16–17, **17**, 36, 37
X-ray tubehead components, 36, **36**

Z

Zygoma
    normal radiographic appearance, **137, 152-155, 197**
Zygomatic arch
    fracture, **406-407**
    normal radiographic appearance, **152-155, 160-161, 166-167, 197**
Zygomatic buttress, **100, 270**
Zygomatic complex, **400-401**
    fracture, **406-408**
    fracture sites and assessment, **404-408**
    radiographic investigations, 401